An Edgar Cayce Encyclopedia of Foods for Health and Healing

“Food Faddists Can Feast

on this hefty, encyclopedic banquet of dietary advice excerpted from the ‘readings’ of clairvoyant-prophet Edgar Cayce. From 1923 to 1944 a faithful secretary recorded Cayce’s trance-readings and since 1945 the Association for Research and Enlightenment has been transcribing, collecting, cross-indexing them . . . This ‘encyclopedia’ catalogs just about every foodstuff and beverage imaginable from ‘Apple Brandy’ to ‘Yogurt.’ ”

PUBLISHERS WEEKLY

An Edgar Cayce Encyclopedia of Foods for Health and Healing

Compiled, edited, and arranged by Brett Bolton

Foreword by William A. McGarey, M.D.

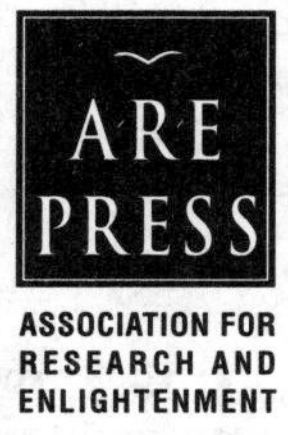

A.R.E. Press • Virginia Beach • Virginia

Formerly published as *Edgar Cayce Speaks*

*I dedicate
this book to the
memory of David Kahn*

Printed in the U.S.A.

First Avon Printing, July 1969
Second A.R.E. Press Printing, October 1998

A.R.E. Press
215 67th Street
Virginia Beach, VA 23451-2061

Library of Congress Cataloging-in-Publication Data
Bolton, Brett.
An Edgar Cayce encyclopedia of foods for health and healing / compiled, edited, and arranged by Brett Bolton : foreword by William A. McGarey.
p. cm.
Originally published as : Edgar Cayce speaks. New York : Avon Books, 1969.
Title of previous ed. : Edgar Cayce speaks.
ISBN 0-87604-378-3 (alk. paper)
1. Diet therapy. 2. Cayce, Edgar, 1877-1945. Edgar Cayce readings. I. Title. II. Title: Edgar Cayce speaks.
RM217.B57 1997
615.8'54—dc21 96-53991

Cover design by Kim Cohen

Grateful acknowledgment is made to the following:

To Mr. Hugh Lyrm Cayce, Director and General Manager of the Association for Research and Enlightenment for granting permission for the compiling and publication of this book.

Especial thanks to one very dear and patient man, Mr. J. Everett Irion, Treasurer and Business Manager of the organization whose cooperation and advice made this book possible.

My thanks to the A.R.E. volunteers for their help.

I humbly and gratefully thank Lucille Kahn for her encouragement over the years *and* her faith in me as I climbed the Glass Mountain toward the Deadline Summit—

And last but not least my deepest appreciation to my untiring leprechauns: Jackie, Bonnie, Jessie, Virginia, and *very* especially to Patricia Morey—the *greenest* of them all—for two thousand eight hundred and eighty-one and 3/4 hours of assistance.

B. B.

(Reprinted from 1969 edition)

Contents

Directory to This Book

Foreword

This is a unique book in an age that has produced the atom bomb, exploration of outer space and photographs of chromosomal abnormalities, to mention but a few of our modern marvels. Indeed, when we find neurophysiologists reporting the biological activity of the brain in terms that describe neurons rapidly rotating and sending out streams of protoplasm as though they were searching for a purposeful direction—then, certainly, we may rest assured that these are memorable and unique times.

Why should an encyclopedia of information compiled from psychic readings given from an unconscious state be of interest and importance to us in the midst of all these wonderful happenings? An appropriate answer would necessarily relate the wonders of the present age in some manner with the nature, the scope and the validity of the information coming from that mind.

Information given by Edgar Cayce to individuals over half a century ago spoke of tubercle bacilli as being causative of some of the skin changes found in scleroderma. It has been in the 1960s that rather interesting studies have been published by Cantwell in the medical literature demonstrating acid-fast bacilli in the skin of scleroderma patients. Cayce has been able, time and again, to "see" or describe conditions or functions in the human organism which predated the scientific demonstration of what is then acknowledged to be fact.

Neuroscientists, for instance, find quite a gap between popular concepts that the brain is a static, precast organ, and findings at the University of California at San Diego. Dr. Robert Livingston reports their work there as showing that nerve endings move as though continually testing their compatibility with the surfaces of other cells, while the glial cells swarm over the neurons. The brain, as a matter of fact, continues to construct itself and modify its structure, sharply influenced by personal and cultural experiences and sensory input of all kinds. Decades before this information came to our attention through the medium of scientific research under highly sophisticated circumstances, Cayce lay down, and under a type of self-induced trance, gave the following information, startingly similar:

> In some respects we find conditions appear to be more aggravated at times than aided, yet—as we will find—when it becomes necessary for a physical body to be builded . . . as of the brain cell's expansion itself, and where scar tissue . . . has formed obstructions . . . in same—that . . . conditions of retraction must necessarily arise . . . that is, the system throwing out that as feelers, or as new lines of activity through that of the voluntary and involuntary nerve reactions from those plexuses in the system, that build for the resuscitating and regenerating of energies from within the system.
>
> . . . The life of a brain cell is only according to the activity of a body physical and mental, and is multiplied according to the activities of same as related to the assimilation of resuscitating forces. 161-3, p. 1

Cayce's ability to understand physical conditions of the body and to suggest means to bring the body back to a state of health has made his name and his work stand out with clarity in a world that recognizes more and more of the use of higher sense perception—psychic ability. His concepts of physiology and therapy are being studied by an ever-enlarging group of physicians for what they may hold of benefit to the medical profession. Clinical studies have been inaugurated to work out the methodology of therapy found in the Cayce readings and serious consideration is being given to specifics in treatment of various disease entities as they are recommended for individuals throughout these more than 14,000 readings.

This provides a bit of a background, then, for a study of the data in the readings related to foods and their utilization in the body. These readings are fascinating in that they not only often state why and in what circumstances a food should be used, but there is also tossed in, for good measure, as it were, a gem of physiology or philosophy, making the reading of these selections an adventure in itself. There are those who will accept from these data only what has since been proved. These people will perhaps not find the same exhilaration from this compilation of material that those find who look with an open mind at the possibility that there might actually be a person such as Cayce who could seek and find accurate information from unconscious minds all over the world. The latter will look for realities not yet scientifically established, much as the prospector used to roam the mountains of the far West in search of gold.

Take yogurt, for example. Yogurt used to be found only in health food stores, but now can be purchased at any good supermarket. Much has been claimed for this food. Cayce had this to say to a 43-year-old woman who apparently was suffering from some sort of general debilitation:

> Also we would add yogurt in the diet as an active cleanser through the colon and intestinal system. This would be most beneficial, not only purifying the alimentary canal, but adding the vital forces necessary to enable those portions of the system to function in the nearer normal manner.

Thus we may bring the abilities for strength and for purifying the circulatory forces, upon which depends the strength to resist physically the inroads of the infectious forces that disturb the locomotion as well as the pulmonary and the circulatory system and the strength through the depleting of the nerve energies of the body.

1542-1 F. 43 yrs. 2/23/38

Several functions are suggested as occurring within this particular body as the result of taking yogurt as part of her diet, few of which are even considered by the manufacturers of the food itself. One traces the effects of the yogurt from the alimentary canal through the bloodstream and lymphatics to the neuromuscular and respiratory systems, affecting each as it passes. Little is given, of course, about what happens specifically, or the details of how these functions are affected. The nagging thought remains, of course—what if Cayce is right, even though he doesn't explain it?

And here is a very unusual food, the Jerusalem artichoke. This is a tuber, and not to be confused with the California artichoke. It stores its carbohydrates as inulin or inulides, which yield levulose on hydrolysis; different from starch, which on hydrolysis yields glucose. The levulose is not as harmful to a body in diabetes as is glucose. Medical opinion has been divided as to the artichoke's use or value in diabetes, however. It has not been used much in this country but is suggested numerous times in the readings. The following extract is interesting:

And at LONG intervals, say once every ten days, give the body a small raw artichoke (Jerusalem artichoke). This will tend to make for a better coordination in the activities of the pancreas as related to the kidneys and pelvic organs; that produce an irritation upon the nervous system.

We will BEST see the indications of the EFFECT of this—particularly—in the eradicating of the tendencies for the little dark circles that come occasionally under the eyes. 1179-5 F. 10 yrs. 2/18/39

The romance to be found in this particular section—at least for the physician—is to be discovered in the concept here that one organ must coordinate its activities with another for the body to be healthy. It is almost as if these organs have consciousness, as if they are aware that they have an individuality and can act differently from the manner in which they are so obviously intended to act. That one small portion of food every ten days can cause dark circles to disappear from under the eyes—this indeed is strange, particularly if it helps the kidney to assume a better community relationship with the pancreas, as they both work to better the condition of the body as a whole. These are strange concepts.

Natural food adherents may not like many of the ideas that come out of the readings in this book. Carrot juice has been used to excess by literally thousands of people in this country of ours. I have seen the color of carrot in the palms and faces of people using this juice as a therapy. Cayce, however, sees carrot juice as a food to be sipped in very small amounts. He says to take an ounce of carrot juice, not "this whole quantity at once, to be sure, but sip it—take fifteen to twenty minutes to take this amount; or it may be sipped in smaller quantities but often through the day." And he sees this particular food helping to control the kidneys and acting to eliminate poisons.

Such a theory of the use of food—small amounts, well mixed with the saliva, and frequently given in cycles—is contrary to the manner in which food extracts or whole foods are often used in large amounts to bring about gross changes in the body. It does fit in with Cayce's concepts of a normal diet, however, and makes for interesting reading and mental questionings.

As I studied these readings I found myself faced with a constant challenge to rethink the relationships that exist between the body itself as a living group of integrated functions and the food which we put into our mouths. I found myself gaining new insights into this body of mine, its workings, and its destiny—the body that has been called the temple of God.

Brett Bolton has done an excellent job of putting together this information which is certainly unique in these unusual times and which can lead the reader gently into a deeper appreciation of one's daily bread.

William A. McGarey, M.D.
A.R.E. Clinic
Phoenix, Arizona

Introduction

The Man

Edgar Cayce was born in 1877 in a small, isolated rural community in Kentucky, where he grew up. He is said to have been a troubled, rather "backward" child—a condition that must have been aggravated, if not caused, by the early discovery by his family and neighbors that he had odd "powers." For, while they surely found it useful to have at hand a boy who could profitably be asked where a lost object would be found, these people—especially young Edgar's peers—were suspicious and mistrustful of these powers, and considered him to be "touched."

Under the influence of his beloved mother, a devoutly religious woman, young Edgar found solace and refuge in the Bible. He read in it constantly and believed in it absolutely. When, later in life, insights gained in his trances convinced him of the truth of reincarnation, his religious philosophy broadened somewhat. Though his belief in the teachings of the Bible and of Christianity remained steadfast, reincarnation is nowhere provided for in that body of belief. Some indication of the broader shape of Cayce's belief is to be discerned in the "Mind Is the Builder" section of this book, a selection of excerpts from trance readings in which he reflects on the need for inner peace—spiritual and mental health as the foundation for physical health.

Edgar Cayce discovered at about the age of 12 some of the remarkable powers he possessed while asleep, but made little use of them until he was a young man of 21. The first public reaction to his gifts was largely skepticism and even abuse, and his early career was mostly unhappy—always excepting the saving grace of his deeply devoted wife Gertrude. They were married after a long courtship in 1903. During this difficult period, her patient love and trust sustained him; later, she would be of incalculable assistance in perfecting the form of the trance readings.

At first full of self-doubt and confusion as to the use and effectiveness of his gifts, Cayce willingly gave himself to grueling tests by medical doctors. Over the next few years, the skepticism of the medical profession yielded very little; but Cayce himself became convinced of the efficacy of his powers and set aside for the time being any hope of convincing organized medicine.

In 1915, now 38 years old and in command of his gifts, confident they were a blessing from God and that great good would be done through them, Edgar Cayce met a young man named David Kahn, who was to give over his life to the furthering of Cayce's work. Excepting only Cayce's beloved wife, David Kahn is the one person most responsible for the survival and burgeoning of Edgar Cayce's works today.

When the Association for Research and Enlightenment was founded in 1931, Cayce's eldest son, Hugh Lynn, undertook the management of it. Edgar Cayce had seen early on in his career that for skepticism finally to be laid to rest, an orderly and thorough documentation and organization of his trance readings would have to be made. The work of the A.R.E. has consisted in the important part of indexing the transcriptions of Cayce's readings and documenting their results, providing research facilities for accredited scientists and medical doctors—in short, solidifying the foundation under the elaborate and beautiful structure of Edgar Cayce's inspiration. This purpose is steadily and surely being realized; as properly hard-headed men of science are provided with the documentation they require to make orderly and convincing tests and comparisons, Edgar Cayce's vision is no longer so categorically rejected as it often was in his lifetime.

In 1923 Gladys Davis became Edgar Cayce's secretary. Every word he uttered in trance from then until his death was recorded by this paragon of patience and devotion.

Edgar Cayce died on January 3, 1945, three months short of his 68th birthday. His readings on himself had indicated repeatedly that his substance would deteriorate rapidly if he undertook more than two readings a day. But by then, his fame having spread through the world, he was besieged by requests for readings, and consistently ignored his own best advice to himself in attempting to fill as many as possible. He was doing as many as 8 readings a day until September, 1944, when exhaustion overcame him. He did no more readings as his health faded steadily until his death.

Gertrude Cayce began to fade with her husband's death, and followed him on April 1, 1945.

David Kahn died on December 7, 1968, a week after completing the dictation of his book on Edgar Cayce's life.

Until her death in 1986, Gladys Davis supervised the complex and meticulous indexing of the approximately 14,000 readings she recorded, working tirelessly in the basement of the A.R.E. Library in Virginia Beach, Virginia.

Hugh Lynn Cayce, until his death in 1982, continued the work of the foundation with undiminishing vigor.

The Vision

Edgar Cayce, in his self-induced hypnotic trance state, had the gifts of a psychic: clairvoyance and precognition. His "healing" powers consisted in diagnosing and suggesting treatment; he did not actually "heal" or "cure" by means of laying on hands or any such miraculous methods. As he described his trance states, they seemed to consist in his mind's traveling to the location of the body which was the subject of the reading—and it might be thousands of miles distant—and entering that body and mind. He seemed able to communicate with each cell of the body, and in his trip would perceive the entity's total state—physical, mental and emotional.

He saw the body and mind as a single entity, whose overall balance was to be maintained: *coordination* among all functions was the key. Remedies which he recommended encompassed physical therapy, surgery, medicine, diet, exercise, and psychological guidance. One striking facet of his fantastic abilities was his gift for locating and recommending to the subject the attentions of a particular medical doctor of whose existence he had no way of consciously knowing. One such doctor whom Cayce recommended repeatedly headed the physiotherapy department at A.R.E. headquarters.

It is beyond the scope of this already sizable book to document the seemingly miraculous cures that were worked by Cayce's recommended treatments of cases which had been thought hopeless before his readings. Similarly, the dozens of treatments which were scorned by medical science when they were recommended but which have since been come upon through medical research and accepted, are endlessly impressive. Hundreds remain that have been spectacularly successful in the specific cases where they were applied, but which have not yet been confirmed by medical research. The beginnings of this confirming research are being made at the Association for Research and Enlightenment, where the Edgar Cayce vision points the way for new areas of study, and at laboratories throughout the world.

A comparison between Cayce's general recommendations for a proper diet and the "normal diet" outlined by the Food and Nutrition Board of the National Research Council in 1950—five years after Cayce's death—shows amazing consistency between the two. The importance of a balanced alkaline/acid intake, for example, is now stressed by those who once scorned Cayce's readings.

This Book

The excerpts from readings in this book pertain to foods and beverages. Included are as many recommendations as to the general health-giving properties of various foods and beverages. Also, there are hundreds of extracts where a specific diet or food or drink is recommended as treatment or preventive of a specific affliction. Where symptoms are identical, Cayce's recommendations have often been useful for cases other than that of the subject of the reading. But, though this warning scarcely needs to be made for the thoughtful reader, Cayce's own words (from a reading) ought always to be kept in mind: *"That which might be applicable to this entity should not be forced upon, or even considered for others; unless their own condition is in that state of being parallel with this individual entity."* And, it might be added, the determination that a state of being is "parallel" is a complex and subtle problem and ought not to be made lightly by the reader.

The purpose of this book is to make accessible to the general reader, by encyclopedic arrangement, Edgar Cayce's trance-reading recommendations as to foods and beverages. In many readings several foods are discussed; at the extreme, a single paragraph may mention as many as twenty. I have lifted specific references and posted each under its own heading in most cases; however, there are instances where combinations are advised and no division is called for. These extracts will be found in "General" and "Combinations" headings. I have been at great pains to transcribe the commentary precisely, without any alteration, and to retain the exact sense of combined recommendations when these had been split up. If any error in text or sense occurs anywhere in this book, I apologize for it now. Further, the Association for Research and Enlightenment is in no way responsible for such.

At the beginning of each reading, at the right-hand margin, I have shown the date of the reading, the sex and age of the subject (the age is recorded in a few cases only as "adult"), and the reading's indexing number. These index numbers may be interpreted thus: for reading 5558-1 (the first in this book), the person given number 5558 is here being given her first reading. For 877-28 (the second in this book), Mr. 877 is here having his 28th reading.

At the left-hand margin, also taken from the A.R.E. index, is an entry which indicates something of the condition of the subject or the purpose of the specific recommendation. It must be borne in mind that these are, indeed, *excerpts* from complete readings; a complete reading may well recommend several remedies for the same condition, or may deal with more than one malfunction. These entries are included, then, only for general orientation.

I

Beverages

1—Alcoholic Beverages: General

4/5/29
F. Adult
CIRCULATION: LYMPH: TOXEMIA **5558-1**

Not too much of sweets nor of any that will produce improper fermentation, nor those of alcoholic content. These should *not* be taken.

Following these lines we will find bettered conditions for the system. The tendency of the irritations to relieve the lessening of the acidity in the system will also clarify and cleanse the system for the conditions to be nearer in the proper functioning.

2/2/39
M. 47 yrs.
DERMATITIS **877-28**

In the matter of the diet, keep well to those things that are better balancing in the alkalinity and the acidity of the system. Not that there should be a refraining from strong drinks or wines and the like ENTIRELY, but these in moderation. Use same more as an aid to digestion; or as indicated, take such, preferably only with the meals. This will aid in keeping a better balance through the eliminations, and the ability of assimilations as combined with the outward applications and the corrections.

11/7/24
M. 29 yrs.
ACIDITY **900-11**

For the acidosis the diet as given, and not too much stimulations through any alcoholic forces with fish, or at *any* time. It makes it bad for the blood supply and for the mental forces.

11/25/34
F. Adult
PSORIASIS **745-1**

Q. Are there any special foods that should be eliminated from the diet?

A. Any great quantity of very highly seasoned or highly spiced foods should not be taken.

Q. Can the body take any kind of alcoholic beverages?

A. Wines; but not the stronger drinks—not rum or the like.

9/2/41
F. 50 yrs.
ELIMINATIONS: INCOORDINATION **2581-1**

Q. Does either alcohol or cigarettes, in moderation cause pain?

A. Alcohol and cigarettes in moderation are NOT harmful, but at times they tend to make for irritations—when the system is overcharged. But with the eliminating of the causes of these disturbances, we find that in moderation these are inclined to be rather helpful.

5/27/44
M. 45 yrs.
PROSTATITIS **5162-1**

In the diet, keep to those things which are not highly seasoned. Never any carbonated waters or drinks. Less of any strong drinks, for these do stir those activities in the spleen, pancreas and gall duct to bring a greater distress to kidneys and bladder and the areas indicated.

1/12/44
HEART: ENGORGED **M. Adult**
THROMBOSIS: CORONARY: TENDENCIES **3554-1**

Do refrain from any carbonated drinks. Do refrain from being in the environs of smoke. For these are becoming very hard on the circulation. Do refrain from any of those environs where any sort of intoxicating liquors are taken. Even the smell of these will be harmful for the conditions of the heart and the thrombose areas—for these show engorgements.

11/7/36
M. 45 yrs.
ALCOHOL: GENERAL **877-13**

Q. The effect of alcohol, should it be strong or not?

A. Alcohol in moderation is well for *most* bodies. But not too great a quantity taken as to cause a slow congestion in the liver area. But alcohols taken evenings—very well.

4/2/35
ANEMIA: TENDENCIES **F. Adult**
ACIDITY **875-1**

Q. Is alcohol bad for the body?

A. Alcohol in excess is bad for the body. As indicated, a glass of red wine once a day or twice a day as a food *is* helpful. Excess of hard liquor or combinations are the more devastating to the gastric flow. Any stimuli that makes for a hardening of the secretions of the sympathetic system is harmful.

8/23/27
DIABETES: TENDENCIES **M. 26 yrs.**
ELIMINATIONS: INCOORDINATION **4145-1**

Q. Does a diabetic condition exist in this body?

A. Not that of purely diabetic. That rather of a hindered circulation, and an overstimulation to the digestive system—for when there is too much alcohol produced in the system, either by the addition of alcoholic stimulants or of the diet that produces the improper equilibrium of alcoholic condition, the pancreas and the liver suffer from same, producing—as is seen in the liver proper—*not* cirrhosis, but a tendency toward cirrhosis, or improper eliminationen—gorged liver, yet not functioning perfectly. Hence the overstimulation to the hepatics, and especially to the kidneys in their functioning.

With the correct diet, with the proper attention to the blood supply, and the proper adjustments throughout the cerebrospinal system, we will find better conditions along this line will prevail.

4/18/40
F. 25 yrs.
VITAMINS: GLANDS **2171-1**

Any form of malt or spiritus drinks, should be eliminated from the system. These tend to irritate those very conditions that are a part of the assimilation.

9/15/36
F. 27 yrs.
EPILEPSY **543-25**

Q. Would it injure this body to smoke, in moderation, or to drink beer or any alcoholic drinks?

A. These would only be a means of expression and so long as it is in keeping with these, very good. Wine or beer either would be preferable, and beneficial in moderation—as would the activities of smoke upon the nervous system. Excesses would make for destructive forces or energies turned in directions that would need or require other outlets.

10/17/35
F. 49 yrs.
ANEMIA **1023-1**

Q. Is alcohol injurious to the body?

A. As indicated from the suggestions to not consume sweets and starches at the same meal, such a form of alcohol becomes detrimental. Wines—and even rum at times—are helpful, if taken *as* a body-building meal; that is, a small glass—preferably in the afternoon—*with* black or sour bread. But those forms that are of the hop nature are detrimental, for they produce—to a disturbed condition in the system—activative forces that are harmful.

11/21/34
M. Adult
ASSIMILATIONS: INCOORDINATION **741-1**

Q. Just what alcoholic beverages could the body take without harm?

A. The wines, or those that act less upon the glands of the liver itself. For with the lack of these flows through the system, and especially in the liver secretions, these make for disturbances to the pancreas and the left lobe of the liver.

Q. What alcoholic beverages should the body particularly *abstain* from?

A. *Hard liquors.*

2/15/39
F. 41 yrs.
1713-21

ASSIMILATIONS: ELIMINATIONS: INCOORDINATION

Be very careful, then, in the combining of the foods. Never have any of those forces of alcohol or of hops or of ANYthing that tends to make for the disturbing in the better assimilation for the body-forces. These tend to create an acidity, which already exists.

8/30/27
F. 27 yrs.
37-2

PLEUROPNEUMONIA

Little stimulants, see? These stimulants may consist of any properties that are a stimulation to the excretory system, see? Spirits frumenti in mild form. Champagne, or any of these, just so they do not work a hardship on the body. Gin, mild, see?

3/30/38
F. 36 yrs.
1560-1

TUBERCULOSIS

Take EGGS, RAW—if they can be taken. And if the body can assimilate same, take the WHOLE egg; for the albumin of the white—while it may be severe at one time, it is necessary at other times. And these may be taken in BEER if so desired, or in a little whiskey—but take the whole egg. This once or twice a day will be found to be MOST helpful.

6/14/41
F. 30 yrs.
2390-4

ANEMIA

Q. Is alcohol in moderation harmful to me?

A. All forms of alcohol are HARMFUL; especially anything made with hops!

1)—Apple Brandy

10/26/36
F. Adult
1278-6

DEBILITATION: GENERAL

Q. Is red wine and brown bread recommended for this—body?

A. This body, in the immediate, would respond better to the stimulation in rock candy and pure apple brandy, as indicated. For these are effective upon the pulmonaries and the whole of the respiratory system; while the wine and the brown bread are more effective upon the digestive system. The red wine may be taken a very little, or occasionally. But as we find these would rather come later than in the immediate future.

As a tonic, as we find, those as may be had from a little rock candy with *pure* apple brandy is strengthening, is that which will work with the digestive forces.

6/25/34
M. Adult
ASTHMA **595-1**

Also at times, not always—but when the condition especially is bad in the evenings, or when there is damp weather, or when there is the tendency or the approach of storms or the like—we would use the pure *apple* brandy; not Apple Jack nor cider, but *brandy*—apple brandy. A small quantity of it. Or, to 4 to 6 ounces of same add 1/2 ounce of Rock Candy. Shake this together until it is dissolved. Do not take at a dose more than a teaspoonful, or a good swallow—which would be 2 teaspoonsful. Never more than that much, and let it go down *very* slowly, see?

2)—Beer

4/1/44
M. 36 yrs.
SINUSITIS **4047-1**

Q. Is beer in the amounts I have been drinking it detrimental?

A. Do not use any of those things made from hops!

3/12/37
M. 28 yrs.
ALCOHOL: ECZEMA **1005-16**

To be sure, only use brown bread. Not *any* of the fluids that carry hops in same, as beer or of that nature.

Refrain from alcohols and of beers or things that carry hops or any of its *combinations*; else we will have greater distresses for the body.

These as we find should be kept as consistent with the activities.

6/6/40
ASSIMILATIONS: POOR **F. 19 yrs.**
ANEMIA **2277-1**

Keep away from any compounds of soft drinks that carry carbonated water. Do not drink beer or those things that are of malt fermentation, unless taken AS medicine. Beer that would be prepared—one glass each day with a raw egg in same—the yolk of the egg put into it—would be very well—but not alone.

12/12/33
F. 22 yrs
DEBILITATION GENERAL: TUBERCULOSIS **418-2**

About three or four o'clock in the afternoon, take BEER—with egg in same! Beat well into the activity.

8/27/41
M. 51 yrs.
BLEPHARITIS **2577-1**

As to those warnings concerning the pancreas condition—be mindful that in the diet there are no sugars taken, nor any of those properties that carry carbonated waters OR any product of the hops, or of such natures.

5/7/37
M. 28 yrs.
ALCOHOL: ECZEMA **1005-18**

Do not overtax the system. Be mindful especially of raw or new beer—do not take these.

8/1/41
CIRCULATION: LYMPH **M. 36 yrs.**
BLOOD: HUMOR **2548-1**

Q. Is beer or natural wine harmful to me?

A. Beer or ANY of the brewed or distilled liquors are harmful. For, they only add to the lymph disturbance—by exciting to activity throughout the mucous membranes of the whole body.

We would refrain even from carbonated drinks.

8/27/40
F. 40 yrs.
ATHLETE'S FOOT: ECZEMA **2332-1**

Q. Is beer harmful?

A. Very harmful for the body. For, the hops act upon the glandular forces that are disturbing to the body; especially the NEW—and so little is aged at present.

Especially the combinations of ale and beer are harmful.

3)—Eggnog

5/10/44
F. 28 yrs.
TUBERCULOSIS **5097-1**

As to the diet: Have plenty of eggs, but not the white of the eggs. This may be taken in spirits frumenti with milk about once a day, making what is called eggnog.

2/21/43
F. 33 yrs.
CANCER **2918-1**

Mr. Cayce: Yes, we have the body here.

As we find, conditions are rather serious. While there is still life there is hope, but the advanced conditions as produced by the effects of some applications made, make it a very serious disturbance to be dealt with.

This, we find, is more consumptive in its nature than ordinarily. Thus the effect of lack of ability of coagulation, where there is the breaking of cellular tissue through the pelvic organs, causes the greater distress.

The searing of same, with the effects of the applications, is at present only temporary.

We may add such elements in the diet as to be helpful, but not curative.

As we find, these will add to the ability of the bloodstream to resist, or to build coagulations:

Take about twice daily a drink made with milk, egg, and a very small quantity of whiskey; just enough whiskey to cook the yolk of the egg—or a teaspoonful poured on the yolk, and then all of the white beaten in it; then this stirred in about half to three-quarters of a glass of milk.

We would not hinder those applications that are made to keep the body from severe pain; but do add these properties as indicated.

10/4/35
ANEMIA **M. 41 yrs.**
DEBILITATION: GENERAL **1014-1**

Do not use milk in the morning meal. Use milk rather in the meal that would be *between* the morning and noon meals; that is, in a glass of milk there would be added the *yolk* of an egg with apple brandy. Have the egg "cooked," as it were, with apple brandy; then add the milk. This should be at least a glassful, in the middle of the morning between the two meals.

ACIDITY
CIRCULATION: INCOORDINATION **5/11/42**
COLD: CONGESTION **F. 74 yrs.**
BODY-BUILDING **2074-2**

Mr. Cayce: Yes—this we have had before. This may become rather serious for the body, unless there is the ability to build some more resistance in the system. For, the complications of the disturbance from cold and congestion in the lymph circulation, which arises from superacidity, as combined with the low vitality AND the heart disturbance, may produce distressing disturbances unless this may be aided without overstimulating heart's activity.

Give semi-liquids and liquids, foods that are very stimulating. Every form of better stimulant that is for building strength, as eggnog. These especially, with the fish foods.

10/11/38
F. 56 yrs.
ASTHENIA **1631-2**

Also, it would be well that there be taken malted milk with the yolk of an egg, and a little bit of spirits frumenti or pure apple brandy. This would, of course, be prepared with the egg; a little poured in at the time—and about a spoonful to the yolk of one egg; this beaten well together, then added to the malted milk as it would be prepared with the water for the proper consistency for a drink. But this, too, would be taken in sips—a glassful taken during a whole day, about three to four times, and a quarter of the quantity sipped at one time, see?

12/5/43
ASTHENIA **F. 6 yrs.**
EPILEPSY **3398-1**

Eggnog will be strengthening for the respiratory system and heart activity. Use the yolk of an egg and a little spiritus frumenti, with only a tiny bit of milk, or it may be taken with orange juice.

These will be strengthening for the body. Take sufficient of these each day to keep the strength. These are only additions to the other foods.

3/17/38
F. 52 yrs.
601-29

CANCER

Q. Are eggnogs recommended with a little cognac?

A. Eggnogs with cognac is very well.

9/5/42
F. 27 yrs.
2806-1

TUBERCULOSIS

Do give other pre-digested foods; as the eggnog (very weak), but no heavy foods nor fat foods.

7/26/37
F. 60 yrs.
1409-4

DEBILITATION: GENERAL
TEMPERATURE: FEVER: AFTEREFFECTS

Since the temperature has been allayed, there is the necessity, to be sure, that there are not foods used nor activities that would tend to make for the weakening of the digestive forces, nor the allowing of activities of the assimilating system—the liver, the kidneys or the whole hepatic circulation—to become so congested as to allow the temperature to arise again.

Hence we would keep rather a tendency to the alkaline-producing foods.

Q. Should the whiskey still be burned for the eggnog before taking?

A. This must be burned, and use RYE whiskey.

6/5/34
M. Adult
572-1

TUBERCULOSIS

All the milk having the animal heat in same that the body can drink. This wouldn't be a great deal in the beginning, but it may be increased. And do not take quantities of sweet milk unless it does have the animal heat in same. When milk is taken otherwise, let it be with egg and spirits frumenti or apple brandy instead of the spirits frumenti. This should be taken in small quantities, not gulped. Two teaspoonsful would be much better than two big swallows, for it would work better with the digestive system and keep the activity of the blood supply and the gastric juices of the stomach itself.

The spirits frumenti or apple brandy in the eggnogs would be taken twice each day.

7/11/39
F. 72 yrs.
1553-15

ASTHENIA: SPIRITUAL

Q. Is there anything to build up her strength?

A. A little spirits frumenti would be well occasionally, or cook the yolk of a raw egg by dropping the whiskey over it, and then adding milk. This will aid materially in giving strength and vitality. For one egg use a teaspoonful or more of the spirits frumenti, with about half a glass of milk—and this quantity taken during a whole day, but keep on ice when not being taken, of course.

4)—Liqueurs

1/20/34
F. 30 yrs.
ALCOHOL: ANEMIA: TENDENCIES **493-1**

Q. Is drinking harmful for this body?

A. Until there are changes, or until there is something builded for the body to make for resistances much better in the system, if any is taken it should be rather *small* quantities.

Q. Wines or liqueurs preferable?

A. Liqueurs are preferable to wines, for the body. Wines tend to make for an activity with the gastric forces that is not as well for this body as liqueurs.

5)—Wine: General

1/22/37
F. 39 yrs.
ACNE **1293-2**

While with meats or with black or brown bread, wine or even strong drink is very good at times; provided the proper eliminations are kept in the system.

5/11/42
F. 74 yrs.
BODY-BUILDING **2074-2**

Give semi-liquids and liquids, foods that are very stimulating. Every form of better stimulant that is for building strength, as wine. These especially, with the fish foods.

3/7/35
F. 43 yrs.
COLITIS: TENDENCIES **846-1**

A stimulation occasionally as of wine with bread, not as a drink but just as a potion to bring rest to the body. When taken it should only be with rye or sour or brown bread.

Q. Until I get better, when I have a headache what can I do to relieve it?

A. As we would find, if these are begun we will have very few returns of the headache—which comes from this heaviness upon the colon and the lacteal duct and the strain on the system.

4/8/38
M. 30 yrs.
ASSIMILATIONS: POOR **849-26**

Keep away from drinks that are distilled; save light or very heavy wines.

1/5/36
F. 46 yrs.
COLITIS: TENDENCIES **404-6**

Q. Is the home-made wine made from the blue grapes good for this body?

A. If fermented a sufficient period, very good for the body; if taken as a food, *not* as a drink! Take with sour bread or *brown* bread at those periods when there is needed the stimulation from the general activity of the system; that is, at three, four to five o'clock in the afternoon is the period when an ounce to an ounce and a half may be taken with the bread and be beneficial.

1/7/37
CIRCULATION: POOR **F. 44 yrs.**
ELIMINATIONS: POOR **1315-6**

Do not combine white bread especially at any time when wines or strong drinks are taken.

2/9/35
ANEMIA **F. 50 yrs.**
ASSIMILATIONS: POOR **821-1**

Evenings—Natural quantity of sugar, natural quantity of wines would be *helpful* to the body if taken *only* with bread; for this produces an activity that is body, blood and nerve building, but wine taken in excess—of course—is harmful; wine taken with bread alone is body, blood and nerve and brain building.

Q. Any particular kind of wines that would be best?

A. That which is well fermented, or grape juices or the like; these are the better, not too much of the sour nor too sweet a wine. Tokay, Port, Sauterne.

6/12/34
CANCER: TENDENCIES **F. 42 yrs.**
ASSIMILATIONS **583-8**

And in the early mornings it would be well for the body to be stimulated with very light wine, which would be helpful to the whole assimilating system; such as Tokay, claret or the like—a small quantity; but this in the mornings, *not* in the evenings.

3/11/38
F. 52 yrs.
CANCER **601-28**

Q. Should a tonic be taken to stimulate appetite? If so, what tonic?

A. As we find, if there is given the light wine this should be sufficient stimulant; and do not overtax or overworry or let overanxiety cause greater disturbances.

3/17/38
F. 52 yrs.
CANCER **601-29**

The light wine will tend to make for a better appetite and will not be as hard upon the heart as other stimulants.

11/7/36
M. 45 yrs.
TOXEMIA **877-13**

Q. What about water, the quantity I should take and when?

A. Periods arise as we find when too much water makes for reactions that are unsatisfactory owing to these balances in the bodily structural forces of the body itself. Hence we would find light wines may be taken occasionally in the place of water.

5/17/44
F. 49 yrs.
ARTHRITIS **5129-1**

Do not take carbonated water, no strong drink or those of other types, as malt drink. Wine may be taken if it is light wine, not necessarily white wine, but light wine, not too high in alcoholic content.

2/18/25
F. 33 yrs.
ANEMIA **2457-1**

Quantities of the juices of beef may be taken, *should* be taken, provided small quantities of stimulant in fruit juices are taken with same, such as light wines, taken with the meat juice, or beef juice.

i)—Blackberry Wine

1/5/36
F. 46 yrs.
COLITIS: TENDENCIES **404-6**

Q. Is blackberry wine better?
A. Blackberry wine is *not* good! It's tendency is to produce constipation.

ii)—Champagne

7/7/36
F. 49 yrs.
ACIDITY & ALKALINITY **920-8**

For this particular body, light wines or champagne or those of that nature would be helpful to add a bit of an alcoholic content with the food: that there may be kept those tendencies for a better elimination, a better coordination through those activities in the alimentary canal as well as the gastric flows from the pancreas, the liver and the spleen, as well as the activity of the gall duct for the lacteals' assimilation.

6/22/28
F. Adult
CANCER **125-2**

For the adminstration of that which will give better elements for the physical body, give stimulus of spirits frumenti . . . or small quantities of dry champagne may be given, very cold. These will add to the comfort of the body. Eliminations need to be stimulated. Do that for the better ease of physical forces of this body.

3/30/38
F. 36 yrs.
TUBERCULOSIS **1560-1**

Once or twice or three times a day take about half an ounce of wine; this to be sipped. Champagne, of course, would be better—but light wine, not real heavy wine nor that which is too sour or too sweet—but that which will by the sipping, give the tendency for the increasing of the flow.

iii)—Red Wine

10/4/35
ANEMIA **M. 41 yrs.**
DEBILITATION: GENERAL **1014-1**

Between the noon and evening meals—that is, in the middle of the afternoon—take two ounces of red wine with black bread, or brown bread, or whole wheat bread that is browned. This should only be taken in such combination, for the iron, the copper, the silicon, the blood-building properties that come from such a combination—especially at this hour. Do not take *other* alcoholic *drinks* at other times!

Q. Has the condition caused from so-called erysipelas been relieved entirely?

A. Naturally, this being a lymph disturbance (erysipelas), and the conditions in the body a drain upon the sympathetic nerve forces and a great deal of disturbance in the blood supply, there are—as it were—*traces:* but the general condition builded as indicated will eradicate same, especially through that as will be assimilated by the system from red wine—copperas.

1/4/36
BLOOD-BUILDING: **F. 22 yrs.**
MINERALS: CALCIUM DEFICIENCY **578-5**

Q. Please give in full a blood-building diet for my body.

A. Those as indicated that have a quantity or an excess of the calcium, and those that will make for a balance in the iodines with the potassiums of the system itself.

Wine taken as a *food,* not as a drink. An ounce and a half to two ounces of red wine in the afternoon, after the body has *worn* itself out; that is, two, three, four o'clock in the afternoon or cocktail time. Take it as a food with brown bread. Not beer or ale, nor any of the hard drinks—but *red wine!*

1/31/38
F. 61 yrs.
ARTHRITIS **1474-2**

Do not take any of the foods that make for fermentation. No beer or heavy drinks, EVER; though red wine may be taken of an afternoon AS food—with rye or whole wheat wafers—but take very slowly, AS a food, not as a drink.

4/30/36
F. 42 yrs.
MENU: NEURASTHENIA **1192-6**

Red wine in the late afternoon with black or brown bread is helpful, *not* taken, however, at mealtimes. This, as we find, brings a stimulation that is laxative in its reaction; only the *red* wine, not the white wine.

3/12/37
M. 28 yrs.
ALCOHOL: ECZEMA **1005-16**

Red wine is helpful if taken as a food—*not* as a drink. So an ounce of this in the late afternoon with brown or sour bread, or the Ry-Krisp, or rye bread, or the pumpernickel or the like—and sipped with the bread, but chewing at the same time—will be helpful. These as we find should be kept as consistent with the activities.

11/18/37
M. 33 yrs.
LACERATIONS: STOMACH **1481-1**

Hence as we find in taking into consideration that which will be helpful and beneficial, and to remove the disturbances from the body:

Not only must there be considered the activities for a physical condition but that which will produce a better coordination through the activities of the mental and the SENSITIVE forces—or senses themselves of the body.

These as we find may be reached the better through the application or the use of these:

First, refrain from any high activative forces of highly seasoned foods. None of those foods that produce excesses of alcoholic reactions; as the combinations of too great quantities of starches, or any liquids or foods with high STRONG alcoholic content.

However, red wine taken as a food WOULD be beneficial; especially if this is taken with brown bread, sour bread, or such natures—as the BETTER grades of pumpernickel or the like. Two to two and a half ounces taken in the afternoons with such breads WOULD be most helpful.

12/17/36
M. 56 yrs.
KIDNEYS **1308-1**

And then be most mindful of the diet. These as we find to beware of, and those other things that agree with the body most any of these may be taken—but these leave off:

No strong drink—or any that carry or produce alcoholic reaction. No beer, no strong drink; though red wine as a *food* may be taken occasionally—for this is blood-building and blood-resisting forces are carried in same—as iron and those plasms that make for the proper activity upon the system. But never more than two or two and a half ounces of same, but this only with black or brown bread, and not with sweets.

Use these consistently for thirty to sixty days, and then we would give further instructions.

12/3/35
F. 51 yrs.
OBESITY: TENDENCIES **1073-1**

Wines, or such natures, may be taken more preferably as food; not as those that would be taken *with* food. Hence red wine—that is, Sherry or Port, or such natures, taken with sour bread, or black bread, in the late afternoon—rather than coffee or tea—is much more preferable; and it doesn't put on weight, it doesn't make for souring in the stomach—if taken in that manner; but not with other foods!

Do these, and be patient, be consistent. And we will bring much better conditions.

4/11/35
ARTHRITIS: TENDENCIES **F. Adult**
BLOOD: HUMOR **888-1**

In the matter of the diet, be more mindful that there are less of the acid-producing foods; more of carbohydrates—that is, sweetsbut sweets—such as wine; but only a small quantity of red wine each day, only with black or brown bread—this would make for a stimulating of the whole system.

9/28/35
F. 18 yrs.
PERITONITIS: AFTEREFFECTS **852-8**

Red wine with brown or black bread, soaked in same, would be well—or "dunked," as some would call it. Very little. The sipping or sucking of same, swallowing—though—a portion of the bread. This about once each day.

5/22/39
ELIMINATIONS **F. 31 yrs.**
LIVER: KIDNEY: INCOORDINATION **1889-1**

In the matter of the diet—keep away from those things that tend to produce acidity in the system. Beware of any of those drinks that carry too great a quantity of carbonated waters, or of such natures that produce an alcoholic reaction.

Red wine—taken of late afternoon as FOOD and not as drink—would be helpful; not only in aiding the activity of an already disturbed circulation through the hepatics, but in stimulating the gastric flow as to aid a better activity through pancreas, spleen AND the activity of the kidneys.

6/14/35
F. Adult
GLANDS: INCOORDINATION **935-1**

In following these diets, it is well that no *fermented* drink be taken; nor ginger ale, Coca-Cola, or any of the ferments. However, red wine may be taken; *not* white wines nor rye, corn or cereal drinks of such natures for the body.

1/7/37
CIRCULATION: POOR **F. 44 yrs.**
ELIMINATIONS: POOR **1315-6**

Do not combine white bread especially at any time when wines or strong drinks are taken.

Do not use too much of or too great quantity of alcoholic drinks, though red wine is very good for the body, or light wines—*not* in excess.

8/29/35
ACIDITY: ALKALINITY **M. 51 yrs.**
COMBINATIONS **462-6**

Q. Any kind of intoxicating drinks?

A. *Wine* is good for all if taken alone or with black or brown bread. Not with meats so much as with just bread. This may be taken between meals, or as a meal; but not too much—and just once a day. Red wine only.

5/20/35
M. Adult
ACIDITY **926-1**

Beware of any stimuli as to make for fermentations in the system, as spirits frumenti of any kind. However, one meal each day—or two to three times a week—may include only black bread and wine (red wine); this should not be taken with vegetables or with other foods, save with either cold fowl or black bread or whole wheat bread or rye bread especially, or sour bread.

8/12/37
F. 36 yrs.
LACERATIONS: STOMACH **1422-1**

No strong drinks or any food that makes for a quantity of alcohol in its activity in the system; that is, no cocktails, no beer. Wine may be taken as a food, not as a drink. Red wine in the late afternoon is very well, not more than an ounce and a half to two ounces; preferably with black or brown bread.

11/16/36
BLOOD: COAGULATION: POOR **F. 41 yrs.**
BODY-BUILDING **1100-8**

In the diet include those foods that are blood and body-building, that carry iron in such manners as may be assimilated by the body. Red wine with sour or black bread also is most helpful, for this carries these properties in such measures that resistances may be builded in those activities of the glandular system that are lacking in their effective functioning.

Q. How can the bodily resistance be kept up, especially during the winter months?

A. By following these suggestions that have just been indicated, we find we may build resistances for this body, through the periods of sudden changes or distresses that may come from sudden changes to the bodily temperature.

9/14/37
DEBILITATION: GENERAL **F. 60 yrs.**
ASSIMILATIONS: POOR **1409-5**

Q. Would sherry wine be good for the body?

A. Very well. Heavy red wine would be better, taken as a food, NOT as mere drink. Sherry is very well, but the heavy red wine is the better.

11/25/36
CIRCULATION: POOR **M. 48 yrs.**
ELIMINATIONS: POOR **437-7**

Do not have those combinations where there are too great quantities of any alcoholic-producing foods. Not referring to alcohol itself so much, for as we find RED WINE would be excellent if taken as a meal with black or sour bread, in the evenings or late afternoon.

Red wine in the evening or afternoon is well. Alcohol in other forms, as hard rum, *not* so well. Light wines are very good. Beer *not* good.

Q. What is meant by red wine?

A. Means RED wine! Not white wine, not sour wine; not that that is too sweet but any of those that are in the nature of adding to the body the effect of grape sugar.

There is a variation, to be sure, in the character of sugars and the necessary forces and influences of that carried on in the system in producing assimilation.

Foods must ferment, naturally, from acid, the action of acid and alkalin. These passing into the duodenum, especially, become then certain characters of sugars; as produced by the activity of the pancreas juices upon the effect of juices from the liver and the spleen, in digestive forces.

Then the addition of red wine, which is carrying more of a tartaric effect upon the active forces of the body, is correct; while those that are sour or that draw out from the system a reaction upon the hydrochlorics become detrimental.

We are through for the present.

iv)—Sherry

11/29/43
M. 36 yrs.
ALCOHOL WARNINGS **849-74**

Q. Would a spoonful of brandy taken after swimming be harmful?
A. If this were sherry it would be better than brandy.

v)—White Wine

7/21/44
F. 60 yrs.
CANCER: LUNGS **5374-1**

White wines as a stimuli will be most helpful for the body. These should be very light; that is, the alcoholic content not more than six percent. These would be most helpful.

4/30/36
F. 42 yrs.
NEURASTHENIA **1192-6**

If the sauterne or the light wines are taken, these should always be *with* meals, not separate.

2—Carbonated: General

6/11/43
M. 36 yrs.
ASSIMILATIONS: POOR **3047-1**

Do not take ANY carbonated waters, or carbonated drinks of any kind.

Do not take ANY of the drinks made with carbonated waters, or those prepared from hops. These are bad for conditions that exist, and the tendencies through alimentary canal.

7/30/36
M. 30 yrs.
HAIR: COLOR RESTORER **416-9**

Q. Is there any liquid I could drink, or something else I could do besides eat potato peelings, to restore the color and prevent gray hair?

A. Any of those that are of the nature that carry these same elements. Not too great a quantity as a drink of Coca-Cola (this may be overdone), though occasionally it would be well. And Root Beer is even better than Coca-Cola, though drink same occasionally—for it is helpful, provided there is the proper balance in the kidney activity to be sure.

10/8/38
F. 51 yrs.
DEBILITATION: GENERAL **1703-1**

Any of the drinks where carbonated waters are used are very well, especially Coca-Cola or those of that nature—just so there is NOT used any preservative in the preparation of same. Hence some of the orange drinks and some of grapefruit drinks are NOT well for the body.

5/18/43
M. 63 yrs.
ARTHRITIS **3009-1**

Q. What drink should I adopt or give up to help my condition?

A. DO NOT take any carbonated drinks of ANY kind!

5/22/39
F. 31 yrs.
ELIMINATIONS **1889-1**

Keep away from those things that tend to produce acidity in the system. Beware of any of those drinks that carry too great a quantity of carbonated waters, or of such natures that produce an alcoholic reaction.

4/5/41
ASSIMILATIONS: ELIMINATIONS: **M. 20 yrs.**
INCOORDINATION **2157-2**

Q. Are soft drinks all right for this body?

A. No; for very few bodies, and not for this body either!

ACIDITY **7/22/31**
ASSIMILATIONS: ELIMINATIONS: **F. 28 yrs.**
INCOORDINATION **2261-1**

Of drinks—beware of any of those that are of the soda; no bottle drinks, or very little from the fountain. These will be harmful to the body.

10/28/42
F. 34 yrs.
ELIMINATIONS: POOR **2833-1**

NO carbonated drinks of any character should be taken. While some soft drinks may be taken beneficially, as those that aid in clarifying the circulation between the liver and the kidneys, they should be made with plain water.

8/4/41
F. 47 yrs.
BODY-BUILDING **1013-3**

DO NOT take any form of drinks that carry carbonated waters. The gases of these, as well as all such, are detrimental and only add fire to the unbalanced chemical forces that are segregating themselves in the body.

8/1/41
CIRCULATION: LYMPH **M. 36 yrs.**
BLOOD: HUMOR **2548-1**

We would refrain even from carbonated drinks. Ice cream and ices may be taken, but not carbonated waters. These also excite lymph activity, and with the burr in some of the tissues of the body is irritating.

4/15/38
ASTHENIA: TENDENCIES **M. 20 yrs.**
BODY-BUILDING **487-22**

When carbonated waters or drinks are taken, either Dr. Pepper's or Coca-Cola may be taken; but let such as these be rather as an extra drink and not too regularly—and of soft drinks BEWARE.

1)—Coca-Cola

11/19/43
F. 66 yrs.
ELIMINATIONS: POOR **3412-1**

Here we find that the addition of Coca-Cola, taken in plain water, would be as helpful for the body as anything that could be taken to aid in the activity of kidneys and bladder. A glass of this about twice each day would be sufficient, taken in plain water—with ice, if this is preferable. This will also aid in the general circulation.

11/5/42
ASSIMILATIONS: ELIMINATIONS **M. 36 yrs.**
LIVER: KIDNEYS: INCOORDINATION **416-17**

In interpreting body-forces for this body, there has been a tendency for an incoordination between liver and kidneys, as we have indicated for the body.

Thus, leave out of the diet those things that tend to slow the activity of this coordination, but rather increase the vital energies that make for, in the assimilations, better coordination.

Then, DO NOT take ANY carbonated drinks—of any nature. Coca-Cola, or such, are well to clear kidneys, but make same with plain water.

4/8/38
M. 30 yrs.
ASSIMILATIONS: POOR **849-26**

CARBONATED drinks may be taken, especially Coca-Cola or those of such derivatives. These will aid especially in purifying the activity and coordinating same through the kidneys and the eliminating system.

4/17/41
M. 63 yrs.
DEBILITATION: GENERAL: DIABETES **584-8**

Keep away from any carbonated waters, save at times—or rather regularly—we would take a little Coca-Cola. This, with some of the activities in same, acts upon the kidneys to aid in relieving the tensions there.

12/31/37
DEBILITATION: GENERAL **M. 41 yrs.**
LIVER: KIDNEYS: INCOORDINATION **1476-2**

Those drinks with a little charged water would be very well—as Coca-Cola or the like, if taken once or twice a day; for their reaction upon the system as related to especially the hepatic or the kidney AND liver circulation would be good.

5/12/28
M. 33 yrs.
LIVER: KIDNEYS: INCOORDINATION **900-383**

The body should not take any of foods that would add to the mental activity sympathetically to the kidneys. Coca-Cola would be very well for the body to take as a stimulant once in a while. This will reduce the activity in this direction.

Q. Is the albumin on the decrease or increase in the urine?

A. This on decrease. Or, as would be seen with one bottle of Coca-Cola for two days, none would appear. Leave this off and we would find sedimentary, and some albumin.

6/16/42
F. 23 yrs.
DEBILITATION: GENERAL **2766-1**

Do not take carbonated drinks. Coca-Cola or the like, if it is prepared from the syrup and using plain water (not carbonated water), will be not harmful; in fact, it would be helpful for the kidneys and for the purifying of the blood flow.

8/27/40
F. 40 yrs.
ATHLETE'S FOOT: ECZEMA **2332-1**

Keep free from ANY carbonated waters, for the carbonations cause an effluvium in the blood. To be sure, Coca-Cola is helpful to the kidneys, but if taken, use the Coca-Cola syrup in plain water—and this to the body will not be very palatable.

6/9/44
M. 35 yrs.
LIVER: KIDNEYS: INCOORDINATION: ACNE **5218-1**

Do be careful that there are no quantities of carbonated waters. These, as we find, will be hard on the body; though Coca-Cola, if it is taken without carbonated water, will be beneficial for the body in clarifying or purifying the kidneys and bladder disorder.

5/5/44
M. 39 yrs.
INJURIES: KIDNEYS **5058-1**

Never take any carbonated water, although it will be found that the syrup of Coca-Cola in plain water will be well for the body, for this will react with the circulation between the kidneys and the liver, and will clear off much of the poisons which will be more beneficial for the activity of the sensory system.

7/26/43
M. 2 yrs.
ELIMINATIONS: INCOORDINATION **3109-1**

Here we find that Coca-Cola will be good, even for this baby. This will act to purify the circulation between the kidneys and the liver. Preferably use this in plain water, however, NOT carbonated water. Have the syrup and make it with the plain water, NOT carbonated or charged water. The effect of the tannic forces will be helpful for this condition. Two to three ounces we would take at the time, not necessarily every day—but three to four times a week would be better.

10/11/38
F. 35 yrs.
CYSTITIS: TENDENCIES **540-11**

If desirable drink Coca-Cola—a little Coca-Cola; this will act in purifying or clearing the ducts through the kidneys, and thus reduce the general forces and influences there.

11/29/37
M. 42 yrs.
KIDNEYS: URINE: SEDIMENT: ACIDITY **1334-2**

This is one body that would do well to occasionally take a Coca-Cola; not to become as a habituate action, but occasionally this would be GOOD for the body. There are influences in same that would purify the activities of the lower hepatic circulation, that would be beneficial. Preferably, though, use that perfectly prepared—BOTTLED, rather than from the counter—for they are more uniform.

10/8/38
KIDNEYS: INFECTIONS **F. 58 yrs.**
KIDNEYS: STONES: TENDENCIES **1472-7**

The beverages that are mixed with the carbonated water are rather inclined to be beneficial: especially such as Coca-Cola.

10/7/43
M. 68 yrs.
NEPHRITIS: TENDENCIES **1112-9**

It may be necessary for the body to drink Coca-Cola, (but use plain water, not carbonated) or to put a little lithia tablet in the drinking water.

3/2/43
M. 10 yrs.
INJURIES: BIRTH: AFTEREFFECTS **2780-2**

Q. Is there a kidney or bladder weakness that necessitates getting up at night?

A. There has been rather the inclination for the eliminating channels to eliminate the poisons or excesses in the system. These are tendencies, but as we find are not weaknesses. These may be clarified by taking a drink such as Coca-Cola occasionally, but this made with plain water—for the body—rather than carbonated water. Or, once in two to three weeks a lithia tablet in the water will prevent any sediment from such activities causing distresses or weaknesses in these directions.

5/10/44
TUBERCULOSIS **F. 28 yrs.**
KIDNEYS **5097-1**

Do take Coca-Cola occasionally as a drink for the activity of the kidneys, but do not take it with carbonated water. Buy or have the syrup prepared and add plain water to this. Take about 1/2 oz. or 1 oz. of the syrup and add plain water. This to be taken about every other day with or without ice. This will aid in purifying the kidney activity and bladder and will be better for the body.

12/12/38
F. 51 yrs.
INTESTINES: GAS **1703-2**

Q. Why is Coca-Cola, and carbonated water good for me?

A. To prevent the formation of gases in the system.

10/3/34
ECZEMA **F. 51 yrs.**
GLANDS: INFECTIONS **677-1**

Q. Has Coca-Cola been harmful to the body?

A. It is an irritant to the activities in the hepatic circulation for *this* particular body, though in many cases it is rather helpful in recuperative conditions.

2)—Ginger Ale

9/30/43
M. 43 yrs.
BODY-BUILDING **3044-2**

When the body is on the mend, take once each day at least four ounces of ginger ale with two ounces of top cream in same.

9/15/43
F. Adult
ANEMIA **2843-4**

Also for this body, it would be very beneficial to take ginger ale and cream—but one of morning and the other in the afternoon—but take some every day.

3)—Limeade

7/25/36
F. 32 yrs.
KIDNEYS: PREGNANCY **540-6**

Keep a well-balance between the diets for sufficient calcium and lime. Especially limeades would be well to be taken.

4)—Orangeade

8/28/28
F. 48 yrs.
CANCER 569-16

Beware of meats. This has caused the greater distress at the present time.

Q. How would two orangeades be for her a day?

A. Be *well*, for the reactions of these are good.

12/31/37
DEBILITATION: GENERAL M. 41 yrs.
LIVER: KIDNEYS: INCOORDINATION 1476-1

These drinks with a little charged water would be very well—as orangeade or the like, if taken once or twice a day; for their reaction upon the system as related to especially the hepatic or the kidney AND liver circulation would be good.

5)—Water

7/30/41
M. 26 yrs.
ANESTHESIA: AFTEREFFECTS 1710-6

The affect of the anesthesia is to produce periods or mornings when there are headaches, a bit of dizziness, an upset at times of the digestive forces. All of these, to be sure, are the natural results—under the conditions.

Hence for this body, it is well to take occasionally—a couple of times each day—carbonated water. This does not mean merely soft drinks, but drink carbonated water—half plain and half carbonated water, at the fount. This is well to counteract the effects of general conditions which exist through the lymph in the general blood supply, especially through these periods of hot days or hot weather.

ACIDITY: EYES 1/28/44
ANEMIA F. 63 yrs.
ASSIMILATIONS: ELIMINATIONS: INCOORDINATION 3607-1

In the diet keep away from any carbonated waters.

Q. What can be done for my eyes?

A. Do these things and we will get rid of this acid throughout the system and relieve the stress upon the kidneys, which will help the eyes.

10/27/39
F. 4 yrs.
ANEMIA 2004-2

Q. What causes her many headaches?

A. The poor assimilation, or digestion of foods. This should soon be corrected if the adjustments are given, and the character of diet followed that includes the building properties indicated—or rather than giving nostrums of any nature.

Q. Is she allergic to some foods?

A. As indicated, do not give ANY CARBONATED WATERS!

CYSTS **9/5/41**
TUBERCULOSIS: TENDENCIES **F. Adult**
850-6

Q. Any other foods or drinks of which I should beware?

A. Beware only of carbonated waters. Drink plenty of water at all times.

6/9/44
M. 35 yrs.
ACNE **5218-1**

Do be careful that there are no quantities of carbonated waters. These, as we find, will be hard on the body.

6/16/34
M. 44 yrs.
INJURIES: ACCIDENTS: AFTEREFFECTS **478-3**

Keep those things that are the more easily assimilated by the body; that is, not merely the liquid diet or of such nature but that which carries with same the iron, the silicon, the blood and nerve building influences.

Carbonated waters are very good, if these are used discreetly.

4/18/40
F. 25 yrs.
VITAMINS: GLANDS **2171-1**

All forms of carbonated waters should be eliminated from the system. These tend to irritate those very conditions that are a part of the assimilation.

8/23/27
M. 26 yrs.
ELIMINATIONS: INCOORDINATION **4145-1**

Do not drink any soda fountain drinks—nothing of carbonated waters.

ASSIMILATIONS: **4/29/37**
ELIMINATIONS: INCOORDINATION **M. 45 yrs.**
BLOOD: HUMOR **877-16**

Do not mix too much of varied characters of the carbonated waters with drink, or strong drink. These make for a disturbance to the very portions that are causing reactions. Keep a well balance in the diets for eliminations as well as for assimilations.

3—Non-Carbonated

1)—Cereal Drink

9/21/34
ANEMIA **F. 19 yrs.**
LACERATIONS: STOMACH **667-1**

Mornings—There may be taken a cereal drink; *not* coffee or tea.

After each meal *rest* for at least ten to fifteen minutes, and while resting have your feet higher than your head; lying down in repose but feet higher than the head, that there may be the proper assimilations and proper positions for the stomach itself.

12/19/34
M. Adult
DIABETES **767-1**

Any of the cereal drinks may be taken. Not too great a quantity of those foods that produce an alcoholic *reaction* in the system, as from the fermentations of sweets and of starches.

1/7/34
F. 21 yrs.
GLANDS: INCOORDINATION **480-3**

At each morning meal there may be taken any character of stimulant as tea, coffee, or milk *in moderation* or, preferably still, a cereal drink, see?

10/4/35
ANEMIA **M. 41 yrs.**
DEBILITATION: GENERAL **1014-1**

Mornings—Preferably the drink would be a *cereal* drink, or one which the greater part of the caffein has been extracted.

2)—Ovaltine

6/4/29
F. 59 yrs.
ARTHRITIS: TENDENCIES **5525-1**

Instead of the use of coffee or tea, use those of the Ovaltine, or of such preparations. Not too much of the sweets!

5/1/38
F. Adult
ARTHRITIS **932-1**

Mornings—A little whole wheat toast may be taken if desired with a little butter and cocoa or better still use Ovaltine at this meal.

Evenings—A little coffee occasionally, preferably, though, use Ovaltine.

2/10/30
M. 41 yrs.
LACERATIONS: STOMACH **5545-1**

Ovaltine may be taken as a drink at times. No tea, no coffee.

9/6/33
ASSIMILATIONS: POOR **F. 3 yrs.**
MALARIA: TENDENCIES **402-1**

Mornings—A little Ovaltine or milk that has been heated—not boiled, but heated, may be taken.

12/18/30
M. 24 yrs.
BACILLOSIS: POLIOMYELITIS **135-1**

Mornings—Ovaltine or cereal grain extract may be used as a drink.

8/11/31
ELIMINATIONS: POOR **F. 42 yrs.**
BLOOD-BUILDING **484-1**

In the matter of the eliminations, be well that the diet as may be taken—Now, in adding those of the drinks . . . Ovaltine or any of the *cereal* drinks, these may be taken—but be sure there is the evacuation of the bowel at least once each day. We want to increase the flesh, increase the weight, as is gradually being diminished by the eating up or the absorption of these fluids as make for gluten, or as make for that element that is as of the emunctory and lymph circulation. Ready for questions.

Q. Should the Ovaltine be taken with the meals?

A. If so desired. Better that it *not* be taken with meals. Ovaltine is *always* better taken as an intermediate, or halfway stage, than at meals.

7/28/34
F. 54 yrs.
RHEUMATISM **133-4**

Mornings—Preferable to coffee would be Ovaltine or any *cereal* drink, though if coffee is taken it should be without cream or milk.

3)—Cocoa

4/17/31
DEBILITATION: GENERAL **M. 19 yrs.**
CHOREA **1225-1**

Evenings—Much of the sweets may be taken, provided (that is, at this period) these are not of the cane sugar variety, but chocolates—or those of the cocoa bean, these may be taken. Not too much of pastries that carry the cane sugars, but those that make for lime, silicon, magnesia—these will be well.

CHILDBIRTH: AFTEREFFECTS **8/3/26**
DEBILITATION: GENERAL **F. 34 yrs.**
ASSIMILATIONS: ELIMINATIONS: INCOORDINATION **583-4**

No stimulants as tea or coffee. Cocoa or Postum may be taken in small quantities. These would be very good, especially for the condition of the body (which is to be body building for two, you see—the nursing).

11/29/37
M. 42 yrs.
RHEUMATISM **1334-2**

In the drinks—such as . . . cocoa or the like in moderation.

4)—Chocolate

10/27/39
F. 4 yrs.
ANEMIA **2004-2**

Q. What causes her many headaches?

A. The poor assimilation, or digestion of foods. This should soon be corrected if the adjustments are given, and the character of diet followed that includes the building properties indicated, rather than giving nostrums of any nature.

Q. What about chocolate?

A. This should be very, very seldom given. But after these conditions are improved, or removed, this will be helpful in the form of a chocolate drink, rather than in candy.

5)—Coffee and Tea

8/27/35
F. 61 yrs.
ARTHRITIS **983-1**

Keep to those things that are body and blood building. Not great quantities of tea or coffee, but these may be taken in moderation provided they do not carry milk or cream in same when taken. These are as foods without same, and are more nourishing. While the food values in the milk or cream may be considered of an equal value alone, when used together they form a condition in the lactic juices of the stomach itself that does not make for the proper eliminations carried on through the whole of the alimentary canal.

1/6/42
M. 57 yrs.
GENERAL **462-14**

Q. Should coffee be taken?

A. It can be taken if this is desired, but not with milk or cream.

Q. What about tea?

A. Tea might be taken when the body is resting—but this is rather a pick-up for the body and does not last as long with the body even as coffee, and coffee is more of a good tharl tea.

8/29/35
M. 51 yrs.
ACIDITY: ALKALINITY **462-6**

Q. Is coffee or tea good for this body?

A. Coffee is better than tea, though the body may prefer the tea. Coffee without milk and without sugar is preferable; but coffee without cream or milk *is* a food value. There is very little food value in tea, though it is a stimulant. Coffee is preferable.

12/28/38
F. 53 yrs.
ELIMINATIONS: POOR **1770-1**

Do not use milk or cream IN coffee, tea or the like for these also produce activities which become combative within the assimilating forces of the body.

6/29/26
M. Adult
ASTHMA **90-1**

Do not take stimulants to *any* excess in the body—that is, tea or coffee, or any of that nature. Do not overload the kidneys for stimulants as of coffee and tea will, you see. These may be taken in moderation.

3/30/35
M. 52 yrs.
GENERAL **816-5**

Q. Can coffee and tea be used by this body without harmful effects?

A. No one can use them without effecting the body. As to whether they are harmful or not depends upon the extent to which they are used. Use one or the other; don't use them both. Tea is more harmful than coffee. Coffee is a food if it is taken without cream or sugar, and especially without cream; and if taken without caffeine—as Kaffa Hag, or the like—it's really a food for the body.

12/3/35
F. 51 yrs.
OBESITY: TENDENCIES **1073-1**

Coffee or tea should preferably be without milk or cream, for again we find that the combination of the acids—or the tannic forces, the chicory, or the properties that are the food values to the digestive forces—becomes disturbing, when combined outside of the body. However, if milk and coffee are taken at the same meal—but not combined before they are taken—the gastric juices flowing from even the salivary glands in the mouth so taking these *change* the activity so that the food values of both are taken by the system, in the activity through the alimentary canal.

Hence at the morning meals coffee or tea may be taken, but *not* with the milk *in* same. Little sugar, for this—as indicated, of course—makes for an activity upon the pancreas that, unless there is a great deal of physical exertion, creates the tendency for the increase of avoirdupois throughout the whole body itself.

Do these, and be patient, be consistent. And we will bring much better conditions.

2/12/38
F. 61 yrs.
ARTHRITIS **1512-2**

Q. Any more advice regarding my diet?

A. As indicated, do not have those combinations that produce great acid. Do not take coffee or tea with milk in same. A little sugar is not as bad as milk or cream.

8/1/36
M. 55 yrs.
ACIDITY **1236-1**

Do not combine milk with tea or coffee. These make for an acidity, and especially are hard on the digestive forces where acid is superactive in the system from the general disturbances.

8/12/37
F. 36 yrs.
LACERATIONS: STOMACH **1422-1**

No strong drinks or any food that makes for a quantity of alcohol in its activity in the system.

Coffee, if taken at all, should be without cream—though sugar may be used in same. This should be fresh (the coffee), never stale.

Beware of tea.

1/30/28
F. Adult
ELIMINATIONS: POOR: TOXEMIA **81-2**

Not too much stimulation of coffee or tea but tea would be preferable over coffee.

12/15/27
M. 30 yrs.
ASTHENIA **4605-1**

As for the diet, let that be principally of that as almost pre-digested foods. Let no stimulants of any character—either tea or coffee be taken for these would be hard on this portion of the body.

8/19/35
ASSIMILATIONS: POOR **F. 80 yrs.**
MENU: CANCER **975-1**

As to the drinks: Do not take quantities of tea, but a very small quantity once a day may be taken. Coffee may be taken in moderation provided milk or cream is *not* used in same. Without the cream coffee is a food; *with* milk or cream it is very hard on the system.

6)—Coffee

6/3/17
M. Adult
ACIDITY & ALKALINITY: ANEMIA **4834-1**

Q. Is coffee and milk good for the body?

A. Coffee is not good, the tannin in coffee affects the milk which the body needs. The body shouldn't take things that produce acid. We have things that are not acid themselves, but change into acid when taken into the mouth. Normally there are glands in the throat which produce lactic fluid or pepsin, this body is not producing sufficient lactic fluid, so that whatever is taken is carried into acid.

10/17/34
F. 40 yrs.
HYPOCHONDRIA **1000-2**

Q. Should the body drink coffee?

A. In moderation—but do not use that that carries chicory with it.

10/3/34
ECZEMA **F. 51 yrs.**
GLANDS: INFECTIONS **677-1**

Q. Is coffee harmful?

A. The cereal drinks would be preferable to coffee, though—with the habits—if coffee is used it should be that with the tannin removed, such as Kaffa Hag.

9/27/39
BRONCHITIS: TENDENCIE5 **M. 38 yrs.**
ACIDITY **1956-2**

Be careful of the diet, that there is not too much of the foods that are acid producing—that is, as milk in coffee.

2/16/35
M. 45 yrs.
ACIDITY **829-1**

Mornings—A little coffee or preferably Ovaltine. Do not drink milk or cream in the coffee when taken. Small quantities of sugar may be taken, but for the *food* value and the proper strengthening the coffee should be taken without either cream or sugar.

4/20/40
F. 74 yrs.
ARTHRITIS **1224-3**

Mornings—Coffee may be used if desired, but NOT with milk or cream in same for this is hard upon the heart, as well as the digestion. If a little sugar is desired, it is very well, but no milk or cream in the coffee.

10/29/36
M. Adult
ANEMIA **1131-2**

Coffee in moderation is very good; it is a food if taken without cream or milk—especially cream.

3/16/36
ANEMIA **F. 38 yrs.**
DEBILITATION: GENERAL **954-2**

Mornings—Coffee may be taken in moderation, but *without* milk *in* same—even though milk may be used in the cereal or even taken as a drink at the same meal.

1/5/36
F. 46 yrs.
COLITIS: TENDENCIES **404-6**

Q. Is coffee good? If so, how often?

A. Coffee taken properly is a food value.

To many conditions, as with this body, the caffeine in same is hard upon the digestion; especially where there is the tendency for a plethora condition in the lower end of the stomach.

Hence the use of coffee or the chicory in the food values that arise from the *combinations* of coffee with breads or meats or sweets is helpful.

But for this body, it is *preferable* that the tannin be mostly removed. Then it can be taken two to three times a day, but *without* milk or cream.

6/13/44
ARTHRITIS **F. 51 yrs.**
ASSIMILATIONS: POOR **5211-1**

There are conditions surrounding the body, just as there have been those suggestions to the body. There may be, just as is indicated in many an individual consciousness, those who can drink coffee and it never hurts them; there are those whose consciousness is such that this if taken late of an evening would prevent sleep. There are those who would not sleep if they didn't take it, for they would have the headache. For certain properties stimulate certain activities.

2/10/38
CANCER. COXITIS: **F. 25 yrs**
HIP EROSION (HEAD OF FEMUR) **275-45**

Q. Is the chemical reaction of raw milk in coffee the same as cream in coffee in relation to the digestion in the stomach?

A. Well, this depends—to be sure—upon the activity of the system at the time. Cream, to be sure, is less hard, or more easily digested—and produces LESS of that hard to be assimilated by portions of the system. But in coffee it is PREFERABLE for the body to use neither cream nor milk. Of course, cream is less harmful—and of course carries more food value, of a different nature. But there is a portion in same that becomes gradually hard upon the activity of the juices from the pancreas and spleen to the activities upon the system through the lacteals in their absorbing from digestion.

Q. What about sugar in coffee?

A. Brown sugar, of course, is preferable. Sugar is NOT as harmful, provided there is of course not too much sugar taken in other sweets.

12/12/38
F. 51 yrs.
INTESTINES: GAS **1703-2**

Q. Why is coffee good for me?

A. To prevent the formation of gases in the system.

7)—Tea

4/5/29
F. Adult
CIRCULATION: LYMPH: TOXEMIA **5558-1**

Beware of how the diet is used in the eliminants. Keep closer to those of the alkaline forming diet. Not too much of sweets—nor of any that will produce improper fermentation, as of tea, nor of those of alcoholic content. These should *not* be taken.

3/3/42
F. 13 yrs.
KIDNEYS: INFECTIONS **2084-11**

No carbonated drinks at any time, though for this body a little tea may at times be taken—but never with milk or cream in same.

8)—Water

6/25/34
M. Adult
ASTHMA **595-1**

Even in drinking water, *chew* it—or masticate it at least three or four times. That is, sip it—let the activity of the glands in the mouth mingle well with the water; not gulping it but sipping it gently.

6/8/40
ANEMIA **M. 55 yrs.**
KIDNEYS: INCOORDINATION **2273-1**

And above all, drink plenty of water every day, that there may be a flushing of the kidneys, so that the uric acid and the poisons that have been as accumulations may be removed.

2/16/34
F. 40 yrs.
TOXEMIA **515-1**

Drink *plenty* of water at *all* times, and preferably—no matter where the water may be taken from—BOIL the water before it is used; then cool and add ice to same, around it rather than in it.

2/28/24
NEURITIS: TENDENCIES **M. 36 yrs.**
ACIDITY **779-6**

Also more water in the system, systematically taken that the acid in the system may be dissolved.

4/29/38
CANCER: TENDENCIES **F. 77 yrs.**
KIDNEYS: INCOORDINATION **1586-1**

In the matter of the diets, these as we find would become rather specific. And these will make for greater changes in the activities, though naturally—these working through natural sources or activities, through assimilation and the building up of the body in the directions by the assimilations—results will be a bit slow; but these must be kept properly.

First, drink plenty of water each day—six or eight glasses. It is true that this tends to flush the kidneys, and it may at times cause some inconvenience in the evening; but they must be flushed out—and water is the better to use for same, see?

6/20/34
TUBERCULOSIS **M. Adult**
ELIMINATIONS: POOR **572-2**

Q. How much water should I drink daily?

A. Six to eight pints.

6/9/27
F. 20 mos.
TOXEMIA **608-3**

Do not give any water that is not first boiled, see? The water—in its precaution—is to meet those conditions as are seen produced in the assimilating system of the body. Hence when the conditions are *normal* again, this is not necessarily kept up.

CHILDBIRTH: AFTEREFFECTS **8/3/26**
DEBILITATION: GENERAL **F. 34 yrs.**
ASSIMILATIONS: ELIMINATIONS: INCOORDINATION **583-4**

Drink *plenty* of water. No stimulants as tea or coffee. The care of the body in general—keeping plenty of water for the system, internal and external, will build the body to its normal resistance.

5/29/25
F. 36 yrs.
ELIMINATIONS **780-4**

Mr. Cayce: Now, we find the conditions in body much improved from these as we had before. Only needing that the system keep eliminations normal and we will have and give the normal vibrations throughout the whole system. The body shows the change as is produced by the properties to produce the nominal eliminations in system, and the effects of same. Need only system keep well balanced. Plenty of water (pure), and the system will respond to the normal forces of the body.

11/18/33
TOXEMIA **F. 62 yrs.**
ARTHRITIS: TENDENCIES **445-2**

Q. Has there been in this system an overstimulation to the kidneys from drinking too much water?

A. As we would find, and as indicated from the condition, rather has the excess of water taken been most helpful for it has tended to wash the kidneys, and this pressure in the left portion of the body, where it makes for at times the tendency for this activity in kidneys when not an excess water taken or too little, with at times when excess water is taken. Rather has this been beneficial than harmful.

11/7/36
M. 45 yrs.
TOXEMIA **877-13**

Q. What about water, the quantity I should take and when?

A. These conditions arise, or this condition of this body: Periods arise as we find when too much water makes for reactions that are unsatisfactory owing to these balances in the bodily structural forces of the body itself, but water taken night and morning is preferable for the body. Not too much in the noontime but night and morning. This will also tend to make for at times a little irritation by cleansing the kidneys, but this is necessary to prevent any toxic forces arising from changes being wrought by these balances created in the bodily system.

4/15/38
ASTHENIA: TENDENCIES **M. 20 yrs.**
BODY-BUILDING **487-22**

Drink more water; less carbonated waters but more pure water. Of soft drinks BEWARE.

9/9/29
F. 43 yrs.
NEURASTHENIA **2713-4**

Q. What kind of drinking water is best for the body?

A. That as is as near nominal in its reaction as is possible. Too much of lime, or too much of *any* of the properties ordinarily will tend to unbalance, of course, the effects of the system. Lithia occasionally is well, but not too much—just the regular water.

5/25/35
F. Adult
ELIMINATIONS **850-3**

Q. How much water necessary for drinking?

A. All the body may drink; six to eight ounces taken three to four times each day.

7/16/35
F. 64 yrs.
ARTHRITIS **950-1**

It is preferable that the water in this particular surrounding (where the body is)* be boiled with other elements in same and used as the drinking water for the body. That is: To a gallon of water add a pinch (between the thumb and forefinger) of *salt* and a handful (or two heaping tablespoonsful) of corn meal. Let this come to a boil. Then siphon or filter and use as the drinking water, and as the water in which the medicinal properties would be taken. Of course, ice may be added.

*[near Dayton, Ohio]

8/25/41
ARTHRITIS: TENDENCIES **F. 54 yrs.**
TOXEMIA **2067-8**

Q. What health condition always makes me less well summers in N.H.?

A. The water and the effect it has upon eliminations.

ASSIMILATIONS: POOR **10/31/31**
INJURIES: ACCIDENTS: AFTEREFFECTS: **F. 60 yrs.**
FRACTURES **501-2**

Q. Why is body so constipated in the summer time, while in the country?

A. This produced, as we see, from the variations in the water for the system. One acts—that is, in its present location or surroundings—more with the lactic forces of the body; while the other being harder acts as a congesting with the body—see?

INCOORDINATION **5/19/35**
GLANDS: SALIVARY: DIGESTION: GENERAL **F. 27 yrs.**
PREGNANCY **808-3**

Q. How about roughage in the diet?

A. Do not go to excess in this direction; but the proper amount is all right provided what is taken at any time is *well* masticated. For, as we have indicated, for each and every body there should be the thorough mastication. For if this is done the activity of the glands in the mouth and the salivary glands is such as to keep the throat and the bronchi in a much healthier condition. Bolting food or swallowing it by the use of liquids produces more colds than *any one* activity of a dietl Even water should be chewed two to three times before taken into the stomach itself, for this makes for the proper assimilation of the lacteal activity in the system; and when being acted upon by the gastric flow of the hydrochlorics in the duodenum area, it is better assimilated and gives more value in the whole of the body.

7/10/22
ANEMIA **F. Adult**
DEBILITATION: GENERAL **4466-1**

The diet should be of forces that carry the highest protein in the system. Keep plenty of water in the system at all times—the body does not drink sufficient amount of water.

5/3/32
F. 49 yrs.
TOXEMIA **5647-1**

Do not drink water with meals. Take the water between the periods, see?

12/12/38
F. 51 yrs.
ELIMINATIONS: GENERAL **1703-2**

Q. Do I drink enough water or juices to keep the colon and kidneys flushed?

A. Drink WATER rather than so much juices, if you would keep the kidneys and the colon flushed. Not sufficient water taken!

9/15/43
M. 55 yrs.
DENTISTRY: GENERAL **3211-1**

Q. Regarding the universal approach: Is it true, as it is thought, that the intake of certain form and percentage of fluorine in drinking water causes mottled enamel of the teeth?

A. This, to be sure, is true: but this is also untrue unless there is considered the other properties with which such is associated in drinking water.

If there are certain percents of fluorine with free limestone, we will find it is beneficial. If there are certain percents with indications of magnesium, sulphur and the like, we will have one motley, another decaying at the gum.

Q. Does too much fluorine cause decay of teeth, and where is the borderline?

A. Read what has just been indicated. It depends upon the combinations, more than it does upon the quantity of fluorine itself. But, to be sure, too much fluorine in the water would not make so much in the teeth as it would in other elements or activities which may be reflected in teeth; not as the cause of same but producing a disturbance that may contribute to the condition.

But where there is iron or sulphur or magnesium, be careful.

To perfectly understand it would be preferable to understand these:

There are areas within the United States—such as in some portions of Texas, portions in Arizona, others in Wyoming—where the teeth are seldom ever decayed. Study the water there, the quantity of fluorine there, the lack of iron or sulphur or the proportions of sulphur; that is in the regular water.

There are many sections, of course, where fluorine added to the water, with many other chemicals would be most beneficial. There are others where, even a small quantity added would be very detrimental.

Hence it cannot be said positively that this or that quantity should be added save in a certain degree of other chemicals being combined with same in the drinking water.

But there are some places where you have few or none. For, here we will find a great quantity of either iron or sulphur, while in some places in the West—as in the central portion of Texas in certain vicinities, you won't find any decay. Certain cases in the northwestern portion of Arizona, or close within some parts of Cheyenne, Wyoming, will not be found to show decay—if the water that is used is from the normal source of supply. But where there have been contributions from other supplies of water, there will be found variations in the supply of magnesium and other chemicals—as from the flowing over, or arsenic and such—these cause destruction to the teeth.

Q. Could the diet give the required amount of fluorine for prevention of decay?

A. It could aid but depending upon the water and other conditions—there's no definite.

Q. Should drinking water in certain localities be prepared with a percentage of fluorine for prevention of decay and for preventing mottled enamel in teeth? If so, how and where?

A. This would have to be tested in the various districts themselves, much as has been indicated. There's scarcely an individual place in Ohio that it wouldn't be helpful, for it will get rid of and add to that condition to cause a better activity in the thyroid glands; while, for general use, in such a district as Illinois (say in the extreme northern portion) it would be harmful. These would necessarily require testing, according to the quantities of other conditions or minerals or elements in the water.

i)—Elm Water

2/23/21
ADHESIONS **F. Adult**
ULCERS: STOMACH **5421-2**

The water to be used should not be the well water, as has been used, because it caused too much calcium. The water this body uses should be thoroughly boiled and cooled, and to each glass should be added either a stick of slippery elm, or a pinch of the ground elm bark; and keep the water cold that is given to this system.

7/4/43
ANEMIA **F. 18 yrs.**
CIRCULATION: LYMPH **3070-1**

Add two pinches of the slippery elm (powdered elm bark) to a glass of water, stir and keep cool. Take this as the water through the day—one glass of this, see?

6/4/26
M. 54 yrs.
STOMACH **4769-2**

For the condition in the duodenum and the stomach proper, take as this:

All the water that is taken, for at least 2 weeks to 3 weeks, should carry small quantities of elm bark, ground. Preferably, let this stand in water for a while before taken, see? but do not allow to stand so long as to become sour, for this would be detrimental, rather than beneficial.

2/10/30
M. 41 yrs.
LACERATIONS: STOMACH **5545-1**

The water that is taken—*most* of same should carry those of elm, and this should be prepared just before taking, but should *always* be cool, or cold.

7/31/31
ANEMIA **F. Adult**
ASSIMILATIONS: ELIMINATIONS **4472-1**

Q. Do I drink sufficient water?

A. With taking of these properties, and plenty of salt but not peppers in those of the foods that are taken, more water *will* be taken. Not sufficient is taken. As we will find, especially in this district, Columbus, that were there added oftentimes a small pinch of elm to the drinking water this would aid in the digestive forces of the body, just a pinch between the fingers added and stirred into the glass of water about three to four minutes before it is drunk.

ii)—Elm or Saffron Water

ASTHMA: TENDENCIES **3/31/31**
GLANDS: ADRENALS: PITUITARY **F. Adult**
WATER: WELLS **4996-1**

In the physical forces we find there has been for some time back an accumulation in the drosses of the system, produced—as we find—principally from the *water*, or the character in some waters that have been taken by the system. These affect the glands of the system, especially those of the adrenal, and pituitary, in such a way and manner as to cause an improper separation in the cellular forces in system, until we have engorgements in the system, *especially* in the spleen itself; so that in the destruction of, or the taking or replenishing of the red blood cellular force, this has made for those disorders in the *functioning* system, until *many* become (as in the *respiratory* system) as of organic disorders, effecting—as is seen from the first causes—that of the lower hepatic circulation, or the kidneys, as well as the organs of pelvis, reacting through same to those of the circulation through the lungs proper; the liver engorged from same.

The water that will be taken in the interim, or during this first treatment—let each carry either small quantities of elm (ground)—this made fresh as it is taken—a pinch between finger and thumb for each glass, preferably kept cool but not with ice in same—see? or a small quantity of yellow saffron—this may be made one to twenty, or steam or steep as for tea—see? and taken, not too strong—but to change the vibrations for the whole system. Ready for questions.

Q. Does climate have any effect on her condition?

A. More in the waters than in the climatic conditions. These, of course, make for those depressions—as for the asthmatic forces, or those repressions in the *respiratory* system—but this is not *ordinary* asthmatic force—see?

iii)—Elm, Lithia, Saffron Water

2/23/35
M. Adult
PSORIASIS **840-1**

First, we would be very mindful as to the character of the diets for the body, and *most* particular as to the character of the water that is taken for those activities with or to supply the natural flow or flushing for the body. The waters about and around the body are of the nature that are hard for, or hard upon, those conditions in the system where there is already an irritation to the organs of assimilation, the organs of elimination and the respiratory system. Hence we find sort of an accumulation from same. We would not take any water unless it carried either a small quantity of lithia, elm bark, or saffron—or the conditions that make for the correcting of toxic forces along the flow of all the intestinal tract, from the mouth throughout the alimentary canal, or the natures that combine with these to make for better conditions. In this proportion we would use these:

To the normal water that may be had in the surroundings, we would add to each gallon (to be kept for drinking water, you see) a five grain lithia tablet. Dissolve this and it would make about the proper proportion, and it would be added and dissolved in same preferably after the ordinary water had been boiled—or had come to a boil and strained or filtered off before used. Then when this is to be taken, once or twice a day we would have just a pinch of the elm bark (between the thumb and forefinger) in a glass of water—the ground elm bark. If it is more preferable, it may be used with a small piece of ice in same; this would be all the better, but stir same and let it stand for a minute or two before it is taken. We would also, from the same type of water have the yellow saffron—the American saffron is correct, or may be used if so desired. This would be the proportions of about a heaping teaspoonful to a gallon of water. This preferably we would make in an enamel container or in a glass container, preferable to the aluminum. This would be allowed to steep as would tea. Then it may be drawn off and kept as a portion of the drinking water to be taken at the regular intervals when the body desires water. Not that there would never be any of the regular routine or drinking of water outside, but let the most—and as much as possible *all* that is taken either carry one or the other of those properties as indicated. This would be the first precaution, for—while it is, of course, slow acting—it will make for a cleansing of the kidneys, a better activity through the alimentary canal, clear those tendencies for the poisons to accumulate through the lymph and emunctory circulation, and overcome these tendencies for toxic forces to arise in the body that affects the body throughout.

1/22/31
M. 42 yrs.
ULCERS: TENDENCIES **2190-1**

Q. How much water?

A. *Quantities* of water! All the body would drink! Take water rather as medicine! Well that occasionally those properties in the elm or the saffron be given as an easing for the conditions in the stomach proper. Just a pinch of the elm in a glass of water—this not hot, but not ice cold. The saffron may be made into a tea, about one to twenty, steeped for thirty to forty minutes, and a teaspoonful taken in half to three-quarter glass of water. These should be taken at least once each day, either or both of these.

2/24/35
ASSIMILATIONS: ELIMINATIONS: **M. 53 yrs.**
INCOORDINATION **843-1**

Do not take any water unless it carries in same either the elm or the saffron. The elm would be made just a few minutes before it is taken. The saffron may be made and kept. A gallon or so may be made at a time, provided it is kept where it is cool or sufficient to prevent the bringing about of fermentation. This would be in the proportion of a heaping teaspoonful of the saffron (American saffron may be used) to a gallon of water. This should be allowed to steep as would tea, for thirty minutes to an hour. Strain and set aside in a cool place. This would be taken in the place of the regular water.

iv)—Lime Water

7/3/42
F. 76 yrs.
WATER: WELLS **1224-9**

Mrs. Cayce: With particular reference to best form of drinking water for the summer period.

Mr. Cayce: Yes.

To be sure, if it were practical, the having of water shipped in would be the better for drinking water.

But for all intents and purposes, that would prevent any disorders, if the lake water were boiled (of which there is plenty) with slack lime in same, it would be all right for drinking. To every two gallons put about half a teaspoonful of slack lime, but BOIL thoroughly; then let it settle and strain; and then keep it cool, see?

Q. Would the well water at Camp Chase be beneficial to drink?

A. This as we find, unless it were boiled, would not be even so well as the lake water. The lake water, treated in this manner as indicated, would be better for all those who would drink same.

Q. Any other helpful suggestions for a healthful summer?

A. Keep these in this direction as indicated, for the better health—as from the standpoint of the water, anyway.

We are through with this reading.

12/27/41
F. 19 yrs.
PREGNANCY **711-4**

DO NOT get feet wet. Do not give way to general feelings. Do not give way to the tendencies for nausea as they arise, so as to prevent the body from eating or from activity. Take a little lime water and cinnamon water, equal parts, if there is the nausea of morning.

10/3/34
ECZEMA **F. 51 yrs.**
GLANDS: INFECTIONS **677-1**

Q. Is the water I drink harmful to me? Is it pure or impure?

A. There's no such thing as an absolutely *pure* water! In this particular environ, and for this particular body, if there were added a teaspoonful of *lime* to each five gallons of water it would be much better.

Q. How much water should I drink daily?

A. Six to eight tumblers.

v)—Lithia Water

10/15/27
F. 42 yrs.
ACIDITY **482-2**

Drink plenty of water. Occasionally use a lithia tablet in same—once a week or once every two weeks.

6/24/41
ECZEMA **M. 29 yrs.**
ELIMINATIONS: INCOORDINATION **2518-1**

At all times drink plenty of water. Occasionally—say once a week—put a lithia tablet in a glass of water and drink it. This will stimulate better circulation and set up better drainage through the whole of the alimentary canal, especially as related to the hepatic circulation; that is, the circulation between the liver, the kidneys, and the flow through the alimentary areas of the body.

8/8/32
M. Adult
TOXEMIA **4246-1**

As to the activities through the hepatic circulation—that is, the liver and kidneys—these make for at times a pressure in the glands, that causes heaviness in the feet, limbs, and groins. These are sympathetic, rather than organic conditions. The hepatic circulation attempting to adjust itself.

Drink plenty of water at all times, and it will be well at this time for there to be added small quantities of lithia in the water taken; which would make for a cleansing of the ducts that function through the kidneys, in the adrenal glands especially. This will aid in clarifying the condition.

7/20/25
UREMIA **F. 20s**
INJURIES: ANKLE: SPRAIN: SPINE: LUMBAR **49-1**

Rest as much as possible, off of feet, with as little to do and think of, save being entertained by someone else. Light reading, plenty of fruit, abundance of water, especially that which would carry lithia and the inclination to carry the overactivity to the secretions of intestinal tract, or of white or black sulphur water, carrying lithia.

These may be taken in this manner, should the body not desire to take the trip to Shenandoah Springs, Arkansas; French Lick Springs, Indiana, or Crazy Water, Elmer Springs, Texas: May be taken at home taking lithia tablets in the double quantity of water; that is, one tablet to half a gallon of water, and double extract of Dawson water taken as drinking water, until system is cleansed, or cerulean water; that is, having cerulean water that carries sulphur.

5/16/29
F. 33 yrs.
1100-5

DIGESTION: INDIGESTION

Q. Is the drinking water being used at present harmful to this body?

A. Better were there more of the properties of the carbohydrates with that of lithia, than so much of the lime.

2/8/28
F. 56 yrs.
1010-2

TOXEMIA

Q. Are the teeth affecting this body?

A. The teeth affected are those especially in the left upper molar, and attention is made to relieve the pressure.

Q. Does city water have any effect on this trouble?

A. We do not find it so, though change of water would be well when there is any trouble with that of the kidneys, more lithia and more calcium would be well in the water, anything that carries more of this would be better for this portion of the body.

vi)—Spring Water

7/14/24
M. 27 yrs.
1447-1

WATER: HEALING

Gladys Davis: Now, you have before you the water in the spring located on the Finkle Farm, nine miles east of Circleville, Ohio, Pickaway County. A sample of the water from this spring is in this room. You will give us the analysis of this water, telling us if it has any beneficial value to the ailments of the human body. If so, what ailments, and how should it be used?

Edgar Cayce: Now, we find, as to the value of this water for the benefit of the human ills, that there are many that this would be beneficial to. There are conditions in the physical body that this would be detrimental to.

We find this is the analysis, and this is the condition that this water as a body would be beneficial to, and how:

First, we find this a light water in the respect that there are many minerals that will be found in solution in this water. The principle that will be beneficial is the light form of iodine and iron, and magnesia and soda in composition, or being by heat there would be left the basis of salt, of soda, of bicarbonate of soda, of sulphate of soda, and these in composition with lithia gives the lightness in gravity of the water, for we find this comes through the bed of soda and salt in its rise to the surface, and portions of this are from old salt petrolia beds carrying these properties. Many of these are slight, but in action on the system we find many of these in correct solutions for the benefit of ills of the body. Specifically, in this character of cases would be the benefit as should be derived in using the water, though few would be the benefits derived in using the water alone, for nearly all derangements, save mental forces, come from some center being so separated by pressure that another functioning position in body becomes either deranged by lack of nutriment received or by overstimulus and producing too much of another character, but these conditions especially; constipation, especially, that in the character of nerve digestion, or that of dyspeptic digestion. Conditions that have to do with the liver and with the kidneys proper, those that have to do with the kidneys that are affected by conditions in pelvic troubles it would be detrimental. Those that come from the lack of elimination beneficial, and should be used in conjunction with other conditions appiied to the body. Should be taken in quantities and without the interference of other waters. Heated it becomes an excellent bath for all skin diseases, especially that produced by eruptions caused from suppressed elimination or poisons eliminated through capillary circulation.

CIRCULATION: LYMPH: LIVER **7/20/24**
DEBILITATION: GENERAL **M. Adult**
ENVIRONMENT: CLIMATE: LIVER **3762-1**

Then, to give the body the normal forces, and to bring the normal effect in body, little of medicinal properties would be effective. Better that climatic conditions; pure water, high altitude. These, with food values, exercise of the physical body, that the forces may be brought to exertion in the system, that the body may become physically tired, without strain to the system.

In food, and in food values, give and keep those properties that give blood rebuilding values. Be careful of the water as is taken in system. Let that be pure. Not too much lime, not too little, but carrying much silica, lithia, magnesia and soda. That is, be nearer *pure* waters.

7/29/36
PLEURISY **M. 28 yrs.**
WATER: MINERALS **1173-5**

Q. Is it advisable to import bottled water for him to drink, and is it advisable for others here to drink the bottled water?

A. It would be advisable for all.

Q. Would you suggest Buffalo Mineral Springs Water for him to use entirely, or some other plain water such as Poland Water, possibly using one glass of Buffalo Water per day?

A. The Buffalo Springs is the preferable.

3/22/32
F. 42 yrs.
COLITIS **404-2**

Q. Is electrified water or pure spring water better for this body than city water?

A. Electrified water or spring water, especially, which is procurable here—of the Williams' water—would be well for the body.

11/28/22
ANEMIA **F. Adult**
ELIMINATIONS: POOR **4439-1**

To give the strength then necessary, we would create within this body, those factors necessary to give elemental force to the body. We would take then in the system these properties to give the correct forces for this body. We would take first: the water that is used for this body should carry the elements necessary to give the correct incentives to the system. They should have in their makeup, magnesia, iron, sulphur, lithium, siliceous, such as we would find in the spring here, see?

Q. Where would this body get these spring waters, Mr. Cayce?

A. . . . This water would be used for drinking water. Would be found here, you see, on Head's place, Old Indian Spring. Do this and we will remove these conditions, cause the body to have an appetite, the body will put on flesh and will feel many, many years younger within six months. Do that.

Q. Mr. Cayce, which one of the Head Springs would you recommend to be used?

A. We have just given it, the Old Indian Spring. Keep this water and drink no other.

5/30/29
M. 30 yrs.
HYPOTENSION **5453-9**

With the corrections, with the exercise, drinking plenty of water—*plenty* of water—taking it more as medicine—we will find the body will improve.

Q. What is the condition of the kidneys?

A. That's why plenty of water should be given, that no sediments are formed from conditions as have existed through these portions of the body. Well to drink plenty of water that carries—not heavily lithia, but lithia—with much of the lime and of sulphur.

Q. Where can this water be obtained?

A. There's parts of it that have been where he lives!

Q. Will the water that is gotten from Williams be of benefit?

A. Be very beneficial. Be very beneficial to keep for any that suffers from such conditions.

II

Dairy Products and Eggs

1)—Butter

5/28/43
GASTRITIS **F. 45 yrs.**
FLU: AFTEREFFECTS **3033-1**

Q. What is cause for the intense soreness in back of shoulders, the right one especially?

A. As indicated, the incoordination between nerve forces of the digestive system—the sympathetic and the central system, see? Hence the reason why no greases, no fats should be taken. Of course, butter may be taken. And the vegetables should be prepared preferably with butter if any seasoning is to be used.

7/15/43
M. 50 yrs.
MULTIPLE SCLEROSIS **3095-1**

No great quantities of grease should be taken at any time. Season the vegetables with butter, and it would be better if they are all cooked in Patapar paper—so that their salts and juices are mixed with them and not left in the water in which they would ordinarily be cooked. Just cook them in Patapar paper, without water, and season with butter.

12/22/43
DEBILITATION: GENERAL **F. 66 yrs.**
NEURITIS: TENDENCIES **1409-9**

A great deal of fats will be hard on the body, as indicated by the lack of ability for digesting greases in the present. Butter fats and cheeses and such are well to be taken in moderation.

3/4/35
F. Adult
KATABOLISM: METABOLISM **844-1**

Evenings—(if this is the dinner) the well-cooked vegetables, but not vegetables cooked in or with grease; those cooked in their own juices, as in a steamer or in Patapar paper. These may be seasoned well with butter, but not seasoned with bacon or with cooking meats of any kind.

10/28/42
F. 53 yrs.
BODY-BUILDING: ASSIMILATIONS **1770-7**

Q. What causes nerve pain below shoulder blades on right side of spine?

A. This is a part of those disturbances from the digestlve forces. A little fat here needs to be taken; especially as from butterfat or dairy products.

2)—Cheese

10/7/39
M. 58 yrs.
GLANDS: INCOORDINATION **2020-1**

Keep away from too much of the combination of starches; such as cheese with macaroni. These may be taken separately at times, but not as a combination one with another. Not great quantities of fats, ever.

11/3/43
M. 54 yrs.
GLANDS: ADRENALS: THYROID: GLAUCOMA **3276-1**

Q. Cheese?

A. Cheese tabu.

5/6/43
F. 37 yrs.
OBESITY **2988-1**

Do not take much of cheeses of any kind. A little milk may be taken, but not too much of this—until there has been a reduction in the glandular forces tending to make for more weight.

8/20/43
F. 54 yrs.
DIABETES: TENDENCIES **3166-1**

Keep away from combinations of white potatoes with any cheese product. No two of these should be taken at any one meal.

1/17/41
F. 44 yrs.
ELIMINATIONS: POOR **459-11**

Have the better elimination by some changes in the diet.

Do be consistent with the diets—keeping away from too much starches—for instance, spaghetti and cheese; though cheese may be taken in moderation if it is a cream of cheddar cheese.

12/22/43
DEBILITATION: GENERAL **F. 66 yrs.**
NEURITIS: TENDENCIES **1409-9**

A great deal of fats will be hard on the body, as indicated by the lack of ability for digesting greases in the present. Cheeses and such are well to be taken in moderation.

1/7/37
CIRCULATION: POOR **F. 44 yrs.**
ELIMINATIONS: POOR **1315-6**

Do not combine great quantities of cheese too much with breads or sweets; but rather as indicated keep the twenty percent acid to eighty percent alkalin reactions.

11/18/36
CIRCULATION: POOR **F. 46 yrs.**
ECZEMA **1158-3**

Cheeses at times with proteins produce improper fermentation.

3)—Margarine

12/29/41
M. 40 yrs.
ASSIMILATIONS: POOR **826-14**

Use not the vegetable oils in the cooking, but either the peanut oil or the Parkay margarine—for this especially carries D in a manner that conforms with these properties in preparation for assimilation by the body.

4)—Yogurt

12/19/38
F. 58 yrs.
TOXEMIA **1762-1**

Evenings—For the most part leafy vegetables, and not too much of same. Use yogurt in the evening meal.

This is to act as a cleanser for the alimentary canal, as well as a better balance for the fermenting and the eliminations of poisons from the system.

3/5/36
F. 38 yrs.
TUBERCULOSIS **1045-8**

Q. How should the yogurt be prepared for this body?

A. Yogurt is prepared by making a curd that passes through the system to absorb and aid in the eliminations.

Use in milk, then, as a curd—and take very small sips for the body.

Yogurt is a preparation from honeycomb, you see, that acts to take caseins from milk that are injurious to the system and helpful to the intestinal tract.

This is needed more later than in the immediate, you see; for these emergencies must be met—in this lack of oxygen supply for the body.

8/13/43
F. 46 yrs.
TUBERCULOSIS: INTESTINES **3154-1**

Do use, for at least the next four or five weeks, the combination found in yogurt as prepared (Battle Creek), as an antiseptic for the intestinal tract. Take this regularly.

2/23/38
F. 43 yrs.
DEBILITATION: GENERAL **1542-1**

Also we would add yogurt in the diet as an active cleanser through the colon and intestinal system. This would be most beneficial, not only purifying the alimentary canal but adding the vital forces necessary to enable those portions of the system to function in the nearer normal manner.

Thus we may bring the abilities for strength and for purifying the circulatory forces, upon which depends the strength to resist physically the inroads of the infectious forces that disturb the locomotion as well as the pulmonary and the circulatory system and the strength through the depleting of the nerve energies of the body.

6/1/31
F. Adult
ELIMINATIONS **1186-3**

Noons—We would take, *between* this meal and the evening meal, either the Bulgarian milk or those of the lactic acids in milk, or those as are combined in yogurt, see?

1/22/36
F. 38 yrs.
TUBERCULOSIS **1045-5**

And we would procure, as soon as possible, the yogurt as prepared in the tablet form from Kellogg Sanitarium. This would prevent, in its activity through the system, the colon and through the intestinal tract, the formation of bacilli by the non-activity of the lactic forces through the eliminating channels.

3/20/36
F. 38 yrs.
TUBERCULOSIS **1045-9**

The yogurt in its preparation may make for the greater absorbing influences through the intestinal system, and with the general inactivity keep the coordinations of activities between the circulatory forces of the liver, the spleen, the pancreas, the lungs, the kidneys, more in order. For from such disturbances the *breaking down* of the katabolism becomes the *destructive* force in *any* condition of this nature.

12/4/22
F. Adult
TUBERCULOSIS **5703-1**

Take into the system yogurt, one tablet, three times each day.

3/7/35
F. 43 yrs.
COLITIS: TENDENCIES **846-1**

Q. What about cheese?

A. Cheese is not as well for the body, this particular body, as some others; unless it is fresh—and this is not as palatable to the body as others. Yogurt and such combinations, which arise as the basis for cheese, is very good; especially for the colon condition.

Q. Until I get better, when I have a headache what can I do to relieve it?

A. As we would find, if these are begun we will have very few returns of the headache—which comes from this heaviness upon the colon and the lacteal duct and the strain on the system.

8/23/34
CYSTS **M. Adult**
ASSIMILATIONS: ELIMINATIONS: !NCOORDINATION **643-1**

The character of milks taken would be varied; not that carrying too much curd or yet too much of any of those properties that produce too great a quantity of activity in the intestinal tract. Here we find that the tablets as of honeycomb with milk would be well, as prepared by the Kellogg Institute—in that termed yogurt, but the *former* and not the latter preparation is much better you see—in the tablets. These would be taken about one or two a day.

ANEMIA: WOMB: TIPPED **6/14/44**
ASSIMILATIONS: POOR: ANEMIA **F. 22 yrs.**
ASTHENIA **5210-1**

From such accumulations, unless measures are taken, it may require operative measures. This, the effect upon the nervous system, upsets the whole activities of the body. It is anemic; it has little assimilations, most of the foods which would be taken, at one time or another, disagree.

All of these are from nerve depressions which are produced upon the organs of the digestion, so that even the stomach itself is dropped; not in the sense that it is "out of line," but tends in its position to cause food to ferment! There is a great deal of gas, apparently through duodenum and the upper portion of the jejunum; grumblings at times through the bowel. All of these become very disturbing to the body; tired, weakness which may follow the periods, with headaches, with a bit of nausea. All of these are the disorders.

Then, for the strengthening of the body, for the gradual building up of the vitality, use yogurt.

1/5/36
F. 46 yrs.
COLITIS: TENDENCIES **404-6**

Q. Is buttermilk good?

A. This depends upon the manner in which it is made. This would tend to produce gas if it is the ordinary kind. But that *made* by the use of the Bulgarian tablets is good, in moderation; not too much.

6/4/29
F. 59 yrs.
ARTHRITIS: TENDENCIES **5525-1**

Milk—this in some manners is tabu for the body, yet in others is excellent.

Those of the Bulgarian milk, or of the buttermilk would be the *better* for the system. This is acid in its reaction, to be sure, in *some* cases. Not so here! for the bacilli as is created in system through same will produce effects such that we will have a cleansed colon by the use of same.

3/22/32
F. 42 yrs.
COLITIS **404-2**

Those of buttermilk, and other milks—or the Bulgarian milk—will be well to create for the system that bacilli that makes for the proper accumulations in the system.

Q. Is pasteurized milk good for the body, and how about buttermilk made from pasteurized milk?

A. Raw milk, to be sure, is better—but pasteurized milk needs to have that added that will make for a better activity with the gastric juices, under the disorders as have been existent in the system. Those like the Bulgarian forces, as make for the proper reaction of the bacilli that becomes active with the gastric juices.

6/23/34
M. 56 yrs.
ULCERS: STOMACH **556-2**

First we would begin with that almost wholly of a Bulgarian milk diet, which will make for the producing of sufficient of the lactic acids and the gastric juices as they are assimilated for the body, in such a way and manner as to meet the *immediate* needs.

2/19/29
M. 48 yrs.
ELIMINATIONS **91-2**

Milk—this may be taken—preferably, though, should be buttermilk, or the milk that has been treated, as the Bulgarian—this is very good for the body.

1/30/28
F. Adult
ELIMINATIONS: POOR: TOXEMIA **81-2**

Drink Bulgarian milk or milk fresh from the cow with the animal heat. Should this turn the system then take the Bulgarian milk.

6/21/32
F. 48 yrs.
ASSIMILATIONS: POOR **428-7**

In the afternoons—it would be well that the bacilli milk be taken. It makes for the proper fermentation and activity through the intestinal system—as the Bulgarian. These may be altered, or one taken for a few days and then the other for a few days. This is the middle of the afternoon.

SURGERY: TONSILLECTOMY: AFTEREFFECTS **6/30/26**
ANEMIA **M. 27 yrs.**
BLOOD-BUILDING **137-85**

Now the body only needs rest, plenty of food (as soon as the body can take it) that digests well with the system. Milk and any condition that builds fat tissue in the system without taxing the digestive organism, or overtaxing liver or kidneys, see? Any of these. That in the milk will necessarily be of that nature that acts with the digestive system—that is, such as the buttermilk, and such natures as that—the Bulgarian milk, or that nature, better than much of the rich sweet milk, but what is necessary is for the system to gather that necessary in the system for the blood rebuilding forces in the system.

5)—Eggs

2/24/32
M. 44 yrs.
ELIMINATIONS: INCOORDINATION **437-4**

Mornings—Hard-boiled egg well mashed. When this is used, however, principally the yolk should be used—with a cereal drink or coffee.

12/1/30
M. Child
COLD: COMMON: SUSCEPTIBILITY: WORMS **203-1**

Beware of sweets for some time. Preferably would be as this: evenings—a little portion of very crisp bacon with eggs—especially the yolk, not much of the white.

3/22/38
F. 29 yrs.
MINERALS: CALCIUM: TEETH **1523-3**

Q. Suggest diet beneficial to preserving teeth.

A. Eggs—these are particularly given to preserving the teeth; or anything that carries quantities of calcium or aids to the thyroids in its production would be beneficial so it is not overbalanced, see?

12/30/42
M. 21 yrs.
BODY-BUILDING: LOCOMOTION: IMPAIRED **2873-1**

The food values should be those fully well balanced with calcium, iron, and especially the vitamins B-1 and the B-complex. These are much preferable for the body.

At least three times each week, then, supply these from the foods rather than the reinforced vitamins (though these reinforcements may be desirable if there is the inability of the body to assimilate foods that carry excesses or the full quantity of such vital forces).

To be sure, these are not all the foods that are to be taken:

Mornings—the yolk of an egg.

4/2/32
F. Child
ASTHMA **5682-2**

Noons—Do not give at this meal any jams, preserves or the like. There may be used the yolks of eggs, but not the white, in sandwiches. Hard boiled and mashed and mixed with dressings, but not with any acid dressing as of vinegar or acetic acid, or pickles.

1/5/31
ANEMIA **F. 20 yrs.**
ASSIMILATIONS: ELIMINATIONS: INCOORDINATION **421-2**

The egg to be taken in between meals. Stuff, as it were, as if stuffing a turkey! See?

2/20/43
M. 28 yrs.
ACIDITY **1710-10**

Q. Suggest foods to stress and foods to avoid in the diet.

A. Avoid those combinations that produce acidity in the system. Not that these suggestions should be used to such measures as to eliminate acids entirely, but that there be kept a normal balance. Avoid the combination of fats with butterfats, as with the white of an egg, or those that produce that character of starch.

2/24/35
M. 53 yrs.
ASSIMILATIONS: ELIMINATIONS: INCOORDINATION **843-1**

Q. Why do some foods, especially eggs, affect my heart action and cause such a raw feeling?

A. They do not assimilate with the system on account of the quantities of the fluids in the white of the egg. The yolk will *not* work the same way.

4/29/38
F. 77 yrs.
TOXEMIA **1586-1**

Do not eat fried foods of any kind, EVER; especially NOT fried eggs.

7/30/40
F. Adult
OBESITY **2315-1**

Each meal should be preceded by the grapejuice—thirty minutes before eating.
Mornings—The yolk of an egg (soft boiled or poached; NOT fried).

3/15/44
F. 26 yrs.
PARALYSIS **3694-1**

Do not eat the white of eggs but the yolk once or twice a day, however, it may be the more palatable—whether prepared in drink or in foods. Do take at least the yolks of two eggs each day.

10/28/42
F. 53 yrs.
BODY-BUILDING: ASSIMILATIONS **1770-7**

We find that the diets need consideration. There would be a helpful or beneficial effect from the body taking the tonic that carries the B-1 vitamins, the iron and the G vitamin. This particular type of combination is excellent.

Hence, if the tonic is taken with such foods added in the diet, it will be more efficient for the body than the supplementing of the diet with other vitamin preparations. Do not overtake same, but only as a tonic; adding to the diet such foods as the yolk of an egg at least once daily.

3/21/39
F. 49 yrs.
RELAXATION **1158-21**

Q. First, egg yolks?

A. These are good taken about twice or three times a week, but not every day, to be sure.

Q. How much?

A. Whether half a dozen, dozen, one or two! Whatever is the desire or the need for the body! Depends on how much is to be added with it when it is taken!

12/4/22
F. Adult
TUBERCULOSIS **5703-1**

Let the diet be that that will give the vital forces to the body, principally of eggs. Do that. We will bring the proper forces and incentives to this body.

11/3/43
M. 54 yrs.
GLANDS: ADRENALS: THYROID: GLAUCOMA **3276-1**

Q. Eggs?

A. The yolk, not the white for this body.

9/29/34
M. 11 yrs.
DIABETES **674-1**

Coddled egg; the whole egg may be taken—this, while carrying on acid in same, if *coddled*—that is, put on with the water boiling and take it off and let it set for four and a half minutes—it will be all right. Only whole wheat browned bread.

5/24/35
M. 26 yrs.
EPILEPSY **567-8**

Q. Should egg whites still be eliminated from my diet? If so, why?

A. Egg white, unless it is prepared in the form of a coddled egg, makes for a formation of acid by the extra amount of these qualities that we find in same. With the changes that are wrought, it would be very good to use the whole egg—provided it is coddled or soft-scrambled.

9/12/37
BLOOD: COAGULATION: POOR **M. 62 yrs.**
ACIDITY & ALKALINITY **1411-2**

Noons—Use green vegetables, raw, or salads, or sandwiches provided these are preferably of the egg or the like.

2/10/30
M. 41 yrs.
LACERATIONS: STOMACH **5545-1**

In the evenings—these may be altered to those that are blood and nerve building, and may be changed to any of the characters of foods that are *alkaline-reacting!* Eggs may be taken at this time, provided the *yolk* only is prepared, either in the form of hard and *well mashed* afterward, mixed with any of the oils—olive oil, also those of cod-liver oil, should be part of the diet.

5/12/28
M. 33 yrs.
LIVER: KIDNEYS: INCOORDINATION **900-383**

Q. Is the albumin on the decrease or increase in the urine?

A. On the decrease. Beware of eggs!

1/26/27
F. 22 yrs.
TUBERCULOSIS **4236-1**

Keep all the eggs the body will assimilate. Do not overcrowd the system, but taking that that will assimilate, without producing nausea or clogging the system. Better that a small quantity be taken often, that it may be assimilated by the system. Eggs and milk—these may be put together, if possible for the body to take it in this way and manner, see? Fresh eggs. Keep the animal heat—or being eaten while the heat is still there. These are well taken into the system, for these give their vibrations as will produce better assimilation in this condition, and are more digestible to the body and to the lining of the intestinal tract, as well as to the portions of the duodenum and stomach proper.

10/24/30
F. 59 yrs.
ANEMIA **501-1**

Also of mornings, well that the yolk of one or two eggs be beaten either in milk or malt and drunk as the morning meal, *with* whole wheat gruel or oaten gruel—but either or both should be well cooked before taken.

8/31/41
ARTHRITIS: PREVENTIVE **F. 51 yrs.**
BODY: GENERAL **1158-31**

Q. Whole eggs or yolk?

A. Whole eggs about once or twice a week, yolks about three times each week. In most instances, it is best that they NOT be taken raw. If taken raw, take them WITH something else; as in orange juice or beer or the like.

6/16/42
F. 23 yrs.
DEBILITATION: GENERAL **2766-1**

Do take plenty of eggs. Have eggs at least once each day.

10/17/34
F. 40 yrs.
HYPOCHONDRIA **1000-2**

In the matter of diets . . . those of the phosphorus nature, and of those that carry these properties as are necessary—the creation with the chlorine foods carry the gold in its combination— follow these closely.

Q. What foods contain gold, silicon and phosphorus?

A. These are contained more in varieties that are given as same. Yolks of eggs—not the white, or the whole may be taken at times—but when taken should be raw—it may be, of course, burnt with spirits frumenti when taken in that manner.

8/13/30
M. 42 yrs.
DEBILITATION: GENERAL **2335-1**

Use eggs, not with the white, stirred well into malt, as one of the meals.

10/29/36
M. Adult
ANEMIA **1131-2**

Mornings—Principally cereals or citrus fruits, but these should not be taken at the same meal; either may be balanced with a small amount of crisp bacon, or coddled eggs—using principally or altogether the yolk. These will carry with them an abundant amount of resisting forces in the system, and aid in the elimination; also add to the blood-building forces of the body.

1/8/30
VITAMINS: DEFICIENT **F. 29 yrs.**
BLOOD-BUILDING **5615-1**

Eggs, but only the yolks of same should be taken for this body at the *present* period. Later they may be taken more, or the whole—where stimuli is needed for the digestive forces in the system.

7/11/34
F. 40 yrs.
PELVIC DISORDERS **607-1**

Q. Why does she have severe attacks of indigestion after eating eggs in any form?

A. The tendency for the nervous reaction to those elements especially that are found more prevalent in eggs; as phosphorous and the natures that make for the gluten. This trouble will not be experienced if only the yolk of the egg is prepared—coddled; if the treatments as indicated as applied.

7/13/35
F. 59 yrs.
ECZEMA **3823-4**

Q. Are eggs harmful to my condition?

A. Not harmful in moderation, provided they are *not* used with *grease!*

11/23/37
M. 13 yrs.
PSORIASIS **1484-1**

Mornings—Eggs occasionally—but ONLY the yolk of the egg should be taken; NONE of the white, or that which carries so much (under the present conditions of the body) of the activities that are acid-forming.

12/12/38
F. 51 yrs.
FADS **1703-2**

Q. Are eggs the menstruation of hens, as taught by one, and so not fit for food?

A. No. They are the product of the body. No more the menstruation than a body in conception, or after conception, is menstruation of the human body!

1/13/41
F. 27 yrs.
DEBILITATION: GENERAL **2426-1**

Q. Do eggs disagree with me?

A. Eggs disagree with the body at present. In the second week of the osteopathic treatments, when these may be added gradually to the diet, we would take only the yolk—which should be soft boiled, or the like—and little or none of the white, or albumin.

3/30/38
F. 36 yrs.
TUBERCULOSIS **1560-1**

Take EGGS, RAW—if they can be taken. And if the body can assimilate same, take the WHOLE egg; for the albumin of the white—while it may be severe at one time, it is necessary at other times. And these may be taken in BEER if so desired, or in a little whiskey—but take the whole egg. This once or twice a day will be found to be MOST helpful.

5/25/39
M. 5 mos.
BABY CARE **1788-6**

The yolk of an egg would be well to be taken once or twice a week, though half a yolk or the like should be sufflcient for one meal—but if he takes more, it will be very well. Prepare same in this manner: Let the water come to a hard boil, then drop an egg in and immediately set the water off the heat; and when it is possible to take the egg out with the hand (without a spoon), then it is ready to give to the child—but ONLY the yolk, see? This is the manner of preparation, and is what we would call a CODDLED egg, see?

8/25/44
F. 28 yrs.
COLD: COMMON: SUSCEPTIBILITY **5399-1**

Q. Should I avoid eggs?

A. This depends upon supply of other elements. There are some elements in eggs not found in other foods—ordinarily, sulphur. The whites, however, do occasionally cause certain other elements to be bad for the body. These we would take occasionally, but not necessarily avoiding same.

5/5/44
F. 43 yrs.
DIGESTION: INDIGESTION: CATARRH **5046-1**

Q. What foods should be stressed and which avoided?

A. Alkaline-producing foods, for acids do arise from the combination of foods, causing a great distress. Don't take the white of egg when eggs are taken.

10/27/34
F. 11 yrs.
DEBILITATION: GENERAL **711-3**

Coddled egg, and *only* the yolk of same—don't fry the eggs! *Coddle* them—which means to put them on when the water is boiling and let them set in the water five minutes; but take off the water, of course, don't leave it on boiling for five minutes—else the eggs would be blue! Give the yolk to the child, and you may eat the white yourself if you want to—it would be very good for you!* (*Gladys Davis's note: Evidently, Edgar Cayce here was making a side remark to the mother, Mrs. [2457].)

12/8/36
ASSIMILATIONS: POOR **F. Adult**
TOXEMIA **1303-1**

Never any fried eggs. Rarely take eggs, but when taken only coddled eggs or those that are cooked in the sweetmeats or of other natures.

3/2/43
M. 10 yrs.
INJURIES: BIRTH: AFTEREFFECTS **2780-2**

Q. Would it be helpful to take some preparation such as cod-liver oil, iron, or vitamins, to aid further development?

A. These are best taken in the regular diet, if there is supplied sufficient of those foods needed. If some good whole grain cereal is taken each day, or any such activity, it should supply sufficient. This, combined with the yolk of an egg each day, should supply sufficient, and be much better assimilated by the body than being reinforced from vitamins.

3/22/32
F. 42 yrs.
COLITIS **404-2**

Mornings—Citrus fruit diet, but altered or changed—and thirty to forty minutes after this is taken, take the yolk—not the white of egg, with a cereal. This would be very well for the morning meal.

3/4/35
F. Adult
KATABOLISM: METABOLISM **844-1**

This (diet) would be the outline, though it may be altered at times:

Mornings: Coddled egg, and *only* the yolk of same, not the white—for this carries too much of those properties that are hard for digestion, or too much albumin that is producing an irritation in the adrenal gland secretion and the glands in the pelvis area.

12/11/38
F. 13 yrs.
GLANDS: INCOORDINATION **1206-9**

Q. What about adding egg yolks?

A. Egg yolks are very well. This may be taken as a part of the morning meal. Especially is this well if they are cooked hard, then mashed or eaten with those things that make it more palatable. The sulphur here is desirable.

6/14/35
F. Adult
GLANDS: INCOORDINATION **935-1**

Noons—Principally (very seldom altering from these) raw vegetables made into a salad. Even egg may be included in same, preferably the hard egg (that is, the yolk) and it worked into the oil as a portion of the dressing.

9/27/37
F. Adult
DEBILITATION: GENERAL **1419-5**

Q. Should anything else be taken at breakfast when the citrus fruit juices are taken?

A. Preferably not. At times at breakfast, or at times in the evening meal, a coddled egg may be included—but not WITH the others; make rather a meal of same in itself, with the whole wheat or milk toast.

6—Milk: Cow's Fluid

1)—Cow's Milk: General

5/1/35
M. 1-1/2 yrs.
WORMS: PINWORMS: AFTEREFFECTS **786-2**

The regular preparations of milk would be well; not the raw milk, but the prepared milks may be used occasionally for the regular developing.

Q. Should he have sugar in any form?

A. He will get sugar from the vegetables and from the milk itself.

7/12/35
BODY-BUILDING **F. 23 yrs.**
DIS-EASE: CONTAGION: PREVENTIVE **480-19**

The diet should be more body-building; that is, less acid foods and more of the alkaline-reacting will be the better in these directions. Milk and all its products should be a portion of the body's diet now.

4/2/36
BRAIN: CLOTS: TENDENCIES **F. 60 yrs.**
MALNUTRITION **1137-1**

While the food values should be body-building, in the first they should not be so rich in vitamins or calories or replenishing forces as not to be able to be handled by the digestive forces or the katabolism of the system. For if these were to produce such engorgements in the beginning, they would be less effective and later very destructive to the better influences through the body.

But use those foods that are rich in the vitamins that make for a stimulation to a lymph circulation.

First we would have the rich vitamins from the milk that is dried, or milk and egg, milk with bread that would be crumbled in same. Have these as a great portion of the diet.

10/26/36
F. Adult

DEBILITATION: GENERAL **1278-6**

As we find, the dry milks or condensed milks or the like are preferable to the animal or raw milk.

Q. How much during the day should be taken?

A. This depends upon the manner in which the body assimilates it. Do not overcrowd the body. For if it is not able to assimilate it, owing to the disturbed circulation, it becomes a dross and a heaviness upon the eliminating system. And the sourness of those conditions produced by milk are just as poisonous as any other condition where assimilation does not take place. Depends upon how the body assimilates it. One day it may take two, three, four glasses. Possibly the next day one or two small portions. Be governed by the appetite, the exercise and the reactions.

4/24/26
F. 7 yrs.

COLD: CONGESTION **4281-12**

Q. Should she take milk from cows tested for tuberculosis or diphtheria?

A. Those that are inoculated the body should not take milk from. Those that may be tested would be a different condition. Those that are inoculated give an undue effect to one that is easily swayed by even suggestions through the milk, see? All milk, as has been given, should be heated and boiled or sterilized.

Q. How soon can she have sweet milk on her cereals now?

A. When there is no trace of the malaria in the blood.

11/3/43
M. 54 yrs.

GLANDS: ADRENALS: THYROID: GLAUCOMA **3276-1**

Q. What about milk?

A. Very rarely, except in the preparation of other foods.

12/12/38
F. 51 yrs.

CATARRH **1703-2**

Q. And milk, I find, makes more mucus, the basis for catarrh.

A. This if taken properly is NOT the basis of mucus. If this is thy experience, then there are other conditions producing same. For milk, whether it is the dry or the pasteurized or raw, is near to the perfect combination of forces for the human consumption.

Q. Please explain what "feel" I should be conscious of regarding milk?

A. As to its constituents as related to body elements in their necessity for the balance in the system of the whole activity of assimilation and elimination.

1/25/37
M. Adult

TUBERCULOSIS **1324-1**

Give all the cool, fresh milk that may be taken. Be sure that it is from tested kine or cows, however.

6/9/27
F. 20 mos.
TOXEMIA **608-3**

Do not give any milk unless it is first heated—not necessarily boiled, but heated, see? The milk—in its precaution—is to meet those conditions as are seen produced in the assimilating system of the body. Hence when the conditions are *normal* again, this is not necessarily kept up.

4/30/31
F. Adult
ELIMINATIONS: POOR **4178-l**

Evenings—A well-balanced meal, but don't eat too muchl No stimuli—that is, of alcoholic content nor those of coffees or teas—but any of the milks may be taken.

12/10/37
ADHESIONS: CHILDBIRTH: AFTEREFFECTS **F. 37 yrs.**
ANEMIA: TENDENCIES **1498-1**

Milk should be taken between the morning and the noon meals; these drinks preferably with the chocolate or the vanilla, not only to make same more palatable but to supply strength for the body.

5/6/43
F. 37 yrs.
OBESITY **2988-1**

A little milk may be taken, but not too much of this—until there has been reduction in the glandular forces tending to make for more weight.

5/19/35
GLANDS: SALIVARY: DIGESTION: GENERAL **F. 27 yrs.**
PREGNANCY **808-3**

Bolting food or swallowing it by the use of liquids produces more colds than *any one* activity of a diet! Even milk should be *chewed* two to three times before taken into the stomach itself, for this makes for the proper assimilation of the lacteai activity in the system; and when being acted upon by the gastric flow of the hydrochlorics in the duodenum area, it is better assimilated and gives more value in the whole of the body.

5/3/32
F. 49 yrs.
TOXEMIA **5647-1**

Q. Should milk of any kind be taken?

A. Better that the foods be prepared with the milk than the milk taken.

5/5/44
F. 40 yrs.
TUBERCULOSIS **5053-1**

This may be taken in the present environ, as the weather improves, though in the country, not in a sanatorium or city, in the open country where there may be good care, plenty of running water and plenty of the foods as may be indicated. Also there should be plenty of good whole milk that has been tested, and this to be used not only in the regular diet, but use this with an egg and malt beaten in same and take about every other day, or more often, if it agrees with the body. The milk should be whole milk, warm from the body heat of the cow, see?

8/23/27
M. 26 yrs.
ELIMINATIONS: INCOORDINATION **4145-1**

Milk should be the principal drink—sweet milk—cream—when taken when it is *warm,* if possible, from the body from which the milk is taken, or with the heat of the animal in same, see?

The increased circulation—the lack of stimulation to those that *cause* irritation, through the drinks, through the meats, through these other conditions in system—will bring the natural rebuilding forces for the body.

6/17/37
F. 29 yrs.
TUBERCULOSIS **528-9**

As to the diet: Keep that which is not only palatable but that is in a proper relationship as to acids and alkalines. Not all acid; for as is indicated, the very nature of the tubercle reaction is acid, yet at times the throwing off of the reactions tends to make for congestions in eliminating areas—as the liver, the kidneys and the alimentary canal.

Hence the necessity for a little more of the alkalines than the acids. We will find that milk is not so good at times as other drinks; as even water, as wine, as those things that make for a variation in the activity through the eliminations of the bodily forces themselves.

6/1/28
ASSIMILATIONS: ELIMINATIONS: LIVER **F. 23 yrs.**
ASTHENIA: LIVER: CHOKED **288-22**

Milk very good, but more of those properties that will add in strength-building. This may be peculiar, that milk not carrying all necessary, but the casein in same not well with the *present* condition existent.

1/9/35
M. 1 yr.
WORMS **786-1**

Evenings—Principally either milk that is combined with buttermilk or that which is made into same with the use of the tablets for making same, you see; or the hot milk, or the warm combinations of milk, whole wheat toast, and the like.

10/29/43
ASSIMILATIONS: ELIMINATIONS: INCOORDINATION **F. 13 yrs.**
HEADACHE: MIGRAINE **3326-1**

Q. Is milk one of the foods that affects this condition? (She has not had any for about six months, but I would like her to go back to it, if possible.)

A. Depends upon the combinations with which it is taken. If with wheat germ—that is, even puffed oats, puffed rice or puffed wheat, and wheat germ with it—milk may be taken; also with oatmeal that is cooked a long time, not the oats cooked only a few minutes—that isn't very good for anyone. These are much better if they are of the whole grain and not rolled or so treated chemically as to cause them to cook easily. These whole grain cereals may be taken with milk in same.

i)—Evaporated

9/15/43
F. Adult
ANEMIA **2843-4**

Q. Is milk good for me?

A. Not very good in its ordinary form. The prepared milk, as any compound that is already prepared, would be much better, use here, for this body, any of those—for instance, Nestle's foods prepared in and with the milk; using such as the Carnation brand to prepare same. This will prove most effective for the body.

7/11/38
F. 20 days
BABY CARE **1635-1**

Now as we find, with this body, there are rather the effects of heat, disagreement of the food in the digestive system by its carrying too much casein or fat and not sufficient of that as is digestible by the body itself.

Hence we have the effects of an upset digestive system, with an added condition in the heat making a very violent rash in portions of the body; and it will become or grow to be more and more disturbing unless there is a relief not only by the ability for foods to be assimilated but by purging or purifying of the system in such a manner as to eliminate the excess, already indicated through the various activities of the bodily function- ings.

As we find, we would change from the mother's milk to the Carnation Milk, with this rather weak; and in each bottle as it is given add an extra two or three drops of the Lime Water, see?

3/17/40
COLITIS: TENDENCIES **M. 2 mos.**
BABY CARE **2148-1**

The thing to be more fearful of here is colitis, and the activity of the congestion upon the assimilating system.

We would change the diet to those combinations which are not so strong, but that may be altered more from time to time by the addition of the calcium or lime in same. We would use the Carnation Milk, with the dextrin in same, see? Use the regular formula for the age, but WEAKEN same in the present.

Q. Why won't he take his milk?

A. It's very well he doesn't! Owing to the condition which has been indicated in the digestive system!

ii)—Homogenized

5/25/43
F. 35 yrs.
PREGNANCY **457-12**

Q. Does the homogenized Vitamin D milk have greater advantages or disadvantages for this body during pregnancy?

A. It's advantageous.

Q. How much should be taken?

A. That to satisfy the body's appetite.

Q. Is there no possibility that the milk will produce dangerous fat making delivery difficult?

A. Not if other conditions, that have been indicated for the body, are kept intact.

Q. Would milk have the tendency to make the baby larger which in turn would make a Caesarean necessary for this body?

A. Not necessarily.

Q. Is there any way to keep down the size of the baby without causing any detrimental effects on either mother or child?

A. Who knows how to create the body better, the Creator or the man?

iii)—Pasteurized

5/1/36
ANEMIA: TENDENCIES **F. 46 yrs.**
CIRCULATION: INCOORDINATION **1158-1**

Q. Should I take milk at the meal when I am taking raw vegetables?

A. Milk may be taken; preferably not raw milk. That is, rather milk that has been prepared, or milk that has been heated sufficiently for the curdling of certain food forces—the caseins that are hard upon the system.

8/25/39
F. 39 yrs.
TOXEMIA **1985-1**

Plenty of milk should be taken, but most certainly this should always be pasteurized and not the raw milk.

iv)—Raw

3/30/38
F. 36 yrs.
TUBERCULOSIS **1560-1**

For THIS body, drink MILK direct—body heat from the cow! In the surroundings let the cow be one that not only has the fresh pasture but also the dry food. Let there be tests made, to be sure, for the character of milk from the cow chosen for this condition. But drink it at least twice a day with the body heat of the animal in same, see? This may be a little disturbing at first but will soon be found to be MOST helpful, MOST beneficial.

7/10/22
F. Adult
ANEMIA
DEBILITATION: GENERAL **4466-1**

Milk should be taken into the system preferably warm with animal heat which will add fatty portions in the system and will produce better forces in the chyle.

Q. How much milk should be taken?

A. One half pint night and morning.

8/13/30
M. 42 yrs.
DEBILITATION: GENERAL **2335-1**

Milk, but only milk that is warm with animal heat should be taken; not that that is chilled, or that has set in any container which has been opened or exposed to where bacilli—either of the milk itself or outside—may have been active with same.

12/4/22
F. Adult
TUBERCULOSIS **5703-1**

Let the diet be that that will give the vital forces to the body, principally of milk but warm milk with the heat of the animal and not of the fire. Do that. We will bring the proper forces and incentives to this body.

9/29/36
F. 33 yrs.
PREGNANCY **540-7**

As we find, the general conditions are developing in a nominal way and manner. There should be those precautions that there be plenty of calcium in the system for developing of bone and muscle tissue. Most of this, of course, may be had from raw milk.

11/13/33
M. 28 yrs.
APPETITE: BODY-BUILDING **436-4**

Q. Do I drink too much milk at times?

A. If the milk is nearer fresh, not too much. Much preferable would be milk with the animal heat still in same; and then you may not drink too much.

4/22/36
F. 28 yrs.
DEBILITATION: GENERAL **1126-2**

Q. Is milk good for the body?

A. In moderation, and *not* raw milk. This should be heated, or let come to a boil—and yet modified for this body; that is, to a quart of milk that has been—or before heating, put to the quart of milk a teaspoonful of limewater and a teaspoonful of soda—level teaspoonful you see, of the limewater and of the baking soda; and let come to the boil. With these additions, we take out of the raw milk much that is harmful for the body. Do not take too much at a time. About two glasses a day should be sufficient. Of course, it should be taken after it has cooled—or after being prepared and allowing to cool.

1/17/44
BABY CARE **F. 2 yrs.**
DERMATITIS **2752-3**

Be cautious that there is sufficient of vegetable forces in one manner or another added to the diet, so as to prevent incoordination in any of the eliminating channels. For we find, there is a tendency for the alimentary canal not to coordinate with the eliminations through the circulation, to the lymph or the exterior or perspiratory circulation, (you see the body seldom sweats), or the kidneys and the lungs.

Hence there is needed a stimulation by massages and the occasional adding to the system of those laxatives, if the same form of milk or diet is kept. Raw milk—provided it is from cows that don't eat certain characters of food. If they eat dry food, it is well, if they eat certain types of weeds or grass grown this time of year, it won't be so good for the body.

1/26/27
F. 22 yrs.
TUBERCULOSIS **4236-1**

Keep all the milk the body will assimilate. Do not overcrowd the system, but taking that that will assimilate, without producing nausea or clogging the system. Better that a small quantity be taken often, that it may be assimilated by the system. Eggs and milk—these may be put together if possible for the body to take it in this way and manner, see? Keep the animal heat—while the heat is still there from the animal in the rnilk. These are well taken into the system, for these give their vibrations as will produce better assimilation in this condition, and are more digestible to the body and to the lining of the intestinal tract, as well as to the portions of the duodenum and stomach proper.

3/14/32
M. Adult
TOXEMIA **5672-1**

Noon—Milk may be taken at this same period. Much better that the milk is heated, but not boiled—or better still with the animal heat in same when taken. Bad time to milk a cow, but be very well to give it at that period.

6/7/40
M. 49 yrs.
ASSIMILATIONS: POOR **2183-2**

Drink plenty of milk; preferably the milk should be taken while still warm from the body-heat of the cow—or as soon after it is taken from the cow as possible—provided such an animal or cow is tested well, and there is no germ or no tubercle in same.

11/16/22
BLOOD: OXIDIZATION **F. Adult**
BLOOD-BUILDING **4810-1**

Q. Mr. Cayce, the body wants to know if sweet milk should be given for her diet?

A. If warm and carrying the animal heat—cold or sterilized milk do not use.

8/31/41
F. 51 yrs.
1158-31

ARTHRITIS: PREVENTIVE
BODY: GENERAL

Q. Raw milk?

A. This should be a part of each day. At least a glass, or six ounces.

4/18/29
M. 2 yrs.
5520-6

BABY CARE
DERMATITIS: ACIDITY

Q. What causes the itching and breaking out on face and limbs? What can be done to remedy it?

A. This is produced by too much protein in the system, and a tendency towards acid reaction in the digestive system. We would use the modified raw milk.

Q. How many ounces of milk does he need in 24 hours?

A. Twelve.

Q. Does he need 3 or 4 feedings in 24 hours?

A. Better that they are 4, divided properly, with *modified* milk.

Q. Just what proportion should the milk be?

A. Use that of lime water for the weakening of same, and make two tablespoonsful to one of water, see?

Q. Did the raw milk cause the serious illness of his bowels last July?

A. The condition of the system at the time, and the condition of the milk also.

v)—Skim

3/21/39
F. 49 yrs.
1158-21

RELAXATION

Q. Skimmed milk?

A. This is NOT so good for the body, though it is desirable, four to five ounces a day would be very well.

2)—Buttermilk

7/26/37
F. 60 yrs.
1409-4

DEBILITATION: GENERAL
TEMPERATURE: FEVER: AFTEREFFECTS

Since the temperature has been allayed, there is the necessity, to be sure, that there are not foods used nor activities that would tend to make for the weakening of the digestive forces, nor the allowing of activities of the assimilating system—the liver, the kidneys or the whole hepatic circulation—to become so congested as to allow the temperature to arise again.

Hence we would keep rather a tendency to the alkaline-producing foods.

To be sure, buttermilk (if it is homemade)—may be gradually added; not all at once, but just sufficient that the body gains the strength physically. And keep the eliminations well.

11/9/39
M. 48 yrs.
DIABETES **2040-1**

Let plenty of buttermilk be taken at one of the meals each day, you see; for this (preferably fresh buttermilk) carries in same those properties that would aid in creating that effluvium that is preferable to be in the intestinal system under the existent conditions.

9/29/39
F. 59 yrs.
ASSIMILATIONS: ELIMINATIONS: INCOORDINATION **538-57**

ANY form of yeast or a yogurt for the body will be well. Of course, this is a portion of that as will be had from buttermilk. It is those germicidal influences in same that will be effective upon the intestinal system.

6/29/26
F. Adult
ASTHENIA **67-1**

The diet should be that as will best assimilate in and for the system, which of necessity then should be changed often. As much buttermilk as the body will assimilate will always be good for the system.

9/27/37
F. Adult
DEBILITATION: GENERAL **1419-5**

In the evening meal, these may be also varied: Not at the same meal but at times half a glass or a glass of NEW buttermilk (not that that is too old) may be taken; with which there may also be included the crumbs of whole wheat bread or of such natures, or the whole wheat crackers.

2/17/31
F. 22 yrs.
OBESITY **2096-1**

Buttermilk may be taken occasionally, but be mindful that it is not taken with too many vegetables.

1/10/41
APPENDICITIS: TENDENCIES **M. 33 yrs.**
ULCERS: DUODENAL **481-4**

Use rather buttermilk with bread—such as corn bread or whole wheat toast—crumbled in same.

5/1/38
F. Adult
ARTHRITIS **932-1**

A little buttermilk may be taken at times, *between* meals—*not with* the meals.

7/25/39
M. 24 yrs.
CANCER **1967-1**

Do not eat meats of any great quantity. Plenty of buttermilk.

4/2/32
F. Child
ASTHMA **5682-2**

At the evening meal there may be also taken buttermilk, if fresh, or the Bulgarian milk. These would be well.

3)—Clabber

7/5/34
APPETITE: ASSIMILATION: ELIMINATIONS: **M. 56 yrs.**
INCOORDINATION **556-3**

Q. Why does milk seem to disagree?

A. Never been prepared just perfectly in the right way, but—as has been given—use this now only as the basis for the diet.

Q. If the milk is to be continued, just how should it be prepared?

A. As is stipulated on the directions in making same, with those additions to other milk—or if preferable, change entirely and use only buttermilk, or churned milk, you see—or clabber, which would be preferable of all.

7)—Goat's Milk

4/12/27
ASSIMILATIONS: ELIMINATIONS **F. 22 yrs.**
ASTHENIA **5714-2**

Goat's milk or mare's milk may be taken by the body in small quantities, *provided* same *agrees* with the body, see? for this will agree in small quantity, yet if too much is crowded into the system, the system will not be able to handle same.

7/30/27
DERMATITIS **M. 5 mos.**
BABY CARE **5520-1**

Q. Did this body have whooping cough, or was the cough caused from bad milk?

A. Whooping cough, as it is known. Those manipulations and those conditions accorded for the body's eliminations have kept the body well, and the germ—or that producing whooping cough, as yet, has not been *entirely* eliminated from the system. The effects of same are greatly diminished in the system. Hence goat's milk and modified Mellin's Food the better for the body.

2/22/44
F. 26 yrs.
CIRCULATION: LYMPH: TUBERCULOSIS **3687-1**

Plenty of milk whenever possible. Also goat's milk in the beginning might be especially helpful for the body.

4/20/31
M. 20 yrs.
DEBILITATION: GENERAL **4320-3**

Q. How much milk should he drink each day?

A. This should be goat's milk or mare's milk and if this *cannot* be obtained—*we* would prefer those of Dryco or malted milk. These would be much preferable to those of the raw milk, and these may be taken—as has been given—in *smaller* quantities and often, and if as much as six to eight ounces is taken—or can be taken—during the day, this will be better, or even more if it may be assimilated by the body. If goat's milk or mare's milk may not be obtained, then use the *dry* milk—rather than raw milk, or even that that has been pasteurized. This is not good for these conditions.

2/10/30
M. 41 yrs.
LACERATIONS: STOMACH **5545-1**

In the character of *milks*—this will not always agree with the system, for curds would be produced from same that would be bad. Then, these may be altered by the *character* of the milk at times as may be taken. That of the goat's milk may be used occasionally. This with the cereals, or with the foods, or with the first morning foods.

8)—Milk: Dry

10/17/35
ANEMIA **F. 49 yrs.**
ACIDITY & ALKALINITY **1023-1**

In the place of raw milk it would be well that the compounds be used, or dry milk, either in the preparation of foods or as a drink. For the natural animal reaction is not as well for the body as the more sterile.

These will be found to bring near normal conditions for this body.

8/13/37
F. 25 yrs.
DIABETES: TENDENCIES **480-42**

Q. Can milk and dairy products be included in diet?

A. Milk products may be gradually added, but for the body yet it is much preferable to use dry milks rather than raw milk. There is so easily an overstressing upon milk, by many; for there are many products much more healthful than milk. So few milks are free from tubercle; so few are free from those influences that cause a great deal more irritation than help—unless irradiated or dried milk is used. These as a whole are much more healthful to most individuals than raw milk.

1/24/35
CANCER: TENDENCIES **F. Adult**
DEBILITATION: GENERAL **799-1**

We would be very mindful of the diet; and while it should not be too rich, it should be particularly nourishing. So we find that the dried milks—as Dryco, or as even Mellin's Food for this body would be particularly well; for it, of all such properties, may be so altered by the addition of water—rather than boiled or heated milk—in such ways and manner as to *control* the activity of the liver and its tributary reactions to the whole of the hepatic circulation.

1/18/35
F. 3 yrs.
ASSIMILATIONS: POOR **795-1**

We would be very mindful that the diet consists of those things that are most easily assimilated. Instead of using cow's milk we would use the combinations of the dried milk—as those combinations of milk with vegetable forces; such as may be found in Dryco and the like—or in Mellin's Food, which has a proper combination. These will make for an activity with the digestive system and may be changed by the leaving off or the addition of the combination itself, as to regulate the activities through the system in making for the proper assimilations.

12/12/23
ACIDITY & ALKALINITY **F. 22 yrs.**
DEBILITATION: GENERAL: TUBERCULOSIS **418-2**

In between the morning meal (and eat it early; don't lay in bed till nine, ten or eleven o'clock and then expect to eat in between that and twelve, but eat it early!) and the noon meal, or at ten o'clock, take dried milk with raw egg stirred in well, or a few drops or a teaspoonful of spirits frumenti (that's about 95 or 90 proof) may be added to a whole glassful taken.

4/24/34
M. 43 yrs.
ACIDITY: ALKALINITY: ANEMIA **642-1**

We would also in the middle period (of the day) have *dried* milk, preferable to raw milk, in which there would be carried such as egg or a stimulation that will make for more gastric forces.

11/23/34
ANEMIA **M. 3 yrs.**
COLD: CONGESTION **773-4**

Q. Does milk agree with this body?

A. Dry milks would be better than the animal milk.

Q. Does dry milk have the same value?

A. For this body it would have better values!

Q. How often should the dry milk be taken?

A. Just as it would with the ordinary milk at the meals.

Q. Whose preparation would be the best?

A. Any of these that have the proper content, which would be indicated by the recipes upon same. Dry or malted, provided these carry the proper content.

Q. Should the other type of milk be eliminated entirely from the diet?

A. It may be used in the cooking, or at times it may be taken—but not in great quantities.

10/5/36
CIRCULATION: POOR **F. 42 yrs.**
UREMIA **1016-1**

Q. Is milk a suitable article of diet for me?

A. As we find, the dried milk or malted milk would be more preferable than the raw milk. Or even the raw milk heated would be better. But we find that the milk *preparations* will be more preferable for the body.

5/29/34
F. 19 yrs.
ANEMIA **562-1**

In the middle of the morning take the dried milk in which an egg is beaten with spirits frumenti or beer.

In the middle of the afternoon take again a stimulant as of milk that is not heated, but well beaten with the spirits frumenti, or a malt, or the like.

10/31/31
ANEMIA **F. 60 yrs.**
ASSIMILATIONS: POOR **501-2**

We would also take in the interim—that is, between the morning meal and the lunch hour—those of the milk—*dried* milk, that is mixed *with* those properties that give to the chyle of the lacteal system more lactics to work with—see? These we would take with the properties that may be found in those of the *addition* to it in the yolk (not the white)—the *yolk*—of an egg.

6/3/28
F. 2 yrs.
COLITIS **608-5**

As for the diet—this should consist principally of . . . milk—but preferably use dry milk rather than cow's milk. This necessarily will need to be regulated according to the conditions as arise. These, as we find, would bring the normal forces—reducing the conditions in system.

6/18/37
F. 22 yrs.
ASSIMILATIONS: POOR: ANEMIA **667-8**

Do not take again the malted milk. Do not take raw milk. Preferably if milk is to be taken, use Dryco or the like—this may be taken once a day, but if taken should be taken with an egg beat in same—and spirits frumenti with it also—or whiskey—five to ten drops, not spoonsful—this to be put upon the egg, and the egg beat in this before it is put into the milk.

11/28/33
M. Adult
ANEMIA **461-1**

Noons—take dried milk, not raw milk—and especially not that which has been boiled. Hence ice cream is *not* so good.

11/23/37
M. 13 yrs.
PSORIASIS **1484-1**

Evenings—Milk may be taken, but preferably only the dried or prepared milk—rather than the raw.

Q. What about vitamin D milk?

A. Vitamin D milk is very good. BETTER STILL is the Dryco, especially in the beginning. A little later the vitamin milks will be very well. But in the beginnings, if these adjustments are made, only the dry milks are preferable.

4/15/35
F. 56 yrs.
ASTHENIA **895-1**

In the matter of the diet, be very mindful that in the beginning this consists much of pre-digested foods; as the milks that are dried.

2/10/30
M. 41 yrs.
LACERATIONS: STOMACH **5545-1**

In the character of *milks*—this will not always agree with the system, for curds would be produced from same that would be bad. Then, these may be altered by the *character* of the milk at times as may be taken. That of the dried milk, or of such, may be used occasionally. This with the cereals, or with the foods, or with the first morning foods.

6/21/32
F. 48 yrs.
ASSIMILATIONS: POOR **428-7**

In the middle of the morning—nine-thirty or ten o'clock—there should be taken those of the malt with egg, or dry milk with egg. Here the yolk or the whole egg may be whipped or stirred in same. Also there may be added a few drops—not more than ten to fifteen—of spirits frumenti, which will prevent the flat taste, as well as make for better digestion. It will make the drink more palatable, more strengthening, and will give better tone to the general system.

1)—Malted Milk

6/26/39
F. 21 yrs.
ENVIRONMENT: HAY FEVER **1771-3**

Q. Should I refrain from drinking milk?

A. Do not drink raw milk. Not necessarily to refrain from other milk, if it is desired to be taken. Malted milks, especially, are very well, if properly prepared.

1/10/41
APPENDICITIS: TENDENCIES **M. 33 yrs.**
ULCERS: DUODENAL **481-4**

Keep away from soft drinks that carry carbonated waters. Keep away from any drinks that have malt in same. However, malted milk is very well. If the raw egg yolk is taken in malted milk once a day it will be most beneficial.

8/29/40
M. 27 yrs.
PSORIASIS: TENDENCIES **641-5**

Q. Should I continue the malted milk?

A. Malted milks are very well. If you drink two or three of these a day, it will be well for the body; but these are to be taken between meals, not AT the meals, or not having them to supply or take the place of vegetables. These are in addition, so that they work with the gastric flow of the body itself. An egg added to these at times, raw—the WHOLE egg, will be helpful.

1/9/35
M. 1 yr.
786-1

WORMS

We would begin with a body-*building* diet for the body.

Mornings—We would have preferably not cow's milk but that prepared with the *dried* milk, which will make for the better assimilation of the active forces; and may be prepared with the regular combination of malted milk, you see—but may be altered at times from the plain to the chocolate flavored, as they are prepared in both ways and manners. We find also that Coco-Malt would be a good drink at times for the body; well prepared—and when it is prepared, let it be prepared with skimmed milk; not too rich a milk for the body in the beginning of the increasing of the weight and the diet for the activities in this body of [786].

4/9/43
F. 33 yrs.
2959-1

ASSIMILATIONS: POOR
BODY-BUILDING

DO drink malted milk twice each day, and with an egg in same. Let this be rather between meals, if at all possible.

5/18/43
F. 56 yrs.
2956-2

CANCER

Q. Should butter and milk be excluded?

A. Butter and milk are hard on the body; though malted milks may be used in moderation.

3/16/36
F. 38 yrs.
954-2

ANEMIA
DEBILITATION: GENERAL

Between the morning meal and the noon meal (about the middle of the morning) have a malted milk with the yolk of an egg beat in same, and a few drops of spirits frumenti to take the taste off of the egg. A full glass of this should be taken.

1/8/37
F. Adult
1278-7

DEBILITATION: GENERAL

We would find it well to use every character of food that is body- and blood-building. Milk; but preferably the malted milk with an egg and a little spirits frumenti in same; taken once to twice a day rather than solid foods. This, of course, just for three to four days, but still afterward remaining as a greater portion of the diet. The malted milk taken twice a day with a whole egg in same, but thoroughly beaten and made tasty by the addition of spirits frumenti or apple brandy or apple jack. But do not give too great quantities of the stimulants of this nature save as in food values, or in milks or the like, see? Eggs, rather the yolk—if these are cooked at all, but if these are taken in the malted milk it should be sufficient.

8/4/36
F. 29 yrs.
1239-1

ANEMIA
DEBILITATION: GENERAL

Between the morning meal and the noon meal, drink a small glass of malted milk—*malted* milk. Stir this together as the directions are given for making malted milk. The original Horlick's as we find would be the better for this particular body.

In the afternoon, about three to three-thirty o'clock, we would have a malted milk with an egg beat in it—the whole of the egg.

1/23/39
M. 32 yrs.
1798-1

ASSIMILATIONS: POOR

Malted milk with apple brandy may be alternated with beef juice; the proportions being a teaspoonful of the apple brandy to a glass of the malted milk and egg. This quantity may be prepared at the time if it is kept on ice, but NEVER give more than a teaspoonful at the time, you see, and this only in sips.

1/13/41
F. 27 yrs.
2426-1

DEBILITATION: GENERAL

Throughout that period let the diet be of those foods the more easily assimilated. Use rather the prepared milks, or those that are condensed in such a manner that there is the addition of milk to prepare same—as in malted milk; and we will find this should NOT disagree, nor should the body b allergic to same, if the Atomidine is being taken in the manner indicated. Do not overburden the body with this, however, especially in the first five to ten days.

6/10/35
F. Adult
715-3

ANEMIA

Q. Have been taking a quart of milk daily—so tired of it. Can I get along on less?

A. Can get along without any, if you'll use those things that have been indicated!

Be well were this changed to this way and manner of taking the milk:

Between the breakfast and the noon meals, in the middle of the morning, we would take a *small* glass of the *malted* milk in which there would be put a few drops (three to four) of Jamaica Ginger.

Then in the middle of the afternoon we would take a malted milk with *egg* and a few drops of spirits frumenti in same; or half a teaspoonful.

8/13/37
F. 25 yrs.
480-42

DIABETES: TENDENCIES

Q. Can milk and dairy products be included in diet?

A. Milk products may be gradually added, but for the body yet it is much preferable to use malted milks rather than raw milk.

6/6/40
ASSIMILATIONS: POOR **F. 19 yrs.**
ANEMIA **2277-1**

Drink plenty of MALTED milk, which is preferable to the raw milk—or even to the sterilized milk. Malted milks and the like—eggs even in this occasionally would be very well.

3/5/35
F. 3 yrs.
ASSIMILATIONS: POOR **795-2**

We would find also that in the matters of the milk, and especially of the dried milks, if these are changed occasionally to the malted milk with the chocolate flavor, and the like, these will be more palatable for the body—and will be taken much better by the body.

4/15/35
F. 56 yrs.
ASTHENIA **895-1**

In the matter of the diet, be very mindful that in the beginning this consists much of pre-digested foods; as malted milks with a little stimuli of brandy (preferably apple brandy)—a few drops, not great quantities; just enough to stimulate the activities of the system as to make for a reduction in the activity of the secretions from the spleen and the pancreas to the system.

5/23/35
M. 45 yrs.
TUBERCULOSIS **929-1**

We would build the body up. Take the food values that make for *body-building*, but let them be rather alkaline-reacting.

In the middle of the morning we would have a malted milk with a whole egg (white *and yellow*) in same, but this should be beaten very thoroughly, you see.

4/1/44
M. 36 yrs.
ENVIRONMENT: CLIMATE: GENERAL: SINUSITIS **4047-1**

Q. Are daily heavy chocolate malted milks detrimental?

A. Chocolate that is prepared in the present is not best for ANY diet. This, too, the chocolate, is not produced in the vicinity of [4047]. Those foods that may be taken from the vicinity or food values of that nature are the better.

9)—Nut Milk

4/21/36
F. Adult
BEVERAGES: NOT RECOMMENDED **1140-2**

Q. With lacteal area disturbed, shall I continue to drink so much sweet milk?

A. This is not so well, for the casein as well as the quantity of calcium in same makes for a hardening of those activities through the lymph flow in the intestinal system.

If this is altered to the milk that is a natural creation from nuts it would be much better; particularly almonds and filberts will be helpful and carry with same elements that are much preferable to so much milk.

10)—Soybean Milk

3/29/40
F. 14 yrs.
ASSIMILATIONS: ELIMINATIONS: INCOORDINATION **1206-11**

Soybean milk, or soybean products, would be very good for this body, but do not make it overCONSCIOUS of same.

7/26/40
F. 12 yrs.
EPILEPSY **2153-2**

Mornings—Preferably use the soybean milk.

6/10/38
F. 13 yrs.
ASSIMILATIONS: ELIMINATIONS: INCOORDINATION **1206-8**

Q. Is it well for the body to refrain from eating all dairy products, with the exception of butter and cream, and substitute a "soybean milk" for a beverage?

A. For this body in the present, it would be very well. Though the soybean milk product is not well for EVERY body, in these particular conditions here it is very good; especially owing to the reactions through the assimilated forces from same for the heart activity.

7/6/38
M. 8 yrs.
CHILD TRAINING **1188-6**

Q. Would SOYBEAN MILK be preferable in place of cow's milk?

A. For this body it would be very well.

6/4/40
F. 11 yrs.
BODY-BUILDING **1179-6**

Q. Do you recommend Borden's irradiated milk or soybean milk?

A. Soybean milk a part of the time as we find is excellent, and better than irradiated milk.

7/6/38
F. 48 yrs.
MENOPAUSE **1158-18**

Q. Is it advisable for the body to drink SOYBEAN MILK?

A. This will depend much upon the activities of the body. If there is sufficient of the energies used for physical activities to make same more easily assimilated, it is well. If these energies are used for activities which are more mental than physical, it would not be so well.

12/11/38
F. 13 yrs.
1206-9

GLANDS: INCOORDINATION

Q. Should she continue soybean milk and no cow's milk?

A. This would be rather governed by the appetite. If there is a desire for same, in preference to the cow's milk, the system will balance itself.

III

Fowl & Game Birds: Stews & Broths

1—Fowl: General

6/9/44
M. 12 yrs.
ASTHMA **5192-1**

Q. What causes the deep ridges in thumbnail and what treatments should be followed?

A. These are the activities of the glandular force, and the addition of those foods which carry large quantities of calcium will make for bettered conditions in this direction. Take often chicken neck, chew it. Cook this well, the feet and those portions of the fowl, and we will find it will add calcium to the body.

7/31/39
F. 71 yrs.
HYPERTENSION: TOXEMIA **1973-1**

In the diet beware of those foods that carry large quantities of fats—as the fat of fowl, though the lean or bony portions would be very well to supply more calcium; and those bony portions of same that are cooked to such an extent that these may be masticated also. Hence these boiled or broiled or roasted would be preferable for the body.

7/26/32
ANEMIA **M. 25 yrs.**
ASSIMILATIONS: POOR **481-1**

We would be mindful of the diet, that those foods are taken that are easily assimilated. Do not take quantities of grease of any nature. When meats *are* taken, they should be those of fowl—but not fried fowl. It should be either baked or broiled.

Do not eat meat more than three times each week, and don't gorge self when this is done!

12/29/41
M. 40 yrs.
ASSIMILATIONS: POOR **826-14**

Have fowl, but these prepared with the re-inforced vitamins in the flour, the meal or the like.

ANEMIA: TENDENCIES **10/2/43**
ASSIMILATIONS: ELIMINATIONS: INCOORDINATION **F. 37 yrs.**
KIDNEYS **1695-2**

Then take at least once each day the vitamins B-1. Do not take A. Do take D and G, but these more in the foods than supplementing in the combinations. These will bring better forces to the body; that is, in the food values take fowl, not other meats.

9/19/40
M. 33 yrs.
ARTHRITIS **849-53**

Calcium is now needed, in a manner that it may be assimilated, and gradually take the place of that which has been crystallized in the bursa and portions of the structural body. This we would add in the form which we have indicated as the BEST—the chewing of bones or ends of bones of the fowl.

9/19/35
ASSIMILATIONS: POOR **F. 80 yrs.**
CANCER **975-1**

Evenings—When meats are taken let them be preferably either small quantities of fowl or the like. These should never be fried. These would only be those that were prepared very thoroughly, and in most instances after preparation be *chilled* almost, as it were, that they may be the easier assimilated by the gastric forces that have had so much disturbance; but these will be aided by the properties we have indicated in the compound for the body.

5/20/35
M. Adult
ACIDITY **926-1**

Beware of any stimuli as to make for fermentations in the system, as spirits frumenti of any kind. However, one meal each day—or two to three times a week—may include only black bread and wine (red wine); this should not be taken with vegetables or with other foods, save with either cold fowl or black bread . . . or whole wheat bread or rye bread especially, or sour bread.

12/30/42
M. 21 yrs.
BODY-BUILDING: LOCOMOTION: IMPAIRED **2873-1**

The food values should be those fully well balanced with calcium, iron, and especially the vitamins B-1 and the B-Complex. These are much preferable for the body.

At least three times each week, then, supply these from the foods rather than the reinforced vitamins (though these reinforcements may be desirable if there is the inability of the body to assimilate foods that carry excesses or the full quantity of such vital forces).

To be sure, these are not all the foods that are to be taken:

Noons—Have soups, broths or the like, and these should include fowl.

Evenings—At least three times a week have fowl, whole wheat breads and the like.

12/6/43
COLD: CONGESTION: PELVIC DISORDERS **F. 15 yrs.**
BODY-BUILDING **2084-15**

Q. Any changes in her diet other than these vitamins?

A. When fowl is taken choose rather the very small bony pieces rather than what might appear to be the more delicate. Take those that are not supposed to be choice pieces—as the wimblebit, the back, the neck, the feet. All of these are much preferable and have much more vital energies for body building.

9/5/29
SPINE: SUBLUXATIONS **M. 55 yrs.**
MEATLESS **5459-5**

Q. Will the elimination of meat from my diet have a weakening effect temporarily?

A. No. Only so far as the mental forces allow same, for there is as much *vitality* in the outline of those things the body *should* eat as would be with the meats, and when conditions are of the nature as has been given, *meats* aggravate, while vegetables, or characters of meats that build—that is, such as fowl, these do not carry those vibrations that aid in accentuating such pressures as disturb this body—but rather give the tendency to give more strength and endurance to a physical body.

8/25/39
F. 39 yrs.
TOXEMIA **1985-1**

The activities of red meats would become more disturbing to the body. Fowl should be a portion of the diet as the meats, if there is any of these taken.

5/20/39
M. 38 yrs.
ARTHRITIS: TENDENCIES **1888-1**

Do not eat great quantities of fat of any kind. With roasts, do not eat the fat of the lamb or the fowl. Of the fowl, preferably eat plenty of the bony portions—as the thigh, the wing, the neck, the head. Chew these so that the juice from same may be swallowed for these are very well, and the calcium from same will be beneficial to the body; but fats work a hardship upon the kidneys as well as upon the upper hepatic circulation, and tend to make the stress greater.

2/22/34
ASTHENIA **F. 65 yrs.**
ACIDITY & ALKALINITY **509-2**

Beware of too much starch and too much fat. But oils, as the olive oil or the fats of any that are taken in the foods—as fowl (provided the same is not the *gross* fat)—will be helpful. But no red meats, nor too much of those foods that will make for sugar reaction in the system.

8/14/36
M. Adult
BLOOD: HUMOR **862-2**

Refrain from most any meats, only those at times of the light portion of fowl and that not fried.

8/24/44
F. 58 yrs.
ASTHENIA **5394-1**

Do take a great deal of fowl—as bird, chicken or the like, see? this well cooked but never fried. Do chew the bones, especially the bony pieces. These are much preferable to the breast or the like; the feet, wings, legs, ends of the bones should be chewed thoroughly, as it is from these that we may obtain the elements needed.

4/23/42
F. 34 yrs.
CONCEPTION **457-8**

Q. Should meat be entirely eliminated?

A. No. Fowl are the character of meats to be taken. Not ham nor hog meat, nor rare beef.

7/30/40
F. Adult
OBESITY **2315-1**

Each meal should be preceeded by the grape juice—thirty minutes before eating.

Evenings—Take a little of one or the other of the raw vegetables as a salad; with baked, broiled fowl, but NOT any fried. ALL cooked vegetables should be cooked in their own juices (as in Patapar paper), rather than with meats or fats.

8/12/40
F. 33 yrs.
ANEMIA: DIGESTION: INDIGESTION **2320-1**

Have fowl—this preferably made into soups; or the bony pieces cooked VERY, VERY well done, so that the feet, the neck, the carcass, the wings, the bones, may be chewed also, and the juices from same swallowed.

Use preferably whole wheat toasted bread with the fowl.

5/22/44
F. 56 yrs.
ARTHRITIS: TENDENCIES **1895-2**

Do decrease any red meats. Fowl we would take but none of any heavy foods, none of these fried.

3/30/44
F. 32 yrs.
SPINE: SUBLUXATIONS **4031-1**

Have plenty of fowl and occasionally lamb. These should be the only characters of meats. Do not change wholly to the vegetable diet, for this would be too weakening for the body conditions.

12/15/43
F. 23 yrs.
PARKINSON'S DISEASE **3405-1**

Not too much meats, nor things that cause gas for the body. Fowl is very good—this would be well.

6/25/40
M. Adult
ARTHRITIS **2288-1**

As to the diet, refrain from any foods carrying any elements as of silicon, lime or the like. Hence not much meats unless fowl. No fried foods of ANY character.

7/25/39
M. 24 yrs.
CANCER **1967-1**

Do not eat meats of any great quantity. Fowl that is very clean or that has been purged, may be taken. Mostly use the leafy vegetables as the diet.

1/17/43
CIRCULATION: IMPAIRED **F. 6 yrs.**
BODY-BUILDING **2883-1**

In the diet—have plenty of calcium, the foods that carry plenty of calcium; especially fowl in small quantities, to be sure, but not large quantities. These should be a part of the diet for the body.

3/16/43
ASSIMILATIONS: POOR **F. 21 yrs.**
BODY-BUILDING **2937-1**

Do give vitamin-rich foods; such as fowl. Season with butter or the like, rather than with other forms of greases.

3/31/43
ASSIMILATIONS: ELIMINATIONS: INCOORDINATION **F. 18 yrs.**
BODY-BUILDING **2947-1**

Keep the diet body building. Plenty of vitamins A and D; plenty of B-1 and the B-Complex or plenty of fowl as a part of the diet. No hog meat of ANY character.

This is not to be all the diet, of course, but these should form a great part of the diet—just so often as not to become obnoxious to the body; altering in the manner of preparation.

Q. What causes pain in arms, shoulders and back, and what can be done for relief?

A. The lack of sufficient energies being supplied to the nerve forces and the stimulation of the nerve plexus calling for more activity. AND at times a pressure in the assimilating system. Thus the need of keeping good eliminations.

Q. How can she best overcome constipation?

A. By the diet; and, as indicated, these are taken into consideration.

8/28/41
CIRCULATION: INCOORDINATION M. 56 yrs.
ASSIMILATIONS: POOR 619-10

Q. Are my teeth causing any ailments?

A. No; these as indicated in the throat and mouth—are more from the disturbances of the glandular forces, or the thyroid activity in relationship to the metabolism. Thus the needs for the supplying those foods that carry quantities of iodine and calcium.

. . . Much of these influences as helpful forces will be found in fowl, especially the bony pieces and these taken as part of the food values—the bony pieces chewed for the marrow and the activity of that about the bones of such that carry the calcium.

2/5/36
M. 28 yrs.
ARTHRITIS 849-13

Be most careful that there are not shell fish. Not too great a quantity of meats, and when meats are taken let same be roast fowl. These, we find, with *quantities* of the green vegetables, would supply greater quantities of those elements to create this balance in *conjunction* with the indicated manipulative and electrical treatments and the baths.

4/18/35
M. Adult
ANEMIA 898-1

Evening meal—In the meats have those especially, whenever possible, of fowl.

Keep these consistently, persistently; we will gain weight, we will put off this dullness, this tendency for catching cold, this weakness throughout the whole system; and bring the body—in six to eight months—to its normal weight of about a hundred and fifty pounds.

4/1/43
POLIOMYELITIS F. 11 yrs.
KIDNEYS: BODY-BUILDING 2948-1

Have plenty of fowl. And when the fowl is eaten, do crunch the small bones as the wing, or the joints in the thigh or the like; for these properties in same will add strength and vitality to this body.

2/11/37
F. 40 yrs.
CIRCULATION: POOR 1337-1

Do not have any fried foods, especially as of steak or things of that nature—but broiled, boiled, of the like; and especially fowl should be used if meats at all are taken.

11/23/37
M. 13 yrs.
PSORIASIS 1484-1

Evenings—Fowl—these would be taken in moderation, with any of the vegetables that are grown UNDER the ground, with one or two of the green variety or nature that grow above the ground.

7/26/40
F. 12 yrs.
EPILEPSY **2153-2**

Evenings—A little fowl (not fried), with mashed potatoes, sweet potatoes, squash or the like.

8/12/37
F. 36 yrs.
LACERATIONS: STOMACH **1422-1**

No food that makes for a quantity of alcohol in its activity in the system.

Meats—never rare meats. Rather use those that are broiled or roasted; preferably only fowl.

5/19/35
GLANDS: SALIVARY: DIGESTION: GENERAL **F. 27 yrs.**
INCOORDINATION: PREGNANCY **808-3**

The meats should be such as fowl. Occasionally the *broiled* steak or liver, or tripe, would be well. A well balance between the starches and proteins is the more preferable, with sufficient of the carbohydrates. And especially keep a well balance (but not an excess) in the calciums necessary with the iodines, that produce the better body, especially through those periods of conception and gestation.

11/16/22
BLOOD: OXIDIZATION **F. Adult**
BLOOD-BUILDING **4810-1**

Q. Should this body eat any meats, Mr. Cayce?

A. Very little meats. When meats are eaten, preferably those of fowl and those not in large quantity, but something of those that carry the sinew and vital forces—no hog meat.

7/6/43
F. 32 yrs.
INJURIES: MINERALS **3076-1**

In the matter of the diet for the body—eat plenty of fowl, and especially the bony pieces. Preferably prepare such pieces as the neck, the head, the wing, the feet, and the bony pieces, so that the small bones may be very well masticated by the body, or the juices chewed out of these. For, the juices from these carry more of the calcium that is needed. This, the calcium, may not be supplied as well in other ways as it may be by taking the bony pieces of fowl or chicken.

12/8/39
M. 32 yrs.
PINWORMS **1597-2**

As to the diet, following the three-day apple diet, let there be more of the supplying forces as will create iron, silicon and the like for the system.

Not too much of meats, though fowl may be taken.

2/5/42
F. 24 yrs.
INJURIES **2679-1**

In the diets, also, much may be accomplished. Necessarily, there must be plenty of those properties that aid in keeping a correct balance in the production of Iymph, leucocyte AND the red blood supply.

Then, have especially those foods that carry more of the calcium and the vitamins A, D, B-1 and other B Complexes.

Hence we would have plenty of fowl.

7/1/26
F. 37 yrs.
BLOOD-BUILDING **5739-1**

The diet should be kept in accord with the rebuilding of a cleansed blood system. Not over amount of meats. Fowl may be taken in small quantities.

7/28/43
ANEMIA **F. 56 yrs.**
MULTIPLE SCLEROSIS **3118-1**

Keep to those things that heal within and without.

Have seafoods often and fowl. These we would give as the main portion of the diet, or the things to be stressed.

12/9/36
ARTHRITIS: TENDENCIES **F. 63 yrs.**
BODY-BUILDING **1302-1**

In the matter of the diets: Here we need body-building foods but those that tend to be more alkaline-producing than acid. For the natural inclinations of disturbed conditions in a body are to produce acidity through the bloodstream. Hence we need to revivify same by the use of much of those that produce more of the enzymes, more of the hormones for the blood supply; yet not overburdening the body with those unless the balance in the vitamin forces is carried.

Hence as we will find, not heavy foods or fried foods ever, nor combinations where there are quantities of starches or quantities of starches with sweets taken at the same time. But fowl preferably as the meats.

4/14/43
M. 5 yrs.
CHILDREN: ABNORMAL **2963-1**

As to the foods—keep a normal, balanced diet; not an oversupply of any particular vitamins, but plenty of the iodine-producing or iodine-giving foods—as fowl.

9/2/29
CHILDREN: ABNORMAL **M. 7 yrs.**
NERVOUS SYSTEMS: INCOORDINATION **758-2**

Fowl and *all* of the ones that carry iodine are well, but in moderation. These, and those elements as are for the changes in vibration will bring the near normal and the proper corrections for this body.

3/21/39
F. 49 yrs.
RELAXATION **1158-21**

Fowl, once or twice a week; as to quantity, depending upon what portion of same and how it is prepared—two to three pieces if ordinarily prepared, or such as this, for a meal.

ALLERGIES: METALS: ECZEMA **12/29/43**
DERMATITIS **M. 32 yrs**
ECZEMA **3422-1**

In the diet refrain from any meats other than fowl for at least ten days. Do include in the diet during those periods a great deal of raw vegetables.

8/31/41
ARTHRITIS: PREVENTIVE **F. 51 yrs.**
BODY: GENERAL **1158-31**

Q. What are the best sources of calcium in foods?
A. The ends of bony pieces of fowl or the like.
Q. Fowl?
A. Once or twice a week.

4/15/38
ASTHENIA: TENDENCIES **M. 20 yrs.**
BODY-BUILDING **487-22**

Keep to those foods that are body-building. When there IS the taxation through the physical exercise, have plenty of meats—as fowl, but let these be WELL DONE. Preferably not the fried foods.

8/27/40
F. 40 yrs.
ATHLETE'S FOOT: ECZEMA **2332-1**

If meats are taken, only take such as fowl, broiled, baked, stewed or the like.

i)—Fowl Broth

6/20/34
TUBERCULOSIS **M. Adult**
ELIMINATIONS: POOR **572-2**

Q. Any other advice for the body at this time that would be of benefit?
A. We would follow these, which we find will be the most helpful and we will find strength being gained. Take all the beef juice that may be assimilated. Broths may be taken at times of such as fowl or the like—anything that is *strengthening* to the body and that doesn't strain some organ already involved.

KIDNEYS: INFECTIONS **5/4/39**
LIVER: KIDNEYS: INCOORDINATION **M. 31 yrs.**
MINERALS: CALCIUM **1885-1**

No meats—if any are taken, only the broths of fowl; ESPECIALLY those portions of the neck, the feet, the back or the like, cooked for a LONG period and broths made from same. From these portions we find calcium in an assimilated form, would aid in strengthening the bloodstream through the assimilation of this for further assisting in purifying the blood force and alleviating those inclinations for that to be carried through the system FROM the hepatics to be eliminated.

1)—Chicken

7/6/43
ANEMIA **F. 30 yrs.**
DEBILITATION: GENERAL **2186-3**

Mr. Cayce: Yes, we find the body here, [2186], kind of out of place, but we find it!

As we find, conditions are not good. There continues to be those irritations from the lack of proper carbonization of the blood. While there is not what might be called so active a tubercle in the lungs, the general weakness and the indications towards anemia—though not wholly pernicious at this time—with the lack of the structural bone and sufficient of the calcium and supply of acids for the digestion in its proper relationships—continue to prevent the body from body-building.

Do use a great deal of seafoods and chicken, and especially the bony pieces. Cook it like you would chicken and dumplings, but don't eat the dumplings—feed these to the dogs! Eat the bony pieces—and the greases of same are good for the body.

6/10/38
F. 13 yrs.
ASSIMILATIONS: ELIMINATIONS: INCOORDINATION **1206-8**

Q. Is it well to eliminate chicken?

A. Not necessary to be eliminated from the system. For there are those vital forces and balances kept through the system by the activities of some of these, that are necessary to be kept in the chemical reaction of the body.

If chicken would be prepared in certain manners, it would be MOST beneficial; especially certain portions of same that supply a character or an assimilated force of certain elements that are seldom found in other foods of the nature—that is, calcium and lime calcium. We refer to the bony portions, you see, that may be stewed so that the juice may be chewed from the same, see? but never fried! (Juice chewed from the soft BONES, you see.)

8/26/39
F. 28 yrs.
PREGNANCY **23-15**

Take more of Calcios—or chew chicken feet and chicken neck and you will have the same thing! Cook them well, then chew the bones thoroughly. This will supply calcium not only for the developing of the teeth of the body that is expected, but of the general bone and sinew structure also. For this is easily assimilated.

9/4/41
BABY CARE F. 2-1/2 yrs.
ELIMINATIONS 1521-5

There needs to be those considerations for more of the foods carrying the vitamins B and D, rather than these taken separately

The bony pieces of chicken, that is cooked very, VERY well done—and dumplings made in same of whole wheat, or B-l reenforced flour; these, as forms or manners of obtaining such, would be well for the body.

Q. Any further advice regarding this body?

A. Do these things, and keep the body in that frame of mind of cheerfulness, ever.

1/9/40
F. 31 yrs.
CONCEPTION 1523-8

Plenty of fowl—but prepared in such a way that more of the bone structure itself is as a part of the diet in its reaction through the system; that better reaction for the calcium through the system is obtained for same. Chew chicken necks, then. Chew the bones of the thigh.

5/23/35
BODY-BUILDING M. 45 yrs.
TUBERCULOSIS 929-1

Take the food values that make for *body-building*, but let them be rather *alkaline-reacting*.

Noons—Chicken broth, or chicken, or things of such nature; not too much of same, but those that are body and blood building. These may be had either with the uncut (unpolished) rice or with the other cereals or grains that may be used with such; that is, in the soups or broths. Not too much grease, but plenty of those things that make for the body building.

7/28/34
F. 54 yrs.
RHEUMATISM 133-4

Between the periods of the grape and grapefruit diet, in the beginning use a liquid diet consisting of the citrus fruit juices of mornings and the vegetable juices at other meals; gradually—that is, in eight to ten days—beginning to add the semi-solid foods as in this manner:

Evenings: (These foods only added gradually, after the eight- to ten-day period)—a little chicken or mutton broth, but very little of the meat itself. A little later the body may begin with stewed chicken, or broiled chicken and well-cooked vegetables—but not with too much grease in same. Even these vegetables and the chicken would be better cooked in the Patapar paper or a steam cooker.

3/30/38
F. 36 yrs.
TUBERCULOSIS 1560-1

Eat all of the chicken that is possible—EVERY DAY, but do not fry same! or merely roast. Rather it would be broiled or baked, or cooked in its own juices inside the oven.

Then the foods for weight will aid in caring for the activities through the absorptions and through the digestive forces.

8/4/34
M. 36 yrs.
555-5

BODY-BUILDING

There are only those precautions necessary now in adding to the system those things that will gently build up the resistances and gain the bodily strength.

Begin with the semi-solid foods and gradually the solid foods; and we will find the general conditions will be *greatly* improved.

Roasted or broiled chicken, or the like. Not too much at the time, but satisfy the cravings of the body; not wholly, but so that the assimilating system may take same on properly.

And we will find conditions will continue to improve.

2/22/44
F. 26 yrs.
3687-1

CIRCULATION: LYMPH: TUBERCULOSIS

Chicken and chicken broths—the bony pieces, not the select pieces but small chickens and chew the bones, the neck, the feet, the limbs, the thighs—these should be the pieces, and these are preferable to other portions of the fowl, for such conditions.

2/23/28
F. 21 mos.
608-4

TOXEMIA

Meats—no hog meats! but chicken; the white meat of the chicken, these may be given in moderation.

6/14/41
F. 30 yrs.
2390-4

ANEMIA

Q. Was the skin disease I had in Sept. 1939 caused by nerves?

A. Nerves alone!

Q. Is the little pimple on my left hand from the same cause, and what should be done for it?

A. Once or twice a day apply Atomidine. This is from the nerves and poor blood circulation, and the anemia. Thus in the foods add quantities of vitamin B-1; as well as chewing chicken bones.

6/6/44
M. 11 yrs.
2890-3

BODY-BUILDING

As we find, there are many changes for the betterment with this body. As we find, there needs to be kept some of those suggestions occasionally, and we would add reinforcements in the amounts of calcium which would be taken into the system; as is indicated in some of the structural portions of the body, as teeth and as a condition in the general blood supply.

We would include more of the bony pieces of chicken.

7/28/39
DEBILITATION: GENERAL **M. 27 yrs.**
ASSIMILATIONS: ELIMINATIONS: INCOORDINATION **1970-2**

We would keep close to these in the diet, though not merely these—of course—but plenty of vegetables. Have plenty of broiled or boiled chicken.

These we would have in the diet, as well as fish.

i)—Chicken Broth

5/29/34
F. 19 yrs.
ANEMIA **562-1**

Noons—Preferably entirely green or raw vegetables, or the meal may be changed to the juices of meats—but *not* the meats; as chicken broth, or the like.

10/8/36
ANEMIA **F. 54 yrs.**
ARTHRITIS: TOXEMIA **1269-1**

Noons—Preferably a combination of meat juices or vegetable juices, but do not put the two together! There may be at times chicken broth with rice or barley or there may be combinations of vegetables, but *preferably* only vegetable juices *or* meat juices.

8/27/32
F. 72 yrs.
CIRRHOSIS OF LIVER **2092-1**

Evenings—Well-cooked vegetables. Also there may be the strengthening foods such as broths of chicken—with barley, but not with rice.

2/23/28
F. 21 mos.
TOXEMIA **608-4**

Chicken broth may be given in moderation.

12/22/43
DEBILITATION: GENERAL **F. 66 yrs.**
NEURITIS: TENDENCIES **1409-9**

Begin to build up the body with good soups—not canned soups but make them—chicken broth, chicken broth with dumplings; chicken broth with the bony pieces and eat the bones as well as the pieces of chicken.

9/28/41
CONSTIPATION **M. 8 yrs.**
ASSIMILATIONS: POOR **2595-1**

Noons—Take small quantities of raw vegetables and meat juices—as chicken broth, any of such broths, but be sure they have a cereal in them—such as barley or rice or the like.

2)—Squab

5/9/38
F. 51 yrs.
MENU: RHEUMATISM **920-12**

Evenings—Preferably the meats would be taken at this meal; which should consist preferably of squab with fish or lamb occasionally.

1)—Game: General

5/12/28
M. 33 yrs.
LIVER: KIDNEYS: INCOORDINATION **900-383**

Q. Is the albumin on the decrease or increase in the urine?

A. On the decrease. Little fowl—preferably, as wild duck, partridge, or such—see?

5/5/44
F. 40 yrs.
TUBERCULOSIS **5053-1**

In the diet take strengthening foods.

Have fowl also, and take this in the manner which is most palatable for the body, but not fried. Small chickens, or any wild birds are preferable. Any of these are good for the body. Chew the bones when masticating same, as this will add to the strength and blood building and resistance of the body.

5/1/36
ANEMIA: TENDENCIES **F. 46 yrs.**
CIRCULATION: INCOORDINATION **1158-1**

Meats should be preferably fowl, fish, lamb, rather than beef or other meats. Wild fowl are, of course, the better.

1)—Wild Fowl Broth

3/14/32
M. Adult
TOXEMIA **5672-1**

Noon—Broths of fresh meats, preferably of wild game—of the partridge, of the grouse, or the like—these would be well for the body; but little of the meats would we take—but thick broths.

IV

Fruit

1)—Fruit: General

INCOORDINATION **5/19/35**
GLANDS: SALIVARY: DIGESTION: GENERAL **F. 27 yrs.**
PREGNANCY **808-3**

As indicated, keep a tendency for alkalinity in the diet. This does not necessitate that there should *never* be any of the acid-forming foods included in the diet; for an overalkalinity is much more harmful than a little tendency occasionally for acidity. But remember there are those tendencies in the system for cold and congestion to affect the body, and cold *cannot, does not* exist in alkalines. Hence the diet would be as indicated. Citrus fruits; or the smaller fruits occasionally with the cereals that are dry (do not have citrus fruits and cereals at the same meal).

11/13/23
BLOOD: OXIDATION **F. Adult**
ASTHMA **4810-2**

Much of the condition in the bronchials and lungs is produced by the diet the body takes. This produces much of the distress to the body. No sweets should be taken for this reason, no meats of the nature of pork or of hog flesh, see? Rather that of the fruit diet, carrying more acids that will become the form of alcohol in the digestive forces to carry out in the system that of vital forces necessary in the blood to meet the conditions in the system.

8/17/38
M. 61 yrs.
LIFE: BALANCED **1662-1**

Upon the natural things, then, that replenish and supply energies—as in these; not as the only things eaten, but this as an outline for the activities of the body to preserve and maintain a balance: Mornings—Fruits. All of these in their regular season are to be a portion of the diet; not as a conglomerate mass, not as combining cereals at the same meal with fruits—for these defeat then their purposes.

11/24/24
ANEMIA **F. Adult**
BLOOD-BUILDING **2221-1**

Take care that the system is supplied with those properties of iron and the food values that dilate the system in its course through the system. Fruits. These carry the necessary properties.

8/15/38
M. 54 yrs.
KIDNEYS: STONES **843-7**

Q. Will a substance known as "Mineral Food" be of value for my condition?

A. Not necessarily. While it is necessary for the vitamin activities through the system, these may be obtained by a better balance being kept in the vital forces as may be obtained from fresh fruits than from concentrated forces such as those.

4/13/35
F. 36 yrs.
BLOOD-BUILDING **890-1**

In the matter of the diet, well that this be that which would supply a sufficient quantity of those vitamins necessary for increased blood and nerve energies for the system; and should naturally be of the alkaline type. That is, fruits.

6/8/27
DEBILITATION: GENERAL **F. Adult**
COMBINATIONS: ELIMINATIONS: POOR **4460-1**

This body should never take fruits with meats. The fruit and the nut diet of mornings—or of the evening meals—may be well, yet never use fruits of any character with the meats or vegetables. Much of the fruit and nuts, or iron, or those elements producing iron in the body, taken of morning.

3/15/29
M. 40 yrs.
ACIDITY & ALKALINITY **5567-1**

While acid may be taken in moderation, these would be better—that the sugars were created in the system from fruits, as may be taken in their reaction with the other elements taken.

1/11/35
F. Adult
NERVE-BUILDING **787-1**

As to the building supply for the system through the diets, we would cling rather to that which makes for the reduction of acidity; the building of the white *and* red blood supply, through a consistent activity towards nerve-building foods and values.

Necessity demands that there be the proper amount of the activities through the digestion, that these do not cause or produce an overfermentation without sufficient of the gastric flows through the lacteal activity to produce overacidity.

Hence, there should be a reduction in sugars—only taking those sugars from fruits.

Not meats, then, that are of the red nature; nor greases of meats. These elements should be supplied rather from the fruits.

7/6/41
F. 46 yrs.
ADHESIONS: LESIONS **2529-1**

In the matter of the diet we would constantly add more and more of Vitamin B-1 in every form in which it may be taken. These vitamins are not stored in the body as are A, D, and G, but it is necessary to add these daily. All of those fruits then, that are yellow in color should be taken; oranges, lemons, grapefruit, yellow peaches, all of such as these.

ANEMIA **11/8/35**
ASSIMILATIONS: ELIMINATIONS: INCOORDINATION **F. Adult**
GLANDS **1051-1**

Throughout the period be very mindful of the diets, that these are kept *tending* toward the alkaline-reaction; but of sufficient body and blood building—that may be found through the food values that carry not only the vitamin E but those also of A and B. Or those forces that make for creating of the effluvium that is *productive* in its activity with the glands of the system (the E). Or those activities in the A that would make for an aid in the *draining*, as it were, or the eliminations as related to the activity of all *structural* portions of the body.

Hence one meal each day we would have of raw fruits. And we would have quantities at times of orange juice, grapefruit juice.

4/11/35
ARTHRITIS: TENDENCIES **F. Adult**
BLOOD: HUMOR **888-1**

In the matter of the diet, be more mindful that there are less of the acid-producing foods; more of carbohydrates—that is, sweets—but sweets such as fruit.

11/9/38
ANEMIA: TENDENCIES **M. 7 yrs.**
BODY-BUILDING **773-16**

Q. Please outline diet for each of the three meals daily.

A. Keep these rather generally well-balanced.

Eat that which the bodily forces call for that supply the necessary building; though do not, of course, overbalance same with too much sweets. Keep the natural sweets—as with fruits.

7/26/40
F. 12 yrs.
EPILEPSY **2153-2**

Refrain from any large quantities of sweets. Most of the sweets, if any form is taken, should be in the fruits—that is, the natural fruit sweets.

Mornings—A dry cereal with some fruit. Or, instead of these there may be taken citrus fruit juices (but not at the same meal with the cereal).

9/15/43
F. Adult
ANEMIA **2843-4**

Q. Are all organs functioning fairly well? and how may they be kept so?

A. As indicated there is a form of anemia. Hence the suggestion to have fruits that supply the vitamins missing in the system. Add these that may be gathered at this particular period, and these will contribute to the helpful forces that may come with the keeping consistent with applications suggested.

7/18/42
ASSIMILATIONS: ELIMINATIONS: INCOORDINATION **F. 2-1/2 yrs.**
ASSIMILATIONS: POOR **1521-6**

Rest, and not overload the body; especially not upon raw fruits, but rather using the easily assimilated or pre-digested foods—until there is a thorough stirring of the liver, and then allowing time for a coordination between lungs, liver, heart and kidneys, through the stimulations given.

11/21/34
M. Adult
ACIDITY & ALKALINITY: ASSIMILATIONS: INCOORDINATION **741-1**

As to the matter of the diet, keep rather to the *alkaline-reacting* foods; and where acids of any building foods are used let them be specifically in fruits. Naturally, the normal vegetable reaction would be kept in at least one meal during the day.

Q. Will you outline a specific diet for the body?

A. As indicated. Those foods that have a tendency towards an alkaline reaction, but let the proteins be taken rather in the form of fruits—for the fats and oils, you see; these are much more preferable.

10/17/34
F. 40 yrs.
HYPOCHONDRIA **1000-2**

In the matter of the diets . . . those of the phosphorus nature, and of those that carry these properties as are necessary—the creation with the chlorine foods carry the gold in its combination—follow these closely.

Q. What foods contain gold, silicon and phosphorus?

A. These are contained more in those of the fruits—these should be the character of the diet.

7/18/41
F. 77 yrs.
DEBILITATION: GENERAL **2538-1**

Give all the foods that are rich in the vitamin B-1, with iron, with all the forms of nerve-building energies and blood coagulative properties. These as we find will be found principally in fruits that are yellow in color. All such should be taken in extra quantity.

7/30/41
M. 26 yrs.
ANESTHESIA: AFTEREFFECTS **1710-6**

The general diet should be for body-building. Be sure that most of the foods carry especially vitamin B. These are found in all fruits of the yellow variety.

1/7/34
F. 21 yrs.
GLANDS: INCOORDINATION **480-3**

Lunch—Fresh fruits entirely. The salad may be made from fresh fruits; as oranges, apricots—a *small* quantity of apple—bananas, grapes, pears and the like.

1/15/31
M. 47 yrs.
ACIDITY & ALKALINITY: TOXEMIA **5544-1**

Evenings—Fruits—prunes, apricots, peaches, apples, pears, plums, cherries—but do not *combine* the fruits too much with cooked vegetables. *Alter* them more than *combining* them.

i)—Canned, Frozen, Stewed Fruit

12/29/41
M. 40 yrs.
ASSIMILATIONS: POOR **826-14**

The fruits should not be those that have been frozen but those that are preserved either in their own syrup or in the regular cane syrup and NOT those prepared with benzoate or any preservative—for the benzoate becomes hard on the system.

1/6/42
HEMORRHOIDS **M. 57 yrs.**
INTESTINES: COLON: PROLAPSUS **462-14**

Q. Considering the frozen foods, especially fruits that are on the market today—has the freezing in any way killed certain vitamins and how do they compare with fresh?

A. This would necessitate making a special list. For, some are affected more than others. So far as fruits are concerned, these do not lose much of the vitamin content. Yet some of these are affected by freezing.

1/5/44
DEBILITATION: GENERAL **M. 27 yrs.**
ANEMIA **3535-1**

Don't eat much of cakes or pastries and pies, but stewed fruits of all characters are very good for the body.

2/21/34
M. 20 yrs.
EPILEPSY **521-1**

Mornings—Dried fruits stewed. At such meals not great quantities, but sufficient to satisfy the appetite.

Do not take stewed fruits or fresh fruits *with* citrus fruit.

1)—Apple: General

1/20/24
F. Adult
BLOOD-BUILDING **4120-1**

The diet should be watched closely, taking those properties that will create stimulation to blood supply, especially nerve-building forces in blood. Cereals with fruits, especially apples.

10/21/32
ELEPHANTIASIS: TENDENCIES **F. 18 yrs.**
ARTHRITIS: GLANDS: INCOORDINATION **951-1**

Supply an overabundant amount of those foods that carry iron, iodine and phosphorus in the system.

Beware of apples among the fruits. Beware of any that would carry more of those that would add silicon in the system.

8/8/29
HEART **M. 61 yrs.**
BLOOD-BUILDING **2597-6**

Q. Does he require any special foods, and what food is most beneficial to him?

A. Those that have blood-building, and especially carrying iron. No apples, but fruits of most other natures.

11/2/38
ULCERS **M. 40 yrs.**
ACIDITY & ALKALINITY **1724-1**

Q. What should the diet be?

A. As just indicated, keep a well balanced diet. This will depend upon the ability of the body to assimilate, see? And whenever there is a great anxiety or stress, do not eat especially apples raw nor fruits of that nature which are acid-producing, but rather use the easily assimilated foods.

4/30/35
F. 42 yrs.
INTESTINES: CATARRH **913-1**

At each meal, save the morning meal, have an apple (this may be raw or it may be cooked, for this body), just so it is *well* ripened; not the green nor those that have been stored too long.

7/30/36
M. 30 yrs.
ATTITUDES: GENERAL **416-9**

Q. What foods should I avoid?

A. Rather it is the combination of foods that makes for disturbance with most physical bodies, as it would with this.

Then, do not combine also the reacting acid fruits with starches, other than *whole wheat bread!* that is, with apples.

4/22/11
MALARIA **M. Adult**
MINERALS: IRON **4841-1**

The body in itself, takes care of the whole body. Let nature or the body in itself care for it as far as possible. If we have a body in a weak dilapidated condition, then we produce an effect to overcome these conditions. For this condition of this body, we take that into the system which produces blood of a character that would act on these forces where they are needed. Fruits, especially apples, contain iron, which we need into the blood.

6/3/17
M. Adult
ACIDITY & ALKALINITY: ANEMIA **4834-1**

Q. Is cereal good for the body?

A. Eat apples. There are properties that are not acid themselves but are turned into acids when taken into the mouth, and properties that are acids that are not acids when taken into the mouth. Certain apples are acid, others are not. This body should take apples that have ripened on the tree.

6/10/38
F. 13 yrs.
ASSIMILATIONS: ELIMINATIONS: INCOORDINATION **1206-8**

Q. Is it well to eliminate apples, cider . . . ?

A. As to apples—as we have indicated oft—these are not best for most people, except under conditions where they are advisable to be taken ALONE as a diet for the eliminations, or where certain characters of apples or their products are taken. Hence for this body, these we would leave off.

2/22/34
ASTHENIA **F. 65 yrs.**
ACIDITY & ALKALINITY **509-2**

Beware of too much starch and too much fat. But a well-balanced diet that carries the rebuilding and replenishing forces and influences in the body, and those of the alkaline-*producing* foods, whether fruits or whatnot—rather those that are inclined toward the alkaline, or their combinations. Beware of apples, unless of the jenneting variety.

i)—Apples—Cooked

9/16/41
ELIMINATIONS: INCOORDINATION **F. 2 yrs.**
VITAMINS **2015-8**

Be mindful as to diets; keeping plenty of the vitamins, especially B-1, A and G. These will be found principally in yellow apples. Give the apples only cooked, however, and these in their skins—as roasted, see?

7/22/31
ACIDITY **F. 28 yrs.**
ASSIMILATIONS: ELIMINATIONS: INCOORDINATION **2261-1**

Beware of apples in any form, unless *well* cooked.

7/26/43
M. 2 yrs.
ELIMINATIONS: INCOORDINATION **3109-1**

Apples—these should be cooked, NEVER taken raw.

9/15/36
F. 27 yrs.
EPILEPSY **543-25**

Q. Will it be advisable to eat raw apples?

A. These are not so well, as has been indicated. Though there may be taken a little, these should be well masticated. Preferably those that are roasted or baked.

4/27/35
ASSIMILATIONS: ELIMINATIONS: INCOORDINATION **F. 39 yrs.**
NEURITIS **908-1**

Mornings—Citrus fruit juices. Or to change the diet, there may be stewed fruits or dry cereal. Any of the stewed fruits, even though they be acid, if the system desires same take a little at the morning meal; as apple (that is baked, not raw).

12/31/40
M. 51 yrs.
ASTHMA **2424-1**

No apples save cooked; these may be prepared in sauce, or roasted, baked or the like.

5/30/29
F. 31 yrs.
CONSTIPATION **1713-17**

Q. Does the system require apples?

A. Apples are not good for the system, unless cooked.

11/6/35
ANEMIA: TENDENCIES **F. 26 yrs.**
ACIDITY **1048-4**

Beware of raw apples unless taken *only* as a diet for cleansing the system. Baked or cooked apples may be taken.

12/12/33
MENU: TUBERCULOSIS **F. 22 yrs.**
ACIDITY & ALKALINITY: DEBILITATION **418-2**

Mornings—Stewed fruits, or baked apple, or the like. Any of these may be taken for the morning meal.

10/29/36
M. Adult
ANEMIA **1131-2**

Evenings—Fruits of all kinds are good, whether they be canned or fresh—except apples. The jenneting variety are good; these are all very good that are good for baking—and baked apples are well.

8/15/25
COLITIS **F. 6 yrs.**
MALARIA: TENDENCIES **4281-6**

Baked apples may be given in small quantities as a tonic.

11/8/34
DEBILITATION: GENERAL **F. 12 yrs.**
BODY-BUILDING **632-6**

In the diet, beware of too much starches of *any* kind. No apples, that are raw—though baked or cooked apples may be taken.

11/16/36
BLOOD: COAGULATION: POOR **F. 41 yrs.**
BODY-BUILDING **1100-8**

In the diet include those foods that are blood- and body-building, that carry iron in such manners as may be assimilated by the body. Particularly, then, roasted apples—not baked but *roasted.*

Q. How can the bodily resistance be kept up, especially during the winter months?

A. By following those suggestions that have just been indicated, we find we may build resistances for this body through the periods of sudden changes or distresses that may come from sudden changes to the bodily temperature.

ACIDITY
ANEMIA **10/3/40**
COLD: COMMON: SUSCEPTIBILITY **F. 19 yrs.**
BODY-BUILDING **2374-1**

Evenings—Plenty of vegetables as well as fruits, but do not eat raw apples. Plenty of those that are cooked.

Do these, and as we find we will bring bettered conditions for this body; not only making for the corrections but improving the vitality, the strength, and increasing the weight.

6/14/35
F. Adult
GLANDS: INCOORDINATION **935-1**

Noons—Principally (very seldom altering from these) raw fruits made into a salad. All characters of fruits *except* apples. Apples should only be eaten when cooked; preferably roasted and with butter or hard sauce on same, with cinnamon and spice.

ii)—Apples—Raw

12/1/30
F. 51 yrs.
GASTRITIS **5622-3**

Q. Is raw fruit harmful?

A. *Apples,* but not other fruits.

4/26/35
GLANDS: INCOORDINATION **F. 53 yrs.**
COOKING UTENSILS: GENERAL **906-1**

Apples, raw, should be abstained from.

12/21/43
F. 50 yrs.
ANEMIA **3466-1**

Keep away from sweets and raw apples. These canned, however, are very well.

12/31/34
F. 22 yrs.
ELIMINATIONS: INCOORDINATION **480-13**

Q. Please outline diet to be followed at present.

A. Tend to those foods more of the alkaline reaction, in a general diet; bewaring of too great quantities of sweets at any time, either as at breakfast or at other periods. No raw apples.

2)—Apricot

10/20/32
BRONCHITIS: ELIMINATIONS: POOR **F. Adult**
ELIMINATIONS **4293-1**

Be mindful of the diet, that there are less of the acid-producing foods than have been taken. This means to beware of too much starches, too much of the greater and heavier proteins, or proteins that carry a great amount of dross that is to be eliminated.

In the fruits, especially apricots are well for the body.

3/21/39
F. 49 yrs.
RELAXATION **1158-21**

Q. Sun-dried apricots?

A. These are very well to be taken two or three times during the week. These are PREFERABLE to be taken COOKED; though they may be taken as they are preserved and eaten between or at a meal.

3)—Avocado

11/6/35
ANEMIA **F. 64 yrs.**
TUBERCULOSIS: TENDENCIES **501-4**

Q. Do avocado pears contain much iron and copper and are they good for anemia?

A. They are good for anemia. They contain most iron. Pears are helpful to *anyone,* especially where body- and blood-building influences are needed; for they will be absorbed. These are best to be taken morning and evening; not through the active portions of the day.

4)—Bananas

6/7/37
DEBILITATION: GENERAL **F. 65 yrs.**
ACIDITY & ALKALINITY **658-15**

Do not overtax the system with bananas, unless these are ripened in their natural state; for the activity of these in the beginnings of their deterioration—before they are palatable—makes for a hardship upon the system. But those that are overripe, or that have been gathered or prepared when they have fully matured, may be taken in moderation at certain meals or times.

7/15/41
F. 61 yrs.
DEBILITATION: GENERAL **2535-1**

In the matter of diet—take more of those foods that carry greater quantity of vitamin B-1—such as found in those foods that are yellow in color. Thus, well-ripened bananas, these should form not the whole but a great deal of the diet.

11/19/28
ASTHMA: TENDENCIES **F. 9 yrs.**
COLD: CONGESTION **4281-17**

Keep away from too much sweets. These will irritate the expression manifested in the upper central blood and nerve supply.

Q. Should she eat bananas now, raw or cooked?

A. *Occasionally* these may be taken, *raw.* Let them be well ripened though.

2/27/42
M. 25 yrs.
GLANDS: EYES: COLOR BLINDNESS **820-2**

No bananas, unless you are in the territory where they are grown and ripened there.

11/2/38
M. 40 yrs.
ACIDITY & ALKALINITY **1724-1**

Q. What should the diet be?

A. As just indicated, keep a well-balanced diet. This will depend upon the ability of the body to assimilate, see? And whenever there is a great anxiety or stress, do not eat bananas nor fruits of that nature which are acid-producing, but rather use the easily assimilated foods.

2/22/34
ASTHENIA **F. 65 yrs.**
ACIDITY & ALKALINITY **509-2**

A well-balanced diet that carries the rebuilding and replenishing forces and influences in the body, and those of the alkaline-*producing* foods, whether fruits or whatnot—rather those that are inclined toward the alkaline, or their combinations. Bananas may be taken in moderation and *in their season.*

10/21/32
ELEPHANTIASIS: TENDENCIES **F. 18 yrs.**
ARTHRITIS: GLANDS: INCOORDINATION **951-1**

Supply an overabundant amount of those foods that carry iron, iodine and phosphorus in the system. Beware of bananas among the fruits. Beware of any that will carry more of those that would add silicon in the system.

10/20/32
BRONCHITIS: ELIMINATIONS: POOR **F. Adult**
ELIMINATIONS **4293-1**

Be mindful of the diet, that there are less of the acid-producing foods than have been taken. This means to beware of too much starches, too much of the greater and heavier proteins, or proteins that carry a great amount of dross that is to be eliminated.

In the fruits, do not use any bananas, or of that nature, but other things and other conditions may be taken.

8/8/29
HEART **M. 61 yrs.**
BLOOD-BUILDING **2597-6**

Q. Does he require any special foods, and what food is most beneficial to him?

A. Those that have blood building, and especially carrying iron. No bananas, but fruits of most other natures. Those of the blood building are the better.

10/6/41
F. 64 yrs.
VITAMINS: TOXEMIA **2598-1**

Be careful of the diet, in that there is kept plenty of vitamins of the resistance nature; such as A, D, and B-1. These would take more in the foods than in supplementary extracts themselves.

Bananas for this body, with the cereals, if well masticated, would be well—and these should be THOROUGHLY ripe.

6/14/35
F. Adult
GLANDS: INCOORDINATION **935-1**

Noons—Principally (very seldom altering from these), raw fruits made into a salad. Use in the fruit salad such as bananas.

4/30/35
F. 42 yrs.
INTESTINES: CATARRH 913-1

At each meal, save the morning meal, have a banana, just so it is *well* ripened; not the green nor those that have been stored too long.

5/25/42
M. 58 yrs.
NEURASTHENIA 816-13

Add all of those fruits that are yellow in their nature; that is, bananas occasionally, with cereals. These will aid in stimulating. Not that these should be the things alone taken, but these should form portions of the diet daily.

7/22/31
ACIDITY F. 28 yrs.
ASSIMILATIONS: ELIMINATIONS: INCOORDINATION 2261-1

Beware of bananas. Beware of those fruits that are easily fermented.

4/26/35
F. 53 yrs.
GLANDS: INCOORDINATION 906-1

Bananas should be abstained from.

4/2/35
ANEMIA: TENDENCIES F. Adult
ACIDITY 875-1

Q. Will you outline a specific diet for the body?

A. As we find, those activities of the body are such that to make a specific diet must become rote, which would become disturbing to the better conditions of the body. Then, we would give rather the things of which the body should be warned in regard to its diet, but combinations in other directions may be made. *Do not* eat bananas, either cooked or raw.

11/8/34
DEBILITATION: GENERAL F. 12 yrs.
BODY-BUILDING 632-6

In the diet, beware of too many starches of *any* kind. No bananas!

4/25/40
ACIDITY F. Adult
DEBILITATION: GENERAL 2179-1

No bananas, but plenty of other fruits.

12/31/34
F. 22 yrs.
ELIMINATIONS: INCOORDINATION 480-13

Q. Please outline diet to be followed at present.

A. Tend to those foods of the more alkaline reaction, in a general diet; bewaring of too great quantities of sweets at any time, either as at breakfast or at other periods. No bananas.

5)—Cherries

7/13/35
F. 59 yrs.
ECZEMA **3823-4**

Part arises from the effluvia from certain characters of small fruits or berries. Yet if those vibrations and corrections in the locomotory centers are kept such as to set up the coordination between the eliminating systems and the drainages in the body, as indicated by the supply to the various portions of the emunctory and lymph circulation, these conditions should soon disappear.

Q. Berries or cherries?

A. Cherries are more preferable than berries; that is, than certain characters of berries. Some berries carry a great deal more acid than others; depending a great deal upon where they are grown; that is, they carry too great a quantity of potash and thus require that an equal balance be created by taking sufficient quantities of such natures as carry silicon or iodine.

7/22/31
ASSIMILATIONS: DEBILITATION: GENERAL **F. 28 yrs.**
BLOOD-BUILDING **3842-1**

We would give a diet that is easily assimilated. Let the diet be that as is nerve- and blood-building. Fruits—as cherries.

6)—Dates

12/11/37
M. 30 yrs.
ARTHRITIS **849-23**

Keep to those things that will aid in the eliminations. Build up the body with more of iron, as may be had from dried fruits, dates and the like. Let these form a part of the daily diet.

10/28/42
F. 53 yrs.
BODY-BUILDING: ASSIMILATIONS **1770-7**

We find that the diets need consideration. There would be a helpful or beneficial effect from the body taking the tonic that carries the B-1 vitamins, the iron and the G vitamin. This particular type of combination is excellent.

Hence, if the tonic is taken with such foods added in the diet, it will be more efficient for the body than the supplementing of the diet with other vitamin preparations. Do not overtake same, but only as a tonic; adding to the diet such foods as dates.

5/9/29
F. 64 yrs.
ACIDITY: ASSIMILATIONS: BLOOD-BUILDING **1377-3**

Q. Will natural sweets, such as dates, be detrimental?

A. May be taken in moderation early in the day.

7)—Figs

3/30/32
F. 66 yrs.
5592-1

CONSTIPATION

When it is necessary to take any form of cathartic, that which is of the vegetable nature would be the better, but this will not be necessary if we will have at least one meal each day of wholly the fig, or the syrup of same, or those as carry properties that make for the activity of the muco-membranes from the salivary glands to the jejunum, or the activity of same begins, or to the action of the glands that make for separations in the system—or lacteals. We will find these should carry those sufficient, when the colonics have removed those pressures as produce those in the system of *mucus* in the intestinal tract.

12/11/37
M. 30 yrs.
849-23

ARTHRITIS

Keep to those things that will aid in the eliminations. Build up the body with more of iron, as may be had from dried fruits, figs and the like. Let these form a part of the daily diet . . .

Use those things in the diets that make for the better balance in creating for the activities of the body the better actions BETWEEN the building up and the using of energies in the system.

12/17/38
M. 45 yrs.
1564-3

TUBERCULOSIS

Use all those influences which carry a great deal of the sunshine vitamins, as much as the body assimilates. But whenever there is any food taken that becomes a reactionary influence, ease off in the use of such foods.

A great deal then of . . . figs, or any citrus fruits; either in their combinations or separately, should be the greater part of some meal, or taken during the day.

11/7/38
M. 33 yrs.
1467-4

ASSIMILATIONS: POOR

Precautions should be taken that there is sufficient of the laxative foods, or plenty of such as figs as a part of the diet; so as to make for plenty of iron as well as the activities for resistances through the system.

10/28/42
F. 53 yrs.
1770-7

BODY-BUILDING: ASSIMILATIONS

We find that the diet needs consideration. There would be a helpful or beneficial effect from the body taking the tonic that carries the B-1 vitamins, the iron and the G vitamin. This particular type of combination is excellent. With the alteration that has been made in the Codiron, there is not the assimilation of the type of iron that is processed in same. Hence we would find that the combination of the vitamins in a tonic would be well, if there is the adding in the diet of those things such as the black fig and all of such natures.

These added to some of those activities as may be taken will be found to be more beneficial.

12/13/40
M. 33 yrs.
ARTHRITIS: ELIMINATIONS **849-55**

Q. What type of fruits particularly would aid in eliminations for this body?

A. Figs, prunes, pears, oranges, dates and such. Figs that would be dried and then stewed, you see—both the black and the regular fig. This does not indicate that he is to go on a fig diet, but these are to be taken two to three times a week, as well as prunes and those of such natures as these.

12/11/37
F. 43 yrs.
CONSTIPATION **1446-3**

Use figs. These at various times or in various manners are most beneficial. These are a portion of the NECESSITIES for the body to keep in the physical forces.

3/27/44
DIABETES **M. 38 yrs.**
SPINE: DISK, SLIPPED **4020-1**

No usage of candy, cakes, or things of that kind, though honey may be taken occasionally to supply the sweets, or the natural sweets of vegetables and fruits; such as figs and those things that cause better eliminations.

10/21/32
ELEPHANTIASIS: TENDENCIES **F. 18 yrs.**
ARTHRITIS: GLANDS: INCOORDINATION **951-1**

One meal each day we would supply principally of nature's sugars, nature's laxatives in figs—any of the active principles in such.

4/17/31
DEBILITATION: GENERAL **M. 19 yrs.**
CHOREA **1225-1**

Mornings—We would alter occasionally to those of the stewed fruits, as figs, *any* of the stewed fruits—see? Fresh or those preserved, provided they are not preserved in or with benzoate of soda.

10/20/32
BRONCHITIS: ELIMINATIONS: POOR **F. Adult**
ELIMINATIONS **4293-1**

Be mindful of the diet, that there are less of the acid-producing foods than have been taken.

In the fruits, figs and the like, are good.

10/23/43
F. 60 yrs.
ELIMINATIONS **3314-1**

Have plenty of raw foods such as figs and we will have better eliminations and better conditions for the body.

Q. What causes pain in back and side?

A. As indicated, pressures in those areas that disturb the alimentary canal, the stomach and the eliminations.

3/8/37
F. 55 yrs.
MENU: OBESITY **1183-2**

Two of the leafy vegetables to one of the pod, and three of the leafy to one of the tuberous. And these as we find, if there will be included figs and the like, will aid in assisting in the effect created by the adjustments and by the revitalizing of the vibratory forces for the body.

3/21/39
RELAXATION **F. 49 yrs.**
ELIMINATIONS **1158-21**

Q. Figs?

A. Once to three times during a week, dependent upon what they are mixed with. But either the stewed or the figs of such natures as the dried, once to three to four times a week should be sufficient.

Q. What is best way to insure satisfactory daily bowel movements?

A. By the diet and not by dependence upon ANY of the taking of laxatives or the like. But these are the better taken in the diet in those things indicated, such as figs. These if taken occasionally should keep the bowels in the proper condition.

8/19/41
F. 31 yrs.
ASTHENIA **1688-7**

Q. Are . . . dried figs good for me?

A. Depends upon the manner in which they are prepared. The figs should be stewed, of course, and taken with other food values—to be the most beneficial.

5/9/29
F. 64 yrs.
ACIDITY: ASSIMILATIONS: BLOOD-BUILDING **1377-3**

Q. Will natural sweets, such as figs, be detrimental?

A. May be taken in moderation early in the day.

12/1/30
F. 51 yrs.
GASTRITIS **5622-3**

Q. Is raw fruit harmful?

A. Figs are very beneficial, whether the ripe or those as packed.

1/17/41
F. 44 yrs.
ELIMINATIONS: POOR **459-11**

Aid the eliminations by taking figs, etc., rather than the vegetable compounds, for this body.

ANEMIA **4/15/41**
ASSIMILATIONS: POOR **F. 22 yrs.**
ACIDITY & ALKALINITY **2479-1**

Begin with a corrective diet, which would be one tending towards the alkaline nature, with sufficient of the fruit acids to correct the inclinations for the disturbance in eliminations.

Hence, have plenty of such as figs—stewed, pressed, raw or the like. Take these, in some form, each day.

1/26/35
F. 59 yrs.
INJURIES **3823-2**

Mornings—Citrus fruit juices, figs; or the dried figs stewed.

Noons—During those periods when there is little of the activity, so that there are not the normal eliminations, well that the vegetables or fruits that are the more laxative in form be used as a portion of the meal; such as figs—of course, these should be either fresh or those canned without any superficial or artificial preservative.

9/30/41
M. 11 yrs.
BODY-BUILDING: ELIMINATIONS **1188-10**

Q. What foods should be included in weekly diet and in what amounts?

A. As we have indicated again and again, those that are body building and at the same time keep in the foods the correct balance of the vitamins for body (rather than in chemical additions) building. These are the better foods, and sufficient quantities to satisfy the appetite of the body. A growing body requires plenty of Vitamins A and B and D and C, that the structural portions may also have sufficient from the assimilated foods, rather than supplied from concentrated forms of same.

Do that rather in the body-building diet. Not too much of sugars, yet sufficient. Let the sweets be taken in such forms as of fruits. These are body building, also supply energies that are well for a growing, developing body.

Q. How can bowel eliminations be improved?

A. Include in the diet such as figs, fig juice. All forms of this character of fruit tend to aid eliminations, also carrying the correct character of sugars to supply that needed—and is in a form that is assimilated without becoming too acid forming.

12/27/41
F. 19 yrs.
PREGNANCY **711-4**

Figs, either the preserved or stewed are well, as are raisins. But have these not with sugar—rather in their own syrup, their own sweetening.

12/31/37
DEBILITATION: GENERAL **M. 41 yrs.**
ACIDITY & ALKALINITY **1476-1**

Mornings—Alter at times with stewed fruits as figs . . . These should be taken at one time or another.

12/31/34
F. 22 yrs.
ELIMINATIONS: INCOORDINATION **480-13**

Tend to those foods more of the alkaline reaction, in a general diet; bewaring of too great quantities of sweets at any time. Quantities of fruits—as figs, may be taken.

8)—Grapes

11/8/34
DEBILITATION: GENERAL **F. 12 yrs.**
BODY-BUILDING **632-6**

In the diet, use citrus fruits; all of these may be taken, as also may grapes. Preferably use the fresh fruits, or the nearer fresh fruits; preferably *none* that are canned with any preservative such as benzoate of soda.

3/9/40
ASSIMILATIONS: ELIMINATIONS: INCOORDINATION **F. 50 yrs.**
DEBILITATION: GENERAL **2140-1**

Have as much as the body can possibly assimilate of GRAPES! every character, or all that may be taken of the grapes, and grape JUICE. This will act as an aid in reducing those tendencies for gas.

8/12/40
F. 33 yrs.
ANEMIA: DIGESTION: INDIGESTION **2320-1**

Drink beef juice. Use preferably whole wheat crackers with the beef juice. Then, in conjunction with this, we would have plenty of grapes—not to overload the stomach, but grapes that are well ripened, and those at this season are well for the body.

10/28/42
F. 53 yrs.
BODY-BUILDING: ASSIMILATIONS **1770-7**

We find that the diets need consideration. There would be a helpful or beneficial effect from the body taking the tonic that carries the B-1 vitamins, the iron and the G vitamin. This particular type of combination is excellent.

Hence, if the tonic is taken with such foods added in the diet, it will be more efficient for the body than the supplementing of the diet with other vitamin preparations. Do not overtake same, but only as a tonic; adding to the diet such foods as grapes, and things of that nature.

10/24/30
F. 59 yrs.
ANEMIA **501-1**

No apples, but other fruit—especially grapes, these are well but should be seeded before the portions are eaten.

10/20/32
BRONCHITIS: ELIMINATIONS: POOR ELIMINATIONS F. Adult
4293-1

Be mindful of the diet, that there are less of the acid-producing foods than have been taken.

In the fruits, grapes, and the like, are good.

6/14/35
F. Adult
GLANDS: INCOORDINATION 935-1

Noons—Principally (very seldom altering from these) raw fruits made into a salad. Use in the fruit salad such as grapes, *all* characters of fruits *except* apples.

In following these diets, it is well that no *fermented* drink be taken. However, red wine may be taken.

12/31/34
F. 22 yrs.
ELIMINATIONS: INCOORDINATION 480-13

Tend to those foods more of the alkaline reaction, in a general diet; bewaring of two great quantities of sweets at any time. Quantities of fruits—as grapes, may be taken.

12/1/30
F. 51 yrs.
GASTRITIS 5622-3

Q. Is raw fruit harmful?

A. Grapes, without the seeds are well.

2/27/42
F. 52 yrs.
COLD: CONGESTION 404-10

Q. Fruits—which should be eaten raw and which cooked?

A. As to the raw fruits, fresh grapes and the like.

12/17/38
M. 45 yrs.
TUBERCULOSIS 1564-3

Use all those influences which carry a great deal of the sunshine vitamins, as much as the body assimilates. But whenever there is any food taken that becomes a reactionary influence, ease off in the use of such foods.

A great deal then of grapes, or any citrus fruits; either in their combinations or separately, should be the greater part of some meal, or taken during the day.

2/6/31
F. 22 yrs.
EPILEPSY 543-7

Have fruits—such as grapes (whether canned or otherwise, but if canned be sure they are *not* canned with benzoate of soda).

9)—Guava

6/14/35
F. Adult
GLANDS: INCOORDINATION **935-1**

Noons—Principally (very seldom altering from these) raw fruits made into a salad. Use in the fruit salad such as guava.

10)—Papaya

2/22/44
F. 26 yrs.
CIRCULATION: LYMPH: TUBERCULOSIS **3687-1**

And whenever possible take papayas. These should be prepared for the body whenever possible: not large quantities but small quantities often. These will be well for the body.

11)—Peaches

9/4/41
BABY CARE **F. 2-1/2 yrs.**
ELIMINATIONS **1521-5**

There needs to be those considerations for more of the foods carrying the vitamins B and D, rather than these taken separately.

We find that these would be obtained in the correct proportions, at least two to three times each week, of yellow peaches.

Q. What is causing excessive growth of hair over entire body, particularly in back of neck and across shoulders, and what can be done to correct it? (especially noticeable for last six months).

A. This is a natural development, if we indicate the conditions of the body and its meeting itself. But these will not become unsightly if there is kept the normal balance in especially the B and D vitamins in the foods for the body.

Q. Any suggestions to help increase or make eliminations more normal?

A. The changing in the diet, with fruits of the form and prepared in the manner indicated, will aid in this direction. This is much preferable to taking or giving laxatives, or eliminants.

6/20/40
M. 34 yrs.
BODY-BUILDING **1861-5**

As to the general health—there should be plenty of the food values that are nerve and blood and tissue building. Have plenty of the vitamins, especially that may be had from THESE combined in the diet:

Through the summer have plenty of yellow peaches, plenty of all characters of the fruits—ESPECIALLY those that are yellow in color.

Not that the body is to be abnormal in these directions, but these things carry the character of vitamins necessary for this body.

Of course, take *every* form of food that carries the general body-building influences through the system.

11/29/40
F. 31 yrs.
ANEMIA **2414-1**

Beware of too much of white breads. Have plenty of all characters of foods that carry vitamins B-1 and G. These are found the more in fresh vegetables and fruits that are yellow in their color. Canned peaches—using only the yellow variety.

Q. What can I do to make my hair thicker and more oily?

A. The vitamins and activities supplied that there may be the better glandular forces active in the thyroids—which we have included in these suggestions indicated.

12/21/43
F. 50 yrs.
ANEMIA **3466-1**

Keep away from sweets and raw peaches. These canned, however, are very well.

7/7/23
F. Adult
ANEMIA **4889-1**

Diet for this body will be the greater force, those that carry as much of iron as possible, principally, of fruits in this character and nature such as would be found in some kinds of peaches, though not all.

2/22/34
ASTHENIA **F. 65 yrs.**
ACIDITY & ALKALINITY **509-2**

Peaches, all of these may be taken in moderation and *in their season.*

2/24/35
ASSIMILATIONS: ELIMINATIONS: INCOORDINATION **M. 53 yrs.**
DIET: ACIDITY & ALKALINITY **843-1**

Noons—The fruits should be preferably taken at this meal, such as peaches, with a gluten.

Q. Should the fruit at the noon meal be cooked or raw?

A. It may be raw or preserved, just so it is not preserved in benzoate of soda. Libby's is all right.

2/6/31
F. 22 yrs.
EPILEPSY **543-7**

Have fruits—such as peaches (whether canned or otherwise, but if canned be sure they are *not* canned with benzoate of soda).

8/8/29
HEART **M. 61 yrs.**
BLOOD-BUILDING **2597-6**

Q. Does he require any special foods, and what food is most beneficial to him?

A. Those that have blood-building, and especially carrying iron. Peaches may be taken.

6/6/40
ASSIMILATIONS: POOR **F. 19 yrs.**
ANEMIA **2277-1**

Eat all of the fruits that are especially YELLOW in color; yellow peaches—not white peaches.

5/25/42
M. 58 yrs.
NEURASTHENIA **816-13**

Add all of those fruits that are yellow in their nature; that is yellow peaches with cereals. These will aid in stimulating. Not that these should be the things alone taken, but these should form portions of the diet daily.

8/27/40
M. 39 yrs.
VITAMINS: DEFICIENT **826-13**

Have every form of fruit that carries the yellow coloring matter. These are products that carry the vitamin B in quantities of a helpful nature; also most of these carry G.

It is only necessary that there be the consideration of the proper foods; especially such as yellow peaches and the like. Any and all of these in the varied forms or manners as may be prepared would be most helpful.

7/22/31
ACIDITY **F. 28 yrs.**
ASSIMILATIONS: ELIMINATIONS: INCOORDINATION **2261-1**

In those of peaches, these are all well for the body . . . Be sure that all taken are fresh, firm, and not that that is *overly* ripe; that is, fermentation not already begun.

6/27/41
F. 18 yrs.
ANEMIA **1207-2**

Have the regular foods; those that carry quantities, or an excess, of vitamin B-1, especially such as would be found in all foods that are yellow in nature or color. Eat plenty of yellow peaches and the like. There should be excesses of these in the diet, though—to be sure—other foods would be taken normally.

3/14/32
M. Adult
TOXEMIA **5672-1**

Mornings—Do not mix cereals and fruit juices, though cereals with fresh fruits may be taken—as sliced peaches. Those that are canned may be taken, provided they are not canned—or preserved—with the benzoate of soda. Those of the standard brands, or the Libby, or the LaMonte brands, we find, are the more perfect; though those of the Libby are more perfect than the others.

7/18/40
F. 39 yrs.
ASSIMILATIONS: ELIMINATIONS: INCOORDINATION 2309-1

Take plenty of food values that carry vitamin B-1 and G. These are found especially in yellow peaches. These should be in the diet almost daily. Give these combined in different forms.

5/15/41
F. Adult
ANEMIA: DEBILITATION: GENERAL 2500-1

We would add B-1 in the foods. Yellow peaches (as the canned)—these are well for the body.

7/26/43
M. 2 yrs.
ELIMINATIONS: INCOORDINATION 3109-1

Fruits such as peaches are tabu for the body.

12)—Pears

12/21/43
F. 50 yrs.
ANEMIA 3466-1

Keep away from sweets and raw pears. These canned, however, are very well.

6/3/17
M. Adult
ACIDITY & ALKALINITY: ANEMIA 4834-1

Trouble in the stomach caused by lack of assimilation. This body is a great deal better. Body will improve by time and active forces being supplied by suggestion. This body does not assimilate food properly, it should take food constantly—not every second—but as it is assimilated. This body cannot take a whole lot of food at once but often, but not when in repose. The body should be more out in the air, it needs more red blood, it needs to use itself in the air, use the limbs. Diets should be of iron such as found in a pear, and that of iron itself, it will be hard to assimilate iron, should be taken in small quantities to begin with.

Q. Is cereal good for the body?

A. Fruits are better than cereals. Pears will be better. The body shouldn't take things that produce acid. We have things that are not acid themselves, but change into acid when taken into the mouth. Normally there are glands in the throat which produce lactic fluid or pepsin, this body is not producing sufficient lactic fluid, so that whatever is taken is carried into acid. There are properties that are not acid themselves but are turned into acids when taken into the mouth, and properties that are acids that are not acids when taken into the mouth. Pear, which is acid, forms into iron and loses its acid.

11/6/35
GLANDS: THYROID: HYPOTHYROIDISM F. 63 yrs.
MINERALS 1049-1

In the matter of the diet, this would be rather important. Occasionally use a great deal of those things that carry quantities of iodine, for this the body requires. But for this body it will be most soluble from pears. Two or three pears each day will be *most* helpful in the manner of furnishing iron, silicon; and especially considering the influences such would have with the electrical forces—that is, the pear's activity to produce an activity to the gland forces of the body.

1/20/24
F. Adult
BLOOD-BUILDING **4120-1**

The diet should be watched closely, taking those properties that will create stimulation to blood supply, especially nerve-building forces in blood. Cereals with fruits, especially pears.

12/29/24
M. 26 yrs.
ANEMIA **137-9**

Also let the diet be much fruit, especially pears, well masticated, so that they will not be hard on digestion. These would be well to be taken between meals.

2/27/42
F. 52 yrs.
COLD: CONGESTION **404-10**

Q. What fruits are especially good for my body, considering the condition of kidneys? Which should be eaten raw and which cooked?

A. As to the raw fruits—pears, canned or fresh.

10/24/30
F. 59 yrs.
ANEMIA **501-1**

No apples, but other fruit—especially pears.

4/18/29
BABY CARE **M. 2 yrs.**
DERMATITIS: ACIDITY **5520-6**

The citrus fruits, and pears may be included, provided same are well ripened.

2/22/34
ASTHENIA **F. 65 yrs.**
ACIDITY & ALKALINITY **509-2**

Pears may be taken in moderation and *in their season.*

2/24/35
ASSIMILATIONS: ELIMINATIONS: INCOORDINATION **M. 53 yrs.**
ACIDITY & ALKALINITY **843-1**

Noons—The fruits should be preferably taken at this meal, such as pears or the like—any of these may be taken at this meal—with a gluten. These are adding the strength and the vitality.

Q. Should the fruit at the noon meal be cooked or raw?

A. It may be raw or preserved just so it is not preserved in benzoate of soda. Libby's is all right.

10/21/32
ELEPHANTIASIS: TENDENCIES F. 18 yrs.
ARTHRITIS: GLANDS: INCOORDINATION 951-1

One meal each day we would supply principally of nature's sugars, any of the active principles in such. A great deal of these forces may be found in pears and their derivatives (that is, properties that are made from them, you see, without preservatives).

2/6/31
F. 22 yrs.
EPILEPSY 543-7

Have fruits—such as pears (whether canned or otherwise, but if canned be sure they are *not* canned with benzoate of soda).

4/17/31
DEBILITATION: GENERAL M. 19 yrs.
CHOREA 1225-1

Mornings—We would alter occasionally to those of the stewed fruits, as pears, *any* of the stewed fruits—see? fresh or those preserved, provided they are not preserved in or with benzoate of soda.

Beware of raw fruits in the evenings.

10/20/32
BRONCHITIS: ELIMINATIONS: POOR F. Adult
ELIMINATIONS 4293-1

Be mindful of the diet, there are less of the acid-producing foods than have been taken. This means to beware of too much starches, too much of the greater and heavier proteins, or proteins that carry a great amount of dross that is to be eliminated.

In the fruits, especially pears are well for the body. Beware of too much apples.

4/27/35
ASSIMILATIONS: ELIMINATIONS: INCOORDINATION F. 39 yrs.
NEURITIS 908-1

Mornings—Citrus fruit juices.

Or, to change the diet, there may be stewed fruits or dry cereal. Any of the stewed fruits, even though they be acid, if the system desires same take a little at the morning meal; as pears.

8/8/29
HEART M. 61 yrs.
BLOOD-BUILDING 2597-6

Q. Does he require any special foods, and what food is most beneficial to him?

A. Those that have blood-building, and especially carrying iron. Pears may be taken.

4/30/35
F. 42 yrs.
INTESTINES: CATARRH 913-1

At each meal, save the morning meal, have a pear, just so it is *well* ripened;

not the green nor those that have been stored too long.

7/22/31
F. 28 yrs.
ASSIMILATIONS: ELIMINATIONS: INCOORDINATION **2261-1**

In those of pears, these are well for the body, especially pears—pears that are prepared right, either in can or the fresh fruits.

11/8/34
DEBILITATION: GENERAL **F. 12 yrs.**
BODY-BUILDING **632-6**

In the diet, use pears, or such. Preferably use the fresh fruits, or the nearer fresh fruits; preferably *none* that are canned with any preservative such as benzoate of soda!

4/22/11
MALARIA **M. Adult**
MINERALS: IRON **4841-1**

Fruits, especially pears, contain iron, which we need into the blood.

12/31/34
F. 22 yrs.
ELIMINATIONS: INCOORDINATION **480-13**

Tend to those foods more of the alkaline reaction, in a general diet; bewaring of too great quantities of sweets at any time. Quantities of fruits—as pears, may be taken.

12/1/30
F. 51 yrs.
GASTRITIS **5622-3**

Q. Is raw fruit harmful?

A. Pears and all citrus fruits are *good.*

3/14/32
M. Adult
TOXEMIA **5672-1**

Mornings—*do not* mix cereals and fruit juices, though cereals with fresh fruits may be taken—as pears, or the like. Those that are canned may be taken, provided they are not canned—or preserved—with the benzoate of soda. Those of the standard brands, or the Libby, or the LaMonte brands, we find, are the more perfect; though those of the Libby are more perfect than the others.

10/11/43
F. 26 yrs.
ARTHRITIS **3285-1**

We should have easily assimilated foods, but those very high in the adding of B complex, or the vitamin B—as in pears. These should be a part of the diet daily with plenty of seafoods (not fresh water fish).

1/26/35
F. 59 yrs.
INJURIES 3823-2

Noons—During those periods when there is little of the activity, so that there are not the normal eliminations, well that the vegetables or fruits that are the more laxative in form be used as a portion of the meal; such as pears—of course, these should be either fresh or those canned without any superficial or artificial preservative.

7/7/23
F. Adult
ANEMIA 4889-1

Diet for this body will be the greater force, those that carry as much of iron as possible, principally, of fruits in this character and nature such as thought to be found in pears.

7/22/31
ASSIMILATIONS: DEBILITATION: GENERAL F. 28 yrs
BLOOD-BUILDING 3842-1

We would give a diet that is easily assimilated. Let the diet be that as is nerve and blood building. Fruits—pears, no apples.

13)—Persimmons

5/11/40
M. 25 yrs.
INJURIES: STRAINS 1710-5

Q. What treatment should be followed to restore hair on head?

A. Eat the peelings of Irish potatoes. Eat persimmons as soon as they are in order—even the large persimmons are very well.

14)—Pineapple

2/22/34
ASTHENIA F. 65 yrs.
ACIDITY & ALKALINITY 509-2

And use fruits that are *not* artificially ripened, even though it is necessary to use those that are canned; pineapple and pineapple juices are excellent for the body.

12/11/37
M. 30 yrs.
ARTHRITIS 849-23

Keep to those things that will aid in the eliminations. Build up the body with more of iron . . . AND especially have FRESH pineapple—rather than the canned, for this particular body. And keep mentally in constructive forces, and we should keep the better conditions for the body.

4/25/40
F. Adult
ACIDITY
DEBILITATION: GENERAL **2179-1**

Citrus fruits are well; especially pineapple for this body would be good—but fresh pineapple for this body is better than the canned.

1/26/35
F. 59 yrs.
INJURIES **3823-2**

Hence we would use those foods that carry in a soluble manner that which may be absorbed and become replenishing or rebuilding for the blood; or the calciums, irons, glutens that make for the urea. We would use principally an alkaline-reacting diet.

Mornings—Pineapple and pineapple juice.

3/1/41
F. Adult
ARTHRITIS: NEURITIS: TENDENCIES **838-3**

Starches and roughages should not be so much a part of the diet. Have rather those things that are alkaline-reacting, even though they may be acid in themselves; such as plenty of citrus fruit juices. When using pineapple, squeeze a little lime in same. We would combine these in this manner. Do not ever take these at the same meal with cereals, however, or even during the same day while such properties are working through the system.

This does not mean, of course, that these are to be the ONLY foods taken. We merely give a list of the DO'S and the DON'TS.

Do all of these, and we will make for better conditions.

11/23/37
M. 13 yrs.
PSORIASIS **1484-1**

Pineapple may be taken. These are NOT acid-PRODUCING. They are alkaline-reacting!

But when cereals or starches are taken, do not have the citrus fruit at the same meal—or even the same day; for such a combination in the system at the same time become ACID producing!

Hence those taken on different days are well for the body.

10/27/34
F. 15 yrs.
ACIDITY & ALKALINITY **605-4**

The diet is not being adhered to so well. Add to the morning diet at times pineapple juice—or the sliced or diced pineapple is well to add, too, at this time. Pineapple in the evening is well.

1/9/26
COLD: CONGESTION: FLU: AFTEREFFECTS **F. 7 yrs.**
BABY CARE **4281-10**

Q. Should she have canned pineapple?

A. Pineapple may be, in small quantities.

11/8/34
DEBILITATION: GENERAL **F. 12 yrs.**
BODY-BUILDING **632-6**

In the diet use pineapples or such. Preferably use the fresh fruits, or the nearer fresh fruits; preferably *none* that are canned with any preservative such as benzoate of soda!

15)—Plums

10/29/43
ASSIMILATIONS: ELIMINATIONS: INCOORDINATION **F. 13 yrs.**
HEADACHE: MIGRAINE **3326-1**

Keep away from any sedimentary forces (such as brans or as grains). Prunes will work just the opposite, for these carry another form of activity to the walls of the system itself. It would be well to include prunes in the diet, if they are cooked—or even fresh. Plums of all natures, then, are very well to be taken.

8/8/29
HEART **M. 61 yrs.**
BLOOD-BUILDING **2597-6**

Q. Does he require any special foods, and what food is most beneficial to him?

A. Those that have blood building, and especially carrying iron. Plums may be taken.

7/22/31
ACIDITY **F. 28 yrs.**
ASSIMILATIONS: ELIMINATIONS: INCOORDINATION **2261-1**

In those of plums, things of this nature—these are all well for the body.

12/21/43
F. 50 yrs.
ANEMIA **3466-1**

Keep away from sweets and raw plums. These canned, however, are very well.

2/22/34
ASTHENIA **F. 65 yrs**
ACIDITY & ALKALINITY **509-2**

Plums may be taken in moderation and *in their season.*

2/24/35
ASSIMILATIONS: ELIMINATIONS: INCOORDINATION **M. 53 yrs.**
ACIDITY & ALKALINITY **843-1**

Noons—The fruits should be preferably taken at this meal, such as plums, with a gluten.

Q. Should the fruit at the noon meal be cooked or raw?

A. It may be raw or preserved, just so it is not preserved in benzoate of soda. Libby's is all right.

16)—Pomegranate

10/21/32
ELEPHANTIASIS: TENDENCIES **F. 18 yrs.**
ARTHRITIS: GLANDS: INCOORDINATION **951-1**

One meal each day we would supply principally of nature's sugars—any of the active principles in such. A great deal of those forces may be found in pomegranates and their derivatives.

17)—Prunes

3/15/37
BLOOD: HUMOR **F. 56 yrs.**
TOXEMIA **569-25**

Prunes, to be sure, will assist. These should be taken about once a week, and with the effluvia as produced by their activities and other eliminating properties that are to be a portion of the activity, will work well together if they are taken about this often.

4/5/44
F. 52 yrs.
ASTHMA **4029-1**

Leave off all kinds of sugar. Do take often such as prunes, prune whip, prune juice, prunes prepared in every manner. These would be better for the body for the eliminations, even in the changes that will be necessary if there is to be kept a balance between the sympathetic and cerebrospinal system. For these are producing the mental reactions to the body.

Q. What particular diet is recommended?

A. Let those things indicated be the principal part of the diet daily, then a regular diet that keeps a good balance in supplying the elements for the proper nourishment of the body.

3/21/39
F. 49 yrs.
ELIMINATIONS **1158-21**

Q. What is best way to insure satisfactory daily bowel movements?

A. By the diet, and not by dependence upon ANY of the taking of laxatives or the like. But these are the better taken in the diet in those things indicated, such as prunes. These if taken occasionally should keep the bowels in the proper condition.

These are very well to be taken two or three times during the week. These are PREFERABLE to be taken COOKED; though they may be taken as they are preserved and eaten between or at a meal.

11/7/38
M. 33 yrs.
ELIMINATIONS: POOR **1467-4**

Precautions should be taken that there is sufficient of the laxative foods, or plenty of such as prunes as a part of the diet; so as to make for plenty of iron as well as the activities for resistances through the system.

9/30/41
M. 11 yrs.
BODY-BUILDING: ELIMINATIONS **1188-10**

Q. What foods should be included in weekly diet and in what amounts?

A. As we have indicated again and again, those that are body building and at the same time keep in the foods the correct balance of the vitamins for body (rather than in chemical additions) building. These are the better foods, and sufficient quantities to satisfy the appetite of the body. A growing body requires plenty of vitamins A and B and D and C, that the structural portions may also have sufficient from the assimilated foods, rather than being supplied from concentrated forms of same.

Do that rather in the body-building diet. Not too much of sugars, yet sufficient. Let the sweets be taken in such forms as of fruits. These are body building, also supply energies that are well for a growing, developing body.

Q. How can bowel eliminations be improved?

A. Include in the diet such as prunes, prune juice. All forms of this character of fruit tend to aid eliminations, also carrying the correct character of sugars to supply that needed—and is in a form that is assimilated without becoming too acid forming.

5/30/29
F. 31 yrs.
CONSTIPATION **1713-17**

Q. What should the body do to overcome constipation?

A. We would first, for at least three to five days, beginning now, be on a diet chiefly of prunes, see? Then after three days (for we will find this will tend to cleanse the alimentary canal, especially the colon), we would begin with those of the filling or heavy diet.

10/21/32
ELEPHANTIASIS: TENDENCIES **F. 18 yrs.**
DIET: ARTHRITIS: GLANDS: INCOORDINATION **951-1**

One meal each day we would supply principally of nature's sugars, nature's laxatives in prunes—any of the active principles in such.

10/23/43
F. 60 yrs.
ELIMINATIONS **3314-1**

Have plenty of raw foods such as prunes, and we will have better eliminations and better conditions for the body.

Q. What causes pain in back and side?

A. As indicated, pressures in those areas that disturb the alimentary canal, the stomach and the eliminations.

9/30/41
M. 11 yrs.
BODY-BUILDING: ELIMINATIONS **1188-10**

A growing body requires plenty of vitamins A and B and D and C, that the structural portions may also have sufficient from the assimilated foods, rather than being supplied from concentrated forms of same.

Do that rather in the body-building diet. Not too much of sugars, yet sufficient. Let the sweets be taken in such forms as fruits. These are body building, also supply energies that are well for a growing, developing body.

Q. How can bowel eliminations be improved?

A. Include in the diet such as prunes, prune juice, all forms of this character of fruit tend to aid eliminations, also carrying the correct character of sugars to supply that needed—and is in a form that is assimilated without becoming too acid forming; though many of these fruits are acids in themselves.

10/27/34
F. 15 yrs.
ACIDITY & ALKALINITY **605-4**

Prunes are well to add to the morning diet at times.

9/6/33
ASSIMILATIONS: POOR **F. 3 yrs.**
MALARIA: TENDENCIES **402-1**

Noons—Prunes, with a little cream; or any stewed fruits, provided they are not apples.

10/28/42
F. 53 yrs.
BODY-BUILDING: ASSIMILATIONS **1770-7**

We find that the diet needs consideration. There would be a helpful or beneficial effect from the body taking the tonic that carries the B-1 vitamins, the iron and the G vitamin. This particular type of combination is excellent. With the alteration that has been made in the Codiron, there is not the assimilation of the type of iron that is processed in same. Hence we would find that the combination of the vitamins in the tonic would be well, if there is the adding in the diet of those things such as the activities of prunes and all of such natures. These added to some of those activities as may be taken will be found to be more beneficial.

Hence, if the tonic is taken with such foods added in the diet, it will be more efficient for the body than the supplementing of the diet with other vitamin preparations. Do not overtake same, but only as a tonic; adding to the diet such foods as the prunes.

3/12/37
M. 28 yrs.
ACIDITY & ALKALINITY: TOXEMIA **1005-16**

We find that prunes (they are acid-producing, to be sure) would be well . . .

To be sure, other fruits may be taken.

1/17/41
F. 44 yrs.
ELIMINATIONS: POOR **459-11**

Aid the eliminations by taking prunes, etc., rather than the vegetable compounds, for this body.

ANEMIA **4/15/41**
ASSIMILATIONS: POOR **F. 22 yrs.**
ACIDITY & ALKALINITY **2479-1**

Begin with a corrective diet, which would be one tending towards the alkaline nature, with sufficient of the fruit acids to correct the inclination for the disturbance in eliminations.

Hence, have plenty of prunes in all the different forms. Take some of these each day.

18)—Quince

3/12/37
M. 28 yrs.
ACIDITY: TOXEMIA: ECZEMA **1005-16**

We would find then that especially quince or such fruits—these canned or preserved are very well in small quantities as a portion of the diet.

To be sure, other fruits may be taken.

19)—Raisins

3/8/37
F. 55 yrs.
OBESITY **1183-2**

Two of the leafy vegetables to one of pod, and three of the leafy to one of the tuberous. And these as we find, if there will be included raisins, will aid in assisting in the effect created by the adjustments and by the revitalizing of the vibratory forces for the body.

12/11/37
F. 43 yrs.
CONSTIPATION **1446-3**

Use raisins. These at various times or in various manners are most beneficial. These are a portion of the NECESSITIES for the body to keep in the physical forces.

4/15/41
ASSIMILATIONS: POOR **F. 22 yrs.**
ACIDITY & ALKALINITY **2479-1**

Begin with a corrective diet, which would be one tending towards the alkaline nature, with sufficient of the fruit acids to correct the inclination for the disturbance in eliminations.

Hence, have plenty of raisins in all the different forms. Take some of these each day.

10/3/40
F. 19 yrs.
BODY-BUILDING **2374-1**

Evenings—Plenty of vegetables as well as fruits . . . All characters of foods especially such as raisins, cooked as well as raw.

Do this, and as we find we will bring bettered conditions for this body; not only making for the corrections but improving the vitality, the strength, and increasing the weight.

9/30/41
M. 11 yrs.
BODY-BUILDING: ELIMINATIONS **1188-10**

Q. How can bowel eliminations be improved?

A. Include in the diet such as raisins, raisin juices; all forms of this character of fruit tend to aid eliminations, also carrying the correct character of sugars to supply that needed—and is in a form that is assimilated without becoming too acid forming.

10/23/43
F. 60 yrs.
ELIMINATIONS **3314-1**

Have plenty of raw foods such as raisins and the like and we will have better eliminations and better conditions for the body.

Q. What causes pain in back and side?

A. As indicated, pressures in those areas that disturb the alimentary canal, the stomach and the eliminations.

3/21/39
RELAXATION **F. 49 yrs.**
ELIMINATIONS **1158-21**

Q. Raisins?

A. Raisins also should be taken just about like the almonds.

Q. What is the best way to insure satisfactory daily bowel movements?

A. By the diet, and not by dependence upon ANY of the taking of laxatives or the like. But these are the better taken in the diet in those things indicated, such as raisins.

5/9/29
F. 64 yrs.
ACIDITY: ASSIMILATIONS: BLOOD-BUILDING **1377-3**

Q. Will natural sweets such as raisins be detrimental?

A. May be taken in moderation early in the day.

12/31/34
F. 22 yrs.
ELIMINATIONS: INCOORDINATION **480-13**

Tend to those foods more of the alkaline reaction, in a general diet: bewaring of too great quantities of sweets at any time. Quantities of fruits—as raisins—may be taken.

1/17/41
F. 44 yrs.
ELIMINATIONS: POOR **459-11**

Aid the eliminations by taking raisins, etc., rather than the vegetable compounds, for this body.

20)—Rhubarb (Pieplant)

11/7/24
M. 29 yrs.
ACIDITY **900-11**

For the acid condition that comes at times to the body, the diet will control this, with the manipulation, more than any other condition. Not so much of meats but more of those foods that carry the rougher materials; in rhubarb and such foods should be taken more for the system.

More vegetables of all kinds will give this body the better mental forces, the better physical forces, the better development throughout.

3/30/32
F. 66 yrs.
CONSTIPATION **5592-1**

When it is necessary to take any form of cathartic, that which is of the vegetable nature would be the better, but this will not be necessary if we will have at least one meal each day of wholly the pieplant—as is concentrated.

12/31/37
DEBILITATION: GENERAL **M. 41 yrs.**
ACIDITY & ALKALINITY **1476-1**

Mornings—whole wheat cereals. These may be altered at times with stewed fruits; as the pieplant. These should be taken at one time or another.

5/20/39
F. Adult
ANEMIA: ELIMINATIONS **1779-3**

Q. Should I continue the colonic irrigation?

A. If there is the feeling of an uncomfortableness owing to the formations of gas or the lack of the proper eliminations, use the colonics rather than too much of laxatives or purgatives. However, if there is also used the pieplant as a part of the diet, it should enable the body to greatly correct the condition.

5/4/39
M. 31 yrs.
LIVER: KIDNEYS: INCOORDINATION **1885-1**

Eliminating foods, of course, are preferable—as in any of the vegetable forces, any of the vegetables that are an active force for not too great a stimulation for the lymph and emunctory activity through the alimentary canal, but that are stimulating to same for better activity—as the pieplant, or similar foods that aid in such activity.

10/21/32
ELEPHANTIASIS: TENDENCIES **F. 18 yrs.**
ARTHRITIS: GLANDS: INCOORDINATION **951-1**

One meal each day we would supply principally of nature's sugars, nature's laxatives. A great deal of those forces may be found in the pieplant, or the like; whether those that are preserved or otherwise, provided they are without any of the preservatives.

1/26/35
F. 59 yrs.
INJURIES **3823-2**

Noons—During those periods when there is little of the activity, so that there are not the normal eliminations, well that vegetables or fruits that are the more laxative in form be used as a portion of the meal; such as rhubarb, of course, these should be either fresh or those canned without any superficial or artificial preservative.

3/15/37
BLOOD: HUMOR **F. 56 yrs.**
TOXEMIA **569-25**

Pieplant stewed (that is, rhubarb) to be sure will assist. These should be taken about once a week, and with the effluvia as produced by their activities and other eliminating properties that are to be a portion of the activity, will work well together if they are taken about this often.

10/27/34
F. 15 yrs.
ACIDITY & ALKALINITY **605-4**

Add to the morning diet at times, fresh rhubarb or canned rhubarb.

4/5/44
F. 52 yrs.
ASTHMA **4029-1**

Leave off all kinds of sugar. Do take often such as rhubarb. These would be better for the body for the eliminations, even in the changes that will be necessary if there is to be kept a balance between the sympathetic and cerebrospinal system. For these are producing the mental reactions to the body.

11/20/37
CIRCULATION: INCOORDINATION **F. 30 yrs.**
ARTHRITIS **1482-1**

In the matter of the diets: As has been indicated for the body, naturally the diet is an important factor in the effect produced upon the assimilating forces of the body itself. Keep away from great quantities of starches. Take those things where the activities for the system—as of the pancreas, the spleen, the liver activities—become as a greater portion of the activities to produce desired or effective activity in glandular reaction.

Hence we would find that liquids and semi-liquids, but of a very strengthening character, would be a portion of the diet.

Also pieplant should be a portion, as also the fruits; for these salts contained in such foods should be such as to produce for the system an activity upon the bodily functions in these directions.

12/11/37
F. 43 yrs.
CONSTIPATION **1446-3**

Use the pieplant. These at various times or in various manners are most beneficial. These are a portion of the NECESSITIES for the body to keep in the physical forces.

4/27/35
ASSIMILATIONS: ELIMINATIONS: INCOORDINATION F. 39 yrs.
NEURITIS 908-1

Mornings—Citrus fruit juices.

Or, to change the diet, there may be stewed fruits or dry cereal. Any of the stewed fruits, even though they be acid, if the system desires same take a little at the morning meal; as pieplant or the like.

9/6/33
ASSIMILATIONS: POOR F. 3 yrs.
MALARIA: TENDENCIES 402-1

Noons—Pieplant, or any stewed fruits, provided they are not apples.

12/31/37
DEBILITATION: GENERAL M. 41 yrs.
ACIDITY & ALKALINITY 1476-1

Mornings—Alter at times with stewed fruits; as the pieplant.

2)—Berries: General

7/7/23
F. Adult
ANEMIA 4889-1

To overcome these forces in the body to prevent this retarding of the elements we would take that in the system that will give the balance and equilibrium of all the forces necessary to supply the blood elements. Diet for this body will be the greater force, these that carry as much of iron as possible, principally, of fruits in this character and nature such as would be found in berries, especially, those that grow on the ground, close.

4/27/35
ASSIMILATIONS: ELIMINATIONS: INCOORDINATION F. 39 yrs.
NEURITIS 908-1

Mornings—Citrus fruit juices.

Or, to change the diet, as fresh berries of any kind.

7/12/35
BODY-BUILDING F. 23 yrs.
DIS-EASE: CONTAGION: PREVENTIVE 480-19

The diet should be more body-building; that is, less acid foods and more of the alkaline-reacting will be the better in these directions. Those food values carrying an easy assimilation of iron, silicon, and those elements or chemicals—as all forms of berries. Fruits and the like, should form a greater part of the regular diet in the present—and in the preparations for those activities to come later, whether in relationships in the physical manner or those in the mental forces that are necessary in such activities.

Keep closer to the alkaline diets: using fruits, berries, that carry iron, silicon, phosphorus and the like—and these as we have indicated.

4/7/23
NERVOUS SYSTEMS: INCOORDINATION **M. Adult**
NERVE-BUILDING **4730-1**

The diet—all those that lend energy to nerve-building forces and those that give to the blood force the eliminating properties—berries and fruits, see.

5/7/40
ARTHRITIS **M. 33 yrs.**
BODY-BUILDING **849-50**

Then the dry cereals with fruit may be taken—these either with berries or other fresh fruits. Canned berries may be used if the fresh are not practical.

7/22/31
ACIDITY **F. 28 yrs.**
ASSIMILATIONS: ELIMINATIONS: INCOORDINATION **2261-1**

In those of berries, things of this nature—these are all well for the body.

7/26/40
F. 12 yrs.
EPILEPSY **2153-2**

Refrain from any large quantities of sweets. Most of the sweets, if any form is taken, should be in the fruits—that is, the natural fruit sweets.

Mornings—A dry cereal with some berries.

6/26/39
F. 21 yrs.
ENVIRONMENT: HAY FEVER **1771-3**

Beware of sweets in the diet. Have fruits preferably as the main portion of the diet.

Use fruits, berries of all natures or characters that are grown in the environ of the body, especially.

10/11/43
F. 26 yrs.
ARTHRITIS **3285-1**

We should have easily assimilated foods, but those very high in the adding of B complex, or the vitamin B—as in berries whatever may be obtained. These should be a part of the diet daily with plenty of seafoods (not fresh water fish).

6/4/40
F. 11 yrs.
BODY-BUILDING **1179-6**

Q. Have you any changes in diet to suggest?

A. As we find, only the fruits in season, berries or the like, these are well to become a part of the diet; for they tend not only to purify but clarify general conditions for the body.

7/22/31
BLOOD-BUILDING F. 28 yrs.
ASSIMILATIONS: DEBILITATION: GENERAL 3842-1

We would give a diet that is easily assimilated. Let the diet be that as is nerve and blood building. Fruits—berries—provided they grow off the ground, not *on* the ground—these would be the better.

5/18/43
F. 66 yrs.
ASSIMILATIONS: ELIMINATIONS: INCOORDINATION 3008-1

Beware of berries, or of too much of those things the seeds of which are on the outside.

8/17/31
F. Adult
ULCERS 5619-1

Then, we must be mindful that the diet is such that the gastric forces of the stomach do not become overacid. These we would give as an outline, though these may be altered or changed to meet the conditions as they arise:

Mornings—Would be preferably only those of the citrus fruit juices. Occasionally we would leave these off for a day or two. At such times we would take those of either stewed fruits, or the like—not those of the berries, or those that grow on the smaller vines.

2/8/43
CIRCULATION: INCOORDINATION: ALLERGIES M. 37 yrs.
COMBINATIONS 2772-4

Q. Am I allergic to any other type of food?

A. Only as to combinations, as we find. Certain types of berries, if combined with other foods. Any foods that carry quantities of potash with same, the body would tend to be allergic to; with combinations that are at variance with potash.

1)—Blackberries

7/23/40
F. 37 yrs.
ACIDITY 2310-1

Especially have cereals of morning that carry extra quantities of vitamin B-1. The dry cereals may be taken with fruits if so desired, especially small berries as the blackberry or the like.

7/13/35
F. 59 yrs.
ECZEMA 3823-4

Q. Berries?

A. Blackberries are better than strawberries. Some of these carry a great deal more acid than others; dependent a great deal upon where they are grown; that is, they carry too great a quantity of potash and thus require that an equal balance be created by taking sufficient quantities of such natures as carry silicon or iodine.

1/9/26
COLD: CONGESTION: FLU: AFTEREFFECTS F. 7 yrs.
BABY CARE 4281-10

Q. Should she have canned blackberries?
A. *No* canned blackberries!

2)—Blueberries

7/28/43
ANEMIA F. 56 yrs.
GENERAL: MULTIPLE SCLEROSIS 3118-1

In the diet—keep to those things that heal within and without. And especially use the garden blueberry. (This is a property which some one, some day, will use in its proper place!) These should be stewed, but with their own juices, little sugar but in their own juices.

3)—Currants

10/21/32
ELEPHANTIASIS: TENDENCIES F. 18 yrs.
ARTHRITIS: GLANDS: INCOORDINATION 951-1

One meal each day we would supply principally of nature's sugars, berries of most natures—any of the active principles in such, provided they are without any of the preservatives; currants and their derivatives.

7/13/35
F. 59 yrs.
ECZEMA 3823-4

Q. Berries?
A. Currants or the like, are very good in moderation. Some of these carry a great deal more acid than others; dependent a great deal upon where they are grown; that is, they carry too great a quantity of potash and thus require that an equal balance be created by taking sufficient quantities of such natures as carry silicon or iodine.

4)—Dewberries

7/13/35
F. 59 yrs.
ECZEMA 3823-4

Dewberries are better than the strawberries. Some of these carry a great deal more acid than others; dependent a great deal upon where they are grown; that is, they carry too great a quantity of potash and thus require that an equal balance be created by taking sufficient quantities of such natures as carry silicon or iodine.

5)—Gooseberries

ELEPHANTIASIS: TENDENCIES
ARTHRITIS: GLANDS: INCOORDINATION
10/21/32
F. 18 yrs.
951-1

One meal each day we would supply principally of berries of most natures—any of the active principles in such; a great deal of those forces that may be found in gooseberries in any of their preparations—whether those that are preserved or otherwise, provided they are without any of the preservatives.

HEART
BLOOD-BUILDING
8/8/29
M. 61 yrs.
2597-6

Q. Does he require any special foods, and what food is most beneficial to him?

A. Those that have blood building, and especially carrying iron. Berries—especially gooseberries—may be taken.

ECZEMA
7/13/35
F. 59 yrs.
3823-4

Gooseberries, or the like, are very good in moderation.

GLANDS: INCOORDINATION
4/26/35
F. 53 yrs.
906-1

Gooseberries should be abstained from.

6)—Raspberries

GLANDS: INCOORDINATION
4/26/35
F. 53 yrs.
906-1

Some characters of berries may be taken in moderation, especially those that will soon be in season, as the raspberry—preferably the dark variety rather than the red would be more helpful. These may be taken in the morning meal with the cereals or they may be used in a salad made of fruits occasionally that may be taken by the body.

ACIDITY
7/23/40
F. 37 yrs.
2310-1

Have cereals of morning that carry extra quantities of vitamin B-1. These dry cereals may be taken with fruits if so desired, especially small berries as the raspberry.

7)—Strawberries

4/29/37
ASSIMILATIONS: ELIMINATIONS: INCOORDINATION **M. 45 yrs.**
BLOOD: HUMOR **877-16**

In the diet—of these things beware. Others may be taken very well. Do not eat fresh strawberries. Other berries are tabu also in the early portion of the seasons, or out of season for the surrounding environ of the body. When they are in season in the body's surroundings these are different.

4/27/35
ASSIMILATIONS: ELIMINATIONS: INCOORDINATION **F. 39 yrs.**
NEURITIS **908-1**

Mornings—Citrus fruit juices. Or, to change the diet, there may be fresh strawberries with cream.

2/12/38
F. 61 yrs.
ARTHRITIS **1512-2**

Q. May I eat strawberries?

A. These should be very little, not large quantities of these. A little would be very well, but not very much—and these occasionally.

Q. Any more advice regarding my diet?

A. As indicated, do not have those combinations that produce great acid. Citrus fruits while acid are NOT acid-producing, unless taken with quantities of starch.

4/7/37
F. 29 yrs.
COLD: CONGESTION: AFTEREFFECTS **808-6**

Strawberries may be taken in whatever way is most palatable for the body.

4/26/35
F. 53 yrs.
GLANDS: INCOORDINATION **906-1**

Strawberries should be abstained from.

2/18/23
M. 3 yrs.
CANCER **3751-6**

No strawberries or any other fruits of the acid taste.

8)—Whortleberries

7/23/40
F. 37 yrs.
ACIDITY **2310-1**

Have cereals of morning that carry extra quantities of vitamin B-1. These dry cereals may be taken with fruits if so desired, especially small berries as the whortleberry.

3)—Citrus Fruit: General

1/25/33
F. 44 yrs.
GLANDS: INCOORDINATION **757-3**

First, beware of too great an amount of sugars for the body. So when those things are taken as food values—as in the citrus fruit—do not use sugar; rather use salt, or the other activities that make the food palatable.

Mornings—Citrus fruit juices, or the pulp with citrus fruit, see? with brown toast, whole wheat.

3/30/32
F. 66 yrs.
CONSTIPATION **5592-1**

When it is necessary to take any form of cathartic, that which is of the vegetable nature would be the better, but this will not be necessary if we will have at least one meal each day of wholly citrus fruit.

2/8/41
DEBILITATION: GENERAL **F. 24 yrs.**
ACIDITY & ALKALINITY **2448-1**

First, in the diets, refrain from those things that are acid-producing in the body. And yet there are certain FORMS of acids needed; such as all citrus fruits—these should be kept for the body, but there should be precautions as to their combinations with other foods. For instance, do not have the citrus fruit AND cereals at the same meal. In most of the fruit take the pulp WITH the juices themselves, for the reaction of this BULK is needed in the activity of the lacteals.

3/25/30
F. 45 yrs.
ACIDITY & ALKALINITY: DIGESTION: INDIGESTION **5625-1**

Increase the amount of the salines for the system, so that the drainage throughout the whole system may be increased, so that absorption and coagulation takes place *nominally;* not leaving any of these drosses in system as may accumulate in centers where distresses are seen, yet these acting in their proper drainage will *eliminate* same from the system entirely.

In the food values, then—these being of the salines, or an increased amount of these, we will find these will be in those of a great deal of the citrus fruits. Well were the body in the beginning to take the citrus fruit fast for four to five days, in the beginning. Then, when the foods are given—which would be gruels, cereals—both dry and cooked—with the fruits.

7/15/30
M. 23 yrs.
CATARRH: NASAL: BLOOD: HUMOR **849-7**

Adding those of a great deal of the citrus fruit, especially for the breakfast meal, we will find the blood *cleansed,* and much of that disorder as gives rise to the soft tissue in the head, nasal cavities, and the stomach, or that as is of a catarrhal nature, will be relieved.

We will find then we may give those for *other* corrections. Ready for questions.

Q. Should tonsils be removed?

A. Not under the present conditions. They may be made *necessary,* after we have cleansed the blood. It would be very improper to remove them *under* existent conditions.

4/17/44
F. 34 yrs.
ASSIMILATIONS: ELIMINATIONS: INCOORDINATION 2072-14

Q. What foods can be used with fresh citrus fruits to make a complete meal?

A. Any foods that may be eaten at any time save whole grain cereals.

10/21/32
ELEPHANTIASIS: TENDENCIES F. 18 yrs.
ARTHRITIS: GLANDS: INCOORDINATION 951-1

We would first be very mindful of the diet. Keep away from all forces that supply an overabundance of salines, limes, or silicon, or the like, in the system. Supply an overabundant amount of those foods that carry iron, iodine and phosphorus in the system, for these will act against that already supplied to burn or destroy those tendencies of debarkation or demarcation in the activities of the glands.

One meal each day we would supply principally of citrus fruits, or nature's sugars, nature's laxatives in citrus fruits.

2/6/31
F. 22 yrs.
EPILEPSY 543-7

Have other fruits such as the citrus fruits (whether canned or otherwise, but if canned be sure they are *not* canned with benzoate of soda).

ASSIMILATIONS: ELIMINATIONS: INCOORDINATION 11/9/40
CANCER: TENDENCIES F. 61 yrs.
ACIDITY & ALKALINITY 1697-2

Q. What foods may be taken that will digest properly?

A. Any of those that are easily assimilated; that is, three times as much alkaline-reacting as acid-producing foods. This means the alkaline-REACTING; and not acid-producing. For instance, all citrus fruits that are easily assimilated would be included.

2/12/38
F. 61 yrs.
ARTHRITIS 1512-2

Q. Any more advice regarding my diet?

A. As indicated, do not have those combinations that produce great acid.

Citrus fruits while acid are NOT acid-producing, unless taken with quantities of starch.

8/28/28
F. 48 yrs.
CANCER 569-16

Beware of meats. This has caused the greater distress at the present time.

Q. What would be a correct diet for the body at this time?

A. Pre-digested foods. Those that are not acid. Now there are reactions from fruits that apparently are acid, yet in system are not; such as any of the citrus fruits, see?

1/17/43
CIRCULATION: IMPAIRED **F. 6 yrs.**
BODY-BUILDING **2883-1**

In the diet—have plenty of calcium, the foods that carry plenty of calcium; as plenty of the citrus fruits and the like. These should be a part of the diet for the body.

12/18/30
M. 24 yrs.
BACILLOSIS: POLIOMYELITIS **135-1**

Mornings—Only the citrus fruit diet, *changed,* of course, at times, to the hard cereals. *Do not combine* these with the citrus fruits, or have them taken at the same meal!

7/15/41
F. 61 yrs.
DEBILITATION: GENERAL **2535-1**

In the matter of diet—take more of those foods that carry greater quantity of vitamin B-1—such as found in those foods that are yellow in color. Thus, all citrus fruits. These should form not the whole but a great deal of the diet.

1)—Grapefruit

12/12/28
F. 48 yrs.
ACIDITY **569-18**

Fruits that are non-acid producing as grapefruit are good.

8/31/41
ARTHRITIS: PREVENTIVE **F. 51 yrs.**
BODY: GENERAL **1158-31**

Q. For balanced diet, what quantities should I take per week of grapefruit?
A. About three to four times each week.

10/26/34
ELIMINATIONS: INCOORDINATION **F. Adult**
ACIDITY **710-1**

Grapefruit may be taken, provided they are not taken close with any food that carries *gluten*—which would tend to change these in their activity with the gastric flows of the digestive areas.

12/3/35
F. 51 yrs.
OBESITY: TENDENCIES **1073-1**

As to the matter of the diets, these become naturally—with the general conditions of the body—a necessary element or influence. Do not ever take cereals *and* grapefruit or citrus fruit *at* the same meal. Have the cereal one day and fruit the next. For they form in the system, together, that which is not beneficial—and *especially* not helpful for this body, forming an acid that fattens the body.

2/22/34
ASTHENIA **F. 65 yrs.**
ACIDITY & ALKALINITY **509-2**

Grapefruit may be taken in moderation and *in their season.*

11/23/37
M. 13 yrs.
PSORIASIS **1484-1**

Grapefruit may be taken. These are NOT acid-*PRODUCING.* They are alkaline-reacting!

But when cereals or starches are taken, do not have the citrus fruit at the same meal—or even the same day; for such a combination in the system at the same time becomes ACID-producing!

Hence those taken on different days are well for the body.

4/19/41
F. 51 yrs.
ASSIMILATIONS **1158-30**

Q. Shall I supplement with additional vitamin B tablets?

A. We find that if this vitamin is supplied in the diet it will be better than taking an overquantity of vitamin B, which would be the case if the tablets were taken as a supplement. With the Adirion taken, that is to aid in assimilation, it would be better to supplement the vitamin B in the diet, with such as grapefruit. These taken as we find, with beef and fowl, should carry sufficient vitamins.

6/17/41
NERVOUS TENSION **F. 26 yrs.**
RHEUMATISM **2517-1**

THE BLOOD SUPPLY indicates an unbalanced condition in the chemical reactions, and a lack—in the beginning—of the vitamin or vital forces as might be best adapted to the body—B-1 and F, or B-2.

These produced a nervous reaction, or a lack of nerve vitamin forces. Thus, with the disturbances to the sympathetic system, the high nerve tension or nerve exhaustion that followed, there was a still greater reduction in the chemical forces of the body.

As to the diet throughout the period—keep close to those foods that will supply the greater quantity of B-1 vitamin.

Mornings—Grapefruit may be taken for two or three mornings, then the cereals for two or three mornings.

9/3/41
GLANDS: THYROID **F. 33 yrs.**
BODY-BUILDING **2582-1**

Be mindful that there are the diets that carry full quantities of the vitamins that aid in the strength and body-building. These will be found in grapefruit. These should be a considerable part of the body's diet.

2)—Lemon

1/4/40
ATROPHY: NERVES **M. 32 yrs.**
NERVES: REBUILDING **849-47**

Have plenty (and more than has been taken!) of lemons. These supply salts that should be had by the body. Preferably use the fresh fruit.

8/27/44
F. 43 yrs.
EYES: WEAK **5401-1**

Do add to the diet about twice as many lemons as is a part of the diet in the present. These also supplement with a great deal of carrots, especially as combined with gelatin, if we would aid and strengthen the optic nerves and the tensions between sympathetic and cerebrospinal systems.

10/26/34
ELIMINATIONS: INCOORDINATION **F. Adult**
ACIDITY **710-1**

Lemons may be taken, provided they are not taken close with any food that carries *gluten*—which would tend to change these in their activity with the gastric flows of the digestive areas.

10/22/29
SPINE: SUBLUXATIONS **F. 51 yrs.**
CIRCULATION: POOR **5555-1**

Now, to meet the needs, or to aid in giving ease to the body—the body should first—of diets—have at least for five to six days, *principally* that of a citrus fruit diet—principally lemons, and a few oranges occasionally—occasionally a grapefruit, but little else. Not much sugar used with these, and not too much salt—but quantity of the juices should be taken—even were a dozen a day consumed, not too much.

6/5/34
M. 68 yrs.
CANCER **570-1**

As to the matter of the diet; this should be nerve- and blood-building, a liquid diet through the greater part of the time; citrus fruit juices, a great deal of lemons.

9/3/41
GLANDS: THYROID **F. 33 yrs.**
BODY-BUILDING **2582-1**

Be mindful that there are the diets that carry full quantities of the vitamins that aid in the strength and body-building. These will be found in lemons. These should be a considerable part of the body's diet.

3)—Lime

6/5/34
M. 68 yrs.
CANCER **570-1**

As to the matter of the diet; this should be nerve- and blood-building, a liquid diet through the greater part of the time; citrus fruit juices, a great deal of limes.

8/27/44
F. 43 yrs.
EYES: WEAK **5401-1**

Do add to the diet about twice as many limes as is a part of the diet in the present. These also supplement with a great deal of carrots, especially as combined with gelatin, if we would aid and strengthen the optic nerves and the tensions between sympathetic and cerebrospinal systems.

10/26/34
F. Adult
ELIMINATIONS: INCOORDINATION **710-1**

Limes may be taken, provided they are not taken close with any food that carries *gluten*—which would tend to change these in their activity with the gastric flows of the digestive areas.

7/25/36
F. 32 yrs.
KIDNEYS: PREGNANCY **540-6**

Keep a well-balance between the diets for sufficient calcium and lime. Things of that nature carry these in such quantities that they may be easily assimilated. So let the foods that are prepared occasionally have more and more of limes.

1/4/40
ATROPHY: NERVES **M. 32 yrs.**
NERVES: REBUILDING **849-47**

Have plenty (and more than has been taken!) of limes.

These supply salts that should be had by the body.

4)—Oranges

3/14/41
M. 18 yrs.
LEUKEMIA **2456-4**

Q. What is the effect of the oranges so far?

A. These supply in the activity of the circulation those necessary vitamins, and that element of activities in the system to keep a balance. The principal activity here is the calcium in same.

5/30/29
F. 31 yrs.
CONSTIPATION **1713-17**

Q. What should the body do to overcome constipation?

A. We would first, for at least three to five days, beginning now, be on a diet chiefly of oranges, see? Then after three days (for we will find this will tend to cleanse the alimentary canal, especially the colon), we would begin with those of the filling or heavy diet.

Q. How many oranges should be taken each day?

A. About a dozen.

10/26/34
ELIMINATIONS: INCOORDINATION **F. Adult**
ACIDITY **710-1**

Oranges may be taken, provided they are not taken close with any food that carries *gluten*—which would tend to change these in their activity with the gastric flows of the digestive areas.

APPLES: ELIMINATIONS **12/30/40**
ASSIMILATIONS: POOR **M. 52 yrs.**
COOKING UTENSILS: ALUMINUM: NOT RECOMMENDED **2423-1**

As to the diet after the first cleansing with the apples—we would have plenty of oranges.

2/22/34
ASTHENIA **F. 65 yrs.**
ACIDITY & ALKALINITY **509-2**

Oranges may be taken in moderation and *in their season.*

12/31/34
F. 22 yrs.
ELIMINATIONS: INCOORDINATION **480-13**

Q. Please outline diet to be followed at present.

A. Tend to those foods more of the alkaline reaction, in a general diet; bewaring of too great quantities of sweets at any time. Quantities of fruits—as oranges may be taken.

6/10/38
F. 13 yrs.
ASSIMILATIONS: ELIMINATIONS: INCOORDINATION **1206-8**

Q. Is it well to eliminate oranges?

A. We do not find these necessary to be eliminated from the system. For there are those vital forces and balances kept through the system by the activities of these, that are necessary to be kept in the chemical reaction of the body. Oranges are very well.

11/23/37
M. 13 yrs.
MENU: PSORIASIS **1484-1**

Oranges may be taken. These are NOT acid-PRODUCING. They are alkaline-reacting!

But when cereals or starches are taken, do not have citrus fruit at the same meal—or even the same day; for such a combination in the system at the same time becomes ACID-producing!

Hence those taken on different days are well for the body.

1/4/40
M. 32 yrs.
ATROPHY: NERVES 849-47

Have plenty (and more than has been taken!) of oranges, lemons, limes, grapefruit and the like. These supply salts that should be had by the body. Preferably use the fresh fruit.

11/6/35
GLANDS: THYROID: HYPOTHYROIDISM F. 63 yrs.
MINERALS 1049-1

In the matter of the diet, this would be rather important. Occasionally use a great deal of those things that carry quantities of iodine, for this the body requires. But for this body it will be most soluble from oranges.

6/17/41
NERVOUS TENSION F. 26 yrs.
RHEUMATISM 2517-1

As to the diet throughout the period—keep close to those foods that will supply the greater quantity of B-1 vitamin.

Mornings—Oranges may be taken for two or three mornings, then the cereals for two or three mornings.

9/3/41
GLANDS: THYROID F. 33 yrs.
BODY-BUILDING 2582-1

Be mindful that there are the diets that carry full quantities of the vitamins that aid in the strength and body-building. These will be found in oranges. These should be a considerable part of the body's diet.

2/23/28
F. 21 mos.
TOXEMIA 608-4

Oranges *occasionally*, not too many of same.

6/7/37
F. 65 yrs.
DEBILITATION: GENERAL 658-15

Do not take cereals or toast even, for this body, on the mornings when citrus fruits are taken. Oranges are preferable for this body with a little lemon in same.

12/27/41
F. 19 yrs.
PREGNANCY 711-4

Plenty of citrus fruit juices. Have at least two or three oranges each day. One may be taken in the morning, the other in the evening.

8/27/44
F. 43 yrs.
EYES: WEAK **5401-1**

Do add to the diet about twice as many oranges as is a part of the diet in the present. These also supplement with a great deal of carrots, especially as combined with gelatin, if we would aid and strengthen the optic nerves and the tensions between sympathetic and cerebrospinal systems.

4)—Melons

1)—Watermelon

7/31/43
M. 39 yrs.
CANCER **3121-1**

In the diet—do live mostly, for a while, on watermelon, having these almost daily. The watermelon is for the activity of the liver and kidney.

Most of all, pray. Let the mental attitude be considered first and foremost. Do not promise thyself, nor thy God, nor thy neighbor, that you do not fulfill.

8/8/29
HEART **M. 61 yrs.**
BLOOD-BUILDING **2597-6**

Q. Does he require any special foods, and what food is most beneficial to him?

A. Those that have blood-building, and especially carrying iron. No watermelon. No cantaloupe, as yet, but fruits of most other natures. Those of the blood-building are the better.

8/5/42
F. 37 yrs.
PREGNANCY **1505-4**

Be mindful of the diets that would overexercise the kidneys. For, these are the periods when the pressures begin to indicate the activities there. In the present we find them very well, but this tiredness will cause greater anxiety unless measures are taken and precautions kept as to diets.

Q. What particularly in the diet should she avoid, to prevent this condition in the kidneys?

A. Any of those that tend to carry influences that are overactive on the kidneys; though it is very well that such as watermelon be taken occasionally. Keep on top of the ground more now with all of the vegetables eaten.

7/25/36
F. 32 yrs.
KIDNEYS: PREGNANCY **540-6**

Keep a well-balance between the diets for sufficient calcium and lime; as in watermelon. Things of that nature carry these in such quantities that they may be easily assimilated. So let the foods that are prepared occasionally have more and more of these.

Keep those conditions for the kidneys as indicated through the watermelon taken occasionally, or rather often, three to four times a week, for this keeps sufficient of the properties that will act with the kidneys, keeping them cleansed.

7/13/35
F. 59 yrs.
ECZEMA **3823-4**

Q. Is watermelon all right for me?
A. It's very good.

V

Fruit Diets and Combinations

1)—Banana & Buttermilk Diet

10/4/39
F. 59 yrs.
PRURITUS **538-58**

Q. Would it be better to use bananas or some other fruit for the diet?

A. Use the bananas and the buttermilk. Then continue, of course, with a little of the buttermilk; and don't eat too heavily of ANY foods that are too acid.

Q. Should I continue the yeast tablets during the three-day diet?

A. If necessary for better elimination, continue with same throughout the period of the diet.

8/27/40
F. 60 yrs.
BLOOD: HUMOR **538-65**

Q. Is the buttermilk and bananas a good eliminating diet?

A. The buttermilk and banana diet is very good. The buttermilk and banana diet is rather as a balancing than as an eliminant; for it produces the absorption of certain toxic forces, and the adjustment of other conditions through the system.

11/3/39
F. 59 yrs.
BLOOD: HUMOR **538-60**

While there are the indications of the tendency for the humor or the effluvia in the blood to cause greater disturbances (because of overtaxation of the body physically), we find that these will respond to the adherence to those suggestions as we have indicated—either the yeast, as an eliminant, or the buttermilk and bananas as a builder-up AND a tearer-down in some directions (for these work with the effluvia of the intestinal system for better eliminations).

Q. Should I go on the three-day diet of buttermilk and bananas?

A. Two days should be sufficient, or three days if so desired.

2)—Apple Diet

12/8/39
M. 32 yrs.
PINWORMS **1597-2**

First—we would have a period of at least three days when nothing would be eaten but APPLES! preferably the Jonathan variety, or such natures. Not the wine sap, but any of the Jonathan variety. Of course, water may be taken, but do not drink milk especially through the period; though a little coffee may be taken if desired, or even a cereal drink if desired might be taken; but the diet itself should be just APPLES. Eat just as many as desired.

On the evening of the third day, take half a teacup of olive oil—pure olive oil.

This as we find will remove the causes of the disturbance.

12/15/37
F. 29 yrs.
EPILEPSY **543-26**

As we find in the present, that best is to keep the abilities for eliminations . . . without a general strain upon the body . . . in accord with the activities of the influences that retard or keep down the reactions in portions of the system from the incoordination, and those reflexes that arise from the use of the sedative forces in the body.

For this, then, as we find, occasionally—not too often—take the periods for the cleansing of the system with the use of the APPLE DIET; that is:

At least for three days—two days or three days—take NOTHING except APPLES—RAW APPLES! Of course, coffee may be taken if so desired, but no other foods but the raw apples. And then after the last meal of apples on the third day, or upon retiring on that evening following the last meal of apples, drink half a cup of olive oil.

This will tend to cleanse the system.

Raw apples otherwise taken (except at such cleansing periods) are not so well for the body.

Do not take yeast during that period of the cleansing through the Apple Diet; and this as we find (the Apple Diet) would be very well to be taken at least once a month.

Q. What causes the body to have bilious attacks so frequently?

A. As indicated, the lack of the proper activity through the gall duct and the lacteal duct areas, produced by the reaction of sedative forces upon the system.

5/10/40
F. 32 yrs.
1850-3

ACIDITY

Eat ONLY apples—RAW APPLES—for THREE DAYS! Coffee may be taken with same if so desired, but NOT with milk or cream or sugar in it! Also leave off the milk and bread when the apples are being taken. This is to cleanse the activities of the liver, the kidneys, and the whole system—where there has been disturbance.

On the evening of the third day of the Apple Diet—take internally HALF A TEACUP full of OLIVE OIL!

Then, after that do not overgorge the system when beginning to eat again. Have rather a normal diet, but not too rich nor too highly seasoned foods.

Keep away from cake or pastries or pies or the like.

The principal diet would be rather vegetables, both raw and cooked; with fish, fowl or lamb as the meats, but not beef or hog meat of any kind; and no fried foods at all.

Do these, and we will find that in a few days the ability to talk will return.

Be active in the open, but NOT so as to overstrain the body during the period of the fast and of the apple diet.

2/27/35
M. 26 yrs.
567-7

EPILEPSY

Q. Any other advice for this body?

A. If there is the desire on the part of the body to test self for tape worms, live for three days on raw apples *only!* Then take about half a teacup of olive oil, or half a glass of olive oil. And this would remove fecal matter that hasn't been removed for some time! But it will certainly indicate there is no tape worm!

2/21/44
F. 24 yrs.
3673-1

ELIMINATIONS: INCOORDINATION

Here, one good eliminant for this body would be to go on the apple diet—at least every three months; that is, eat nothing for three days except raw apples, preferably the Jonathan variety or a kindred variety. Follow this with at least two to three teaspoonsful of olive oil; that is, after the three days. This is to change the activity through the whole alimentary canal.

12/22/43
F. 66 yrs.
1409-9

DEBILITATION: GENERAL
NEURITIS: TENDENCIES

It would be well for this body, even after this, to have a three-day apple diet, even in its weakened condition we need to clear the system. For this will get rid of the tendencies for neuritic conditions in the joints of the body. Also take the olive oil after the three-day diet. But don't go without the apples—eat them—all you can—at least five or six apples each day. Chew them up, scrape them well. Drink plenty of water, and follow the three-day diet with the big dose of olive oil.

2/27/42
M. 25 yrs.
GLANDS: EYES: COLOR BLINDNESS **820-2**

No raw apples; or if raw apples are taken, take them and *nothing* else—three days of raw apples only, and then olive oil, and we will cleanse *all* toxic forces from any system! Raw apples are not well unless they are of the jenneting variety. [Gladys Davis's note: Dictionary of obsolete words gives regarding *jenneting:* "A jenneting pear—an early pear resembling the jenneting apple."] Apples cooked, apples roasted, are good.

3)—Grape Diet

4/28/34
F. 45 yrs.
GLANDS: INCOORDINATION **757-6**

We would be mindful that the diet is that which is easily assimilated. Not too great quantities of starch foods, but sufficient to aid in creating the proper balance in those periods of assimilation necessary for proper fermentation. We would not have too great quantities of sugar. Or the body may, under the existent circumstances, go on an entire grape diet—see, *entire* grape diet, for at least three-day periods; then to the regular normal diet that has been indicated. Quantities of grapes! And should there appear any disturbance in the stomach and duodenum through these periods, make a poultice of the grape hull and pulp—between cloths—and apply over those areas; or over the abdomen and liver area, you see. Make this about an inch and a half thick—that large quantity, you see, all over. Plenty of water, but just grapes for three days—*quantities*—all that the body may eat.

10/8/38
F. 51 yrs.
DEBILITATION: GENERAL **1703-1**

Some days, for at least three or four days, eat only GRAPES—morning, noon and night—GRAPES! Not with the seed, to be sure, but preferably those of the purple variety; not the larger but those that are good and NOT those that have been shipped or kept too long.

6/3/41
DEBILITATION: GENERAL **M. 25 yrs.**
APPENDICITIS **1970-1**

Also have the heavy grape poultices each day over the abdominal and stomach area.

And live practically on grapes during that period, or grapes and milk—with a little curd or crackers in same. The Concord grapes are preferable to be eaten also, but not the same ones that are used for poultice, to be sure! Of course, other types of grapes may be eaten also, but preferably and principally the Concord—or the colored grapes rather than the green, see?

9/15/35
F. 44 yrs.
TUMORS **683-3**

We find it would be helpful to have three or four days each month when *only* grapes would be used as the diet. And during those three to four days we would apply the grape poultices across all of the abdomen itself.

Q. The kind of grapes—does that matter?

A. Concord grapes are preferable.

7/28/34
F. 54 yrs.
RHEUMATISM
133-4

The *only* diet would be grapes; not grapefruit, but *at* other times grapefruit juices are to be taken as a one diet—at one meal or a period of the day, see?

The grape poultices across the intestines and bowels have been most helpful. These should be worn each day for periods of three days, and the grape diet should be the whole diet during the three days, you see; letting about three days elapse between each period of such treatments at first, and gradually increase the time elapsing between the use of these until there would be ten days between each period of grape treatment.

Between the periods of the grape diet, in the beginning use a liquid diet consisting of the citrus fruit juices of mornings (such as grapefruit, oranges, lemons and limes).

4)—Figs & Dates

2/10/38
CANCER: COXITIS: HIP EROSION (HEAD OF FEMUR) **F. 25 yrs.**
SPIRITUAL
275-45

At other meals there may be taken, or included with the other at times, dried fruits or figs, combined with dates and raisins—these chopped very well together.

1/7/37
CIRCULATION: POOR **F. 44 yrs.**
ELIMINATIONS: POOR **1315-6**

Q. Are figs and dates good for me?

A. These are very good. Do not combine these, however, with starchy foods.

5)—Figs, Dates & Almonds

9/27/37
F. Adult
DEBILITATION: GENERAL
1419-5

Mornings—At another time use a combination of dates, figs and almonds; these would be cut or ground together; these may be warm or these may be cold; and they may be taken with a little milk—this combination would not be given so often, but it will be found to be most beneficial as an aid to better eliminations.

6)—Mummy Food

In 1937 this recipe was given to Cayce in a dream, by a mummy who came to life and translated ancient Egyptian records for him. Later, in trance, the dream was questioned and again the identical experience took place: the preparation for the food was given exactly as it had been given in the dream and was said to be a "spiritual food."—Brett Bolton

2/10/38
F. 25 yrs.
SPIRITUAL **275-45**

For this particular body, equal portions of black figs or Assyrian figs and Assyrian dates—these ground together or cut very fine, and to a pint of such a combination put half a handful of corn meal, or crushed wheat. These cooked together—well, it's food for such a spiritually developed body as this!

2/10/38
F. 25 yrs.
ELIMINATIONS **275-45**

Q. Give cause and what body should do about occasional impure complexion.

A. For this there is needed better eliminations through the intestinal tract. Now: the raising of the vibratory forces within the body, in the manner indicated, and the use of the figs with the dates, in the combination as indicated, would aid in eliminating these causes.

For it would become more regular with the eliminations, and throw off the greater toxic forces from the natural great QUANTITY of activity as is this body's needs, as well as the production of refuse or ash force or such in the system, see?

9/30/41
M. 11 yrs.
BODY-BUILDING: ELIMINATIONS **1188-10**

It is well for this body, or growing bodies, or elderly individuals also, for strength-building and for correction of eliminations, to use this as a cereal, or a small quantity of this with the cereal, or it may be served with milk or cream:

Secure the unpitted Syrian or black figs and the Syrian dates. Cut or grind very fine a cup of each. Put them on in a double boiler with just a little goat's milk in same—a tablespoonful. Let come almost to a boil. Stir in a tablespoonful of yellow corn meal.

7/11/39
F. 72 yrs.
ASTHENIA **1553-15**

Q. What bulk does she require that can be disguised in food or drink?

A. We would prepare a mixture to be taken as food, in this manner: Chop together a cupful each of black figs and dates. Put this on the stove in a cupful of milk (from which the cream has not been separated). Just before it comes to a boil, stir in same two tablespoonsful of corn meal. This will not only make bulk but will be the character of bulk as a food that will act with those properties for better eliminations, and give food values of a nature most helpful for the body in the present. This quantity might be used three or four meals, and this means it might be taken once or twice a day, dependent upon the ability to get the body to take same.

6/13/44
F. 12 yrs.
DIET: SPIRITUAL **5257-1**

Q. Since babyhood, the mother has been perplexed as to what food is best for this entity. What caused this condition?

A. We haven't the physical condition, but feed the entity oft the foods which were the basis of the food of the Atlanteans and the Egyptians—corn meals with figs and dates prepared together with goat's milk.

11/29/39
F. 40 yrs.
ANEMIA **2050-1**

Then follow the regular diets that aid in eliminations. Use such as figs; or a combination of figs and dates would be an excellent diet to be taken often. Prepare same in this manner:

1 cup black or Assyrian figs, chopped, cut or ground very fine;
1 cup dates, chopped very fine;
1/2 cup yellow corn meal (NOT too finely ground).

Cook this combination in 2 or 3 cups of water until the consistency of mush. Such a dish as a part of the diet often will be as an aid to better eliminations, as well as carrying those properties that will aid in building better conditions throughout the alimentary canal.

Do these.

2/10/38
F. 25 yrs.
SPIRITUAL **275-45**

And for this special body, dates, figs (that are dried) cooked with a little corn meal (a very little sprinkled in), then this taken with milk, should be almost a spiritual food for the body; whether it's taken, one, two, three or four meals a day. But this is to be left to the body itself.

6/22/39
F. 83 yrs.
DEBILITATION: GENERAL **1907-2**

Another strengthening food for this body would be a combination prepared in this manner—that will work with the eliminations, to assist in absorbing those inclinations for the formations of gas owing to the inability of perfect mastication of most foods:

Take a cup of Black Syrian figs and a cup of dates. Seed them. Cut or grind these together. Then add half a cup of water. Let it ALMOST come to a boil. Then add a tablespoonful of yellow corn meal.

This will be almost as a gruel when fully prepared, and would be kept upon ice or in a place for the preservation of its abilities to be active without fermentation. This quantity may last for at least two days. It may be taken at each meal if so desired, and may be taken with milk or cream or without, just as is preferable to the body.

12/5/39
M. 68 yrs.
2055-1

ALCOHOLISM

An excellent food for the body of an afternoon and evening would be this combination:

1 cup Black figs, or packed figs, chopped or ground very fine;
1 cup dates, chopped or ground very fine;
1/2 cup yellow corn meal (not too finely ground).

Cook this in sufficient water (2 or 3 cups), for 15 to 20 minutes, to make it the consistency of mush.

A little of this taken each evening or night will be found to supply energies for the system that will be most helpful—especially combined with the osteopathic corrections.

12/8/39
F. Adult
1779-4

CIRCULATION: POOR
NEURITIS: TENDENCIES

To be sure, keep the eliminations in good order. An aid to this would be found in the use of a food prepared in this manner:

1 cup Black figs, chopped or ground very fine;
1 cup dates (not seeded);*
1/2 cup yellow corn meal (not too finely ground).

Cook this for twenty minutes in sufficient water (2 or 3 cups) for it to be the consistency of mush, or cook until the meal is thoroughly cooked in same. Eat a tablespoonful of this mixture of an evening, not all at once but let it be taken slowly so as to be well assimilated as it is taken. This will be most helpful for the body.

---

*Gladys Davis's note: I think the reference to dates "not seeded" means that you should use the big dates that have not been packed, and take the seeds out yourself just before preparing them.

VI

FRUIT JUICES: GENERAL

7/21/32
NERVOUS SYSTEMS: INCOORDINATION: PRURITUS **F. 81 yrs.**
BLOOD: HUMOR **5431-4**

Q. Are there parasites on the surface of the skin?

A. These are more those conditions *within* the system that *produce* these on the surface, see? If we will keep away from the fats or oils, and not have too much of the starches, but those that are well balanced more with the fruit juices that make for a form of acid and the accumulations of forces in system in fermentation of juices of fruits, nuts, vegetables and the like, these will burn *up*—as it were—those effects that are created.

3/12/36
MUSCULAR DYSTROPHY **M. 43 yrs.**
INTESTINES: GAS **1127-1**

In the diet keep to those things that cause less and less of the gas to form in the digestive system, through a very depleted or very ineffective activity of a peristaltic movement. Hence use fruit juices prepared in their own salts—these would be better for the body.

12/15/36
F. 18 yrs.
ANEMIA **1306-1**

Drink plenty of fruit juices, this preferably during the day rather than at the morning meal.

7/26/37
DEBILITATION: GENERAL **F. 60 yrs.**
TEMPERATURE: FEVER: AFTEREFFECTS **1409-4**

Since the temperature has been allayed, there is the necessity, to be sure, that there are not foods used nor activities that would tend to make for the weakening of the digestive forces, nor the allowing of activities of the assimilating system—the liver, the kidneys or the whole hepatic circulation—to become so congested as to allow the temperature to arise again.

Hence we would keep rather a tendency to the alkaline-producing foods; as fruit juices of all kinds. Quantities of these may be taken, but often rather than a great deal at once.

7/3/36
ASSIMILATIONS: ELIMINATIONS: INCOORDINATION **F. Adult**
COMBINATIONS **1197-1**

Be mindful of the diet, that there are not the combinations of starches with citrus fruit juices. These make for the use of the varied activities and cause a superacidity.

8/23/37
F. 29 yrs.
ACIDITY & ALKALINITY **528-11**

Be sure there is the inclination for the diet to be—whatever is taken—in the proportion of eighty percent alkaline-producing foods to twenty percent acid-producing. Then remember, too, the combinations in this direction as we have so oft indicated. Do not take citrus fruit juices AND cereals with milk during the same day.

ANEMIA **12/8/36**
ASSIMILATIONS: POOR **F. Adult**
TOXEMIA **1303-1**

Have plenty of the juices of fruits, as a portion of the meal; rather than so much meats—and *never* any fried meats, never any fried eggs.

1)—Apple Juice

6/1/28
ASSIMILATIONS: ELIMINATIONS: LIVER **F. 23 yrs.**
ASTHENIA: LIVER, CHOKED **288-22**

Eat that that will be easily assimilated at first, but EAT! And the juices of apples, or such are well to bring about the more normal conditions.

2)—Grape Juice

7/20/43
ARTHRITIS **M. 64 yrs.**
ASSIMILATIONS: POOR **3101-1**

Fresh grape juice, or the juice from the pressed grapes, would be well for the body to take.

This, with whatever foods the body is able to take, should relieve the tensions.

4/23/42
F. 34 yrs.
457-8

OBESITY: TENDENCIES

Q. Why should body take the grape juice?

A. To supply the sugars without gaining or making for greater weight.

Q. Does it really have a direct effect on the reduction of weight?

A. If it hadn't, would it be given?

1/19/44
F. 51 yrs.
3582-1

ASSIMILATIONS: ELIMINATIONS: INCOORDINATION

Hence we would take four times each day, about thirty minutes before each meal and before retiring, three ounces of grape juice in one ounce of plain water (not carbonated). Take this regularly for about four weeks at a time. Then leave off for two weeks and repeat.

3/8/37
F. 55 yrs.
1183-2

OBESITY

If grape juice will be taken in the evening, or just before the evening meal, with Ry-Krisp, this will be found to be not only blood building but reducing also in a consistent manner; and give strength to the vitality of the resistance forces in the body.

9/3/40
F. 52 yrs.
2067-3

ELIMINATIONS: INCOORDINATION

Four times each day, about half an hour before each meal and at bedtime, drink two ounces of grape juice (Welch's, preferably) in one ounce of plain water (not carbonated water). This will make for better assimilation, better elimination, and better conditions throughout the system.

These will bring about an eradication of many of the disturbances apparent as tendencies in the present, that arise as reflex and sympathetic conditions. We will create a better metabolism and katabolism. We will make for the better eliminations. We will find better conditions through the whole of the reactions in the physical forces of the body.

2/18/25
F. 33 yrs.
2457-1

ANEMIA

Quantities of the juices of beef may be taken, should be taken, provided small quantities of stimulant in fruit juices are taken with same, such as grape juice taken with the meat juice or beef juice.

6/27/44
F. 42 yrs.
5290-1

CHOLECYSTITIS

We would take plenty of grape juice, but systematically. This should be taken four times each day. Take the grape juice, three ounces and add one ounce of plain water. A little ice will be well. Take this half an hour before the time for the meal, and don't eat too much. Also take this one-half hour before retiring.

3/5/36
F. 38 yrs.
1045-8

TUBERCULOSIS

For strengthening internal food values we would give the juice of crushed fresh grapes; any character of grapes so long as they are not those fermented or those that have been canned. This, as we find, with little sips of the beef juice as indicated, will be the necessary nourishment in the present.

2/5/36
F. 38 yrs.
1045-6

TUBERCULOSIS

We find that the crushed grapes would still be well. Also we find that the juice of same would be most helpful to the body as a drink; but this should be taken in sips and not in gulps nor swallows.

DEBILITATION: GENERAL — **10/5/38**
OBESITY: TENDENCIES — **F. 40 yrs.**
TOXEMIA — **1657-2**

Also twice each day we would take grape juice (Welch's preferably); one ounce of the grape juice in half an ounce of water, half an hour before the meal—preferably the morning and the evening meals, especially.

With taking these, we find that the appetite will be more readily satisfied, and it will be a REDUCING nature of diet that will NOT disturb an already disturbed glandular system—and also prevent the disturbance through the throat and neck from becoming of greater consequence.

GLANDS: THYMUS: INFLAMMATION — **7/31/40**
LIVER — **F. 49 yrs.**
TEMPERATURE: FEVER — **2314-1**

We would add to the diet the fresh grape juice—the juice from fresh grapes; the purple or pink grapes preferably, instead of the white grapes. Give about half an ounce once or twice a day. Do not give other than the fresh juice, however—or the juice squeezed from fresh grapes, this is helpful; that other than from the fresh grapes would not be so good. This would add sufficient of the properties to aid in creating a better balance with those conditions which have been disturbing to the body.

10/6/42
M. Adult
2826-1

STREPTOCOCCUS

Most of the food taken should be the fresh grape juice (juice extracted from the same character of grapes as used for the poultice).

2/18/43
F. 24 yrs.
2514-11

OBESITY: TENDENCIES

Beware that the body does not become overweight. This might, of course, become an aggravating condition to the body. Use grape juice about four times a day, at least four days of the week; one ounce of grape juice (Welch's, preferably) in one and one-half ounces of plain water (not carbonated water), about thirty minutes before each meal and before retiring at night. This will keep down too much sugar, and will aid better in the eliminations through the kidneys.

5/19/44
OBESITY: TENDENCIES **F. 25 yrs.**
CIRCULATION **2514-15**

That there has been a general or great increase in the weight of the body is not too well, but if we would begin with these by the month, we may reduce the weight without injury to the recuperating forces being set up in the body. Do begin and take for a month, and leave it off for some several weeks and again try, 1/2 hour before each meal and before retiring, 3 oz. of grape juice with 1 oz. of plain water; and do not eat sweets, but more of fresh vegetables cooked and raw, and not too much of any kind of bread, though whole grain cereals may be taken and used as a supplement for bread.

With the taking of grape juice, do take these stipulated exercises as the body is able to handle itself. While the knees and heels still cause a great deal of trouble, do massage the bursae of the feet with the oil, also turn the light on them or draw the feet up under the light.

The exercise: With the body lying on the floor or the bed, take the exercise as of riding the bicycle with the feet in the air. This works the limbs and may be slow at times, but gradually raise the body from the floor on to the shoulders by getting the feet much higher than the head, see? These will change the circulation. Also do these in the morning or evening, but have a regular time, and if this is taken in the morning, then take this in the evening: stand erect, gradually rise on the toes. As the body rises on the toes, gradually raise the hands above the head, bend forward on toes. You can do very little of this at first but this will not only aid the circulation, it will aid in bringing the weight to nearer normal.

3/3/42
KIDNEYS: INFECTIONS **F. 13 yrs.**
OBESITY: TENDENCIES **2084-11**

To produce an equalization in the weight of the body, and to form the proper character of sugars in the body, we would take grape juice at least four times each day (Welch's preferably). Take two ounces of the grape juice, stirred in one ounce of plain water (NOT carbonated), about half an hour before each meal and at about the time of retiring.

Because this reduces the appetite, or the quantity of food taken, do not let this produce anxiety.

Q. Why is she inclined to be heavy for her height?

A. A glandular reaction to the sugars that must be reduced as indicated, by the forming of other characters of sugars or sweets in the body.

5/13/38
M. 47 yrs.
OBESITY: TENDENCIES **1589-1**

Before the morning and the evening meals, about half an hour before, take at least two ounces of grape juice—in one ounce of plain water; not charged water, though such as White Rock may be used in same. This will prevent the body taking on weight, and will make for nearer normal weight for the body.

If there are not too much sugars, nor too much of any drinks that are fermented, these will be the necessary combinations for the correcting of the conditions.

9/30/40
F. 74 yrs.
1224-6

OBESITY: TENDENCIES

Q. Shall I resume taking grape juice? How much, how often?

A. Two ounces with one ounce of plain water four times each day; at least thirty minutes before each meal AND at bedtime. This is the manner in which to take it.

Q. Should I reduce my weight? If so, how much and in what manner?

A. The taking of the grape juice will tend to cut down upon the sugar supplying, and thus maintain a better body ratio throughout the system.

Q. What should I do differently from the present to hasten results?

A. Just be persistent and consistent, and as we find the results will come. These are growths. It is not a hastening that is desired, but the proper corrective forces as related to bodily functionings!

5/20/39
M. 62 yrs.
1170-3

HYPERTENSION: TENDENCIES
OBESITY: TENDENCIES

Q. Is body too fat? If so, how reduce?

A. Keep away from meats, and take grape juice before the meals and at bedtime—about an ounce and a half of Welch's Grape Juice with an ounce—or not quite so much—of plain water, taken just before the meals. This will tend to keep from so much rich foods.

Doing these, we will reduce, as well as making for a more normalcy in the activities of the body. For it will reduce the excess sugar. Though this is sugar in the grape juice, it is a different character and will produce a better reaction through the alimentary canal. Do not take this just once or twice a day—take it three to four times a day, and EVERY DAY for a month! and then see the difference!

12/11/38
M. 49 yrs.
1151-19

OBESITY: TENDENCIES

Q. Any suggestions to help him reduce in weight?

A. Drink grape juice before the meal, and he won't eat near so much!

Q. About how much before each meal?

A. One-third water and the rest grape juice, or one-fourth water and the rest pure grape juice. Four to six ounces about half an hour before the meal.

Q. Three times a day?

A. Three times or even four times a day; before each meal and before retiring! Welch's is the better.

9/14/37
F. 42 yrs.
1100-17

OBESITY: TENDENCIES

Only use as drink, rather than citrus fruits even, for periods at least, the grape juice; preferably the fresh if possible—otherwise that which has no benzoate of soda as a preservative. If this is taken a pint a day—that is, at two periods, morning and evening—it will be found to work well with the body, and while keeping the physical forces down will make for the proper resistance being builded, keeping an attunement in the acidity and the activities of the system and working with the body for body building.

6/20/44
F. 48 yrs.
1100-38

OBESITY: TENDENCIES

We would also indicate that there should be more regular intervals of taking the grape juice, systematically as has been indicated. Not that the body is too heavy, but just don't get too heavy for the bettered conditions of heart, lungs, liver and kidneys.

Q. What length periods should the grape juice be taken?

A. At least for a month or six weeks. Then leave it off a while, then again after two to three weeks, take another six weeks period.

Q. Any further advice or counsel for the body at this time?

A. The attitudes, of course, as the body understands, have much to do with keeping the coordination. When there comes the disturbing conditions in mental relationships or attitudes, just don't let it upset you. Know: that which is, if used, is best.

4/4/41
M. 51 yrs.
470-32

OBESITY: TENDENCIES

As to the increase in weight—this may be controlled by the grape juice way, rather than any particular dieting; just requiring that the body refrain from too much sweets and starches.

6/14/38
M. 48 yrs.
470-21

OBESITY: TENDENCIES

If the body will use the Ry-Krisp or such mostly as the bread, and take before the evening meal at least half to an hour before, two ounces of grape juice with one ounce of carbonated water, this would materially reduce the desire for foods that tend to produce flesh.

10/30/37
M. 48 yrs.
470-19

OBESITY: TENDENCIES

10/22/37 Wife's letter: "We are both feeling fine . . . [470] will not resume the clary water (since we finally obtained the Jerusalem artichokes) unless reading says so . . . Would it be possible to ask a question in his reading? You see, the fresh grapes are beginning to run out (as given in my reading 1100-17) and I would like to know what brand of grape juice is prepared without benzoate of soda. The bottles are not marked and of course they will not tell you."

As we find, to prevent the excesses of weight for this body, we would use also the grape juice. This three-fourths grape juice to one-fourth water, or a small glass of four ounces four times a day. This taken before meals and before retiring. Unless this becomes to the body as heavy upon the system, it will be found to prove beneficial to eliminations, and prevent the use of or desire for starches or sweets; and will give the inclination for the body to keep a normal balance in weight. The Welch as we find is the preferable for this, when the fresh grapes are not available.

Ready for questions.

Q. Is the Welch grape juice prepared without benzoate of soda?

A. Prepared without benzoate of soda. Pure grape juice.

Q. Should starches and sweets be eliminated from the diet, or to what extent may they be eaten?

A. As indicated, if the grape juice is taken it supplies a sugar, the kind of sugar though that works with the system—that which is necessary, see? and then that prevents the system's desire for starches and sweets in excess. Not that these are not to be taken at all, for they supply, of course, the necessary heat units for the body in a great measure: but as these would be supplied through the taking of the grape juice, or the eating of the grapes (if they are taken AS the regular diet, and not just occasionally), there would only be the partaking of others as the appetite calls for same. When the appetite is controlled, it will govern the necessary forces in these directions.

1/22/44
F. 57 yrs.
1612-4

OBESITY: TOXEMIA

The disturbance in the eliminations, the tendency for the lack of removing the poisons and toxic forces from the body is bringing about the effects of pressures in the nerves of the locomotories.

Do continue with the use of the grape juice diet. Try this in series of taking two ounces of the Welch Grape Juice with one ounce of plain water (not carbonated) four times each day, half an hour before each meal and at bedtime. While this will reduce the activities through the appetite, it will supply sufficient sugars without adding avoirdupois.

2/20/38
F. 40 yrs.
1540-1

OBESITY

Twice a day, thirty minutes before the meal, drink at least four ounces of an equal part of grape juice and water. Welch's is preferable. This will only tend to make for the activity upon the glandular forces as related to digestion, and also the activities as related to eliminations will be materially aided.

2/13/37
F. 17 yrs.
1339-1

OBESITY

Use grape juice rather than water; and whether this be two, three, four, five glasses a day, let it be taken with half water (not carbonated water) and half pure grape juice.

Q. Please explain why she should not drink water.

A. This is to meet the needs for the particular forces and influences in the body!

Q. Any special kind of grape juice?

A. Pure grape juice; not that that's fermented.

6/4/40
F. 56 yrs.
1309-3

OBESITY

Q. Is Welch's Grape Juice preferable to Premier unsweetened?

A. If that is more desirable, use same. The Welch's, however, has more of the elements in same that aid in the reduction of the carbohydrates in the system—and thus tends to supply the food values in a way that is in keeping . . . with the purpose for taking same.

7/20/43
F. 37 yrs.
OBESITY **2988-3**

The suggestions for the diet are doing very well. Don't be impatient about losing weight too fast. There has been little or no gain in the weight.

If there will be the continuous taking of the grape juice four times each day, half an hour before each meal and before retiring, this will retard the amount necessary to be supplied for the appetites of the body and will gradually reduce the sugars.

3/24/41
F. 18 yrs.
OBESITY **1431-2**

Q. How can I reduce safely, and how much should I weigh?

A. About a hundred and fifty pounds. Reduce by the Welch Grape Juice way.

Q. Please outline the diet.

A. Eat anything you like, save potatoes and white bread. But take four glasses of Welch's Grape Juice each day—half an hour before the meals and before retiring. This would be three-quarters of a glass of the grape juice and one-quarter of plain water stirred together. Take about five to ten minutes to drink the juice each time, see?

4/10/40
F. 56 yrs.
APPETITE: OBESITY **1309-2**

Take grape juice four times each day; one ounce of plain water and three ounces of grape juice, taken half an hour before each meal and upon retiring. Then in the matter of the diet, it will almost take care of itself, and take those things the appetite calls for, save sweets, chocolate or the like; not great quantities of sugars, nor of pastries; but all other foods, vegetables or meats, provided they are not fats, may be taken according to the appetite; but we will find the appetite will change a great deal.

6/30/41
F. 62 yrs.
ASTHENIA **2521-1**

In the diet—keep strength-building foods; as fresh grape juice, sipped. Press the grapes and save the juice from same. At least an ounce to two ounces of this during the day will be most nourishing and beneficial.

8/20/43
HYPERTENSION **F. 54 yrs.**
DIABETES: TENDENCIES **3166-1**

Four times each day, about a half an hour before each meal and at bedtime, take an ounce to two ounces of grape juice stirred in one ounce of plain water (not carbonated water).

4/20/40
F. 74 yrs.
ARTHRITIS **1224-3**

Q. Is it important to reduce weight? How much and by what means?

A. As we find, the weight may be reduced some WITHOUT disturbances; and as we find, the better manner would be through the refraining from breads or greases of any kind, of course, and by the taking of grape juice—preferably the juice from fresh grapes, this prepared at the time to be taken, three times each day; taking about an ounce and a half to two ounces (diluted with a little water) half an hour before each meal. If the juice from fresh grapes is found to be impractical, then take the fresh Welch's Grape Juice.

4/16/44
M. 44 yrs.
COLITIS **5023-1**

Drink fresh grape juice often.

Thus we will find that we will bring better conditions for this body.

5/20/38
F. 68 yrs.
TOXEMIA **1593-1**

Do not add lemon or lime to grape juice . . .

3)—Pear Juice

6/1/28
ASSIMILATIONS: ELIMINATIONS: LIVER **F. 23 yrs.**
ASTHENIA: LIVER, CHOKED **288-22**

Eat that that will be easily assimilated at first, but EAT! And the juices of pears or such are well to bring about the more normal conditions.

4)—Pineapple Juice

5/1/38
F. Adult
ARTHRITIS **932-1**

Mornings—All the pineapple juice that the body may take.

12/3/35
F. 51 yrs.
OBESITY: TENDENCIES **1073-1**

As to the matter of the diets, these become naturally—with the general conditions of the body—a necessary element or influence. Do not ever take cereals *and* pineapple juices *at* the same meal. Have the cereal one day the fruit the next. For they form in the system, together, that which is not beneficial—and *especially* not helpful for this body, forming an acid that fattens the body.

3/21/39
F. 49 yrs.
RELAXATION **1158-21**

Q. Pineapple juice?

A. Once or twice a week, three to four ounces at a meal.

2/18/35
ASSIMILATIONS: POOR **M. 29 yrs.**
GLANDS: INCOORDINATION **831-1**

Mornings—Citrus fruit juices, including pineapple juice, of course without the sweetening.

2/10/38
F. 25 yrs.
OSTEOCHONDRITIS: PERTHES' DISEASE **275-45**

Q. What kind of fruit juice is best upon rising?

A. Lime may be used with a little of the pineapple. These are well, and the changing occasionally is preferable. Change these, but not too many combinations.

3/15/40
M. 45 yrs.
BODY-BUILDING **2146-1**

This has much to do with the general building up of the body. Have plenty of pineapple juice—preferably with a little lemon in same.

1/24/35
M. Child
COLD: CONGESTION **738-2**

If there will be kept a more alkaline condition in the body, the better will be the general conditions and welfare. With the cold and congestion in the present, almost an entire liquid diet would be the better. Pineapple juice (the canned pineapple is well). These are well for the body, and keeping the strength and vitality without the use of cane sugar, and ridding the system of the cold.

5/1/35
M. 1-1/2 yrs.
WORMS: PINWORMS: AFTEREFFECTS **786-2**

Be very mindful that the diets are body and blood building. Citrus fruit juices of all kinds. Pineapple juice. These are very, very good for the body. They may be taken two or three times a day, provided the body can be induced to take same.

5/20/38
F. 68 yrs.
TOXEMIA **1593-1**

Do not add lemon or lime to pineapple . . .

5)—Prune Juice

5/25/39
M. 5 mos.
BABY CARE **1788-6**

Prune juice may be given provided it is of the small prunes, rather than the "extra special," but little of the pulp with it may be given if it is well cooked and well mashed. This will tend to act with the liver, and the spleen, in making better eliminations.

6)—Citrus Juices: General

11/29/37
M. 42 yrs.
GENERAL: RHEUMATISM **1334-2**

Citrus fruit juices may be taken, and are alkaline in their reaction—UNLESS starches, as especially from cereals, are taken at the same meal. Then they become acid-producing for this body, and in ninety-nine cases out of a hundred become so for any other body!

1/26/35
F. 59 yrs.
ECZEMA **2823-3**

Mornings (this is not all to be taken, but as an outline)—Citrus fruit juices. When citrus fruits are taken, as pineapple or grapefruit, they may be taken as they are from the fresh fruit. A little salt added to same is preferable to make for the activity of same. Yes, and we mean for this body, too—*salt*—sodium chloride, see?

4/2/32
F. Child
ASTHMA **5682-2**

Mornings—Citrus fruit juices preferable to the pulp of the citrus fruits themselves, though this may be taken occasionally, and rather than adding sugar to same add pinches of salt until palatable, and preferably use the *iodized* salt in same.

11/12/35
M. 50 yrs.
ADHESIONS: LESIONS **1055-1**

In the diets, be mindful that we keep those things that add iron, silicon, and gold in the system. It may be necessary later to change some of these, but in the present let the diet consist greatly of citrus fruit juices.

3/20/35
M. Adult
ASTHMA **861-1**

Citrus fruit juices or the pulp of same, and cereals—but do not use cereals *and* citrus fruit juices at the same meal, for these produce an acid that is harmful to such reactions in the system.

3/23/40
F. 12 yrs.
EPILEPSY **2153-1**

Have plenty of the vitamins, especially of foods that carry B, B-1, A, C and D. Such would be included, of course, in plenty of citrus fruit juices.

4/24/34
ANEMIA **M. 43 yrs.**
CATARRH: NASAL **642-1**

Mornings—Citrus fruit, but do not mix this with dry cereals—either use one or the other; neither should there be any quantity of sugars with them, preferably calcium than sugar with the citrus fruits, see?

10/23/43
F. 44 yrs.
ASTHMA **3046-2**

Q. Is there some food that I eat which aggravates my condition?

A. Any sweets will aggravate the condition, or too much starches. Citrus fruit juices are better for the body—whenever there are such symptoms or tendencies.

1)—Grapefruit Juice

2/10/38
F. 25 yrs.
OSTEOCHONDRITIS: PERTHES' DISEASE **275-45**

Q. What kind of fruit juice is best upon rising?

A. Lime may be used with a little of the grapefruit. These are well and the changing occasionally is preferable. Change these, but not too many combinations.

1/4/40
M. 32 yrs.
ATROPHY: NERVES **849-47**

Have plenty (and more than has been taken!) of grapefruit and the like. These supply salts that should be had by the body. Grapefruit juice is preferable to the green fruit, and is more vitamin giving.

1/4/36
BLOOD-BUILDING **F. 22 yrs.**
MINERALS: CALCIUM DEFICIENCY **578-5**

Q. Please give in full a blood-building diet for my body.

A. Those as indicated that have a quality or an excess of the calcium, and those that will make for a balance in the iodines with the potassiums of the system itself.

Quantities then, of the grapefruit. These should form a portion of the diet at most *all* times. *Do not* combine cereals or starches of a great nature with the citrus fruit juices.

8/1/34
M. 36 yrs.
BRONCHITIS **555-4**

Let the diet be only fruit juices, principally grapefruit. And the other periods of diet would consist of vegetable juices.

And you ought to be all right in another day!

2/18/35
ASSIMILATIONS: POOR **M. 29 yrs.**
GLANDS: INCOORDINATION **831-1**

Mornings—Citrus fruit juices, including grapefruit juice or, of course, the pulp of this may be taken (preferably all should be fresh fruit).

5/1/38
F. Adult
ARTHRITIS **932-1**

Mornings—All the grapefruit juice that the body may take; or a large tumbler full of either of these each morning.

3/8/35
F. 37 yrs.
ARTHRITIS **631-6**

Mornings—Citrus fruit juices, or cereals. Grapefruit juice or the pulp and the fruit. Any of these with brown bread, whole wheat or rye, or the combination of these but all toasted.

11/8/35
ANEMIA **F. Adult**
ASSIMILATIONS: ELIMINATIONS: INCOORDINATION **1051-1**

Throughout the period be very mindful of the diets, that these are kept *tending* toward the alkaline-reaction. And we would have quantities at times of grapefruit juice.

8/27/32
F. 72 yrs.
CIRRHOSIS OF LIVER **2092-1**

Mornings—Citrus fruit juices (grapefruit juice). These will be well to be taken, even though they are used from the canned—just so they carry little of the preservatives. Libby's brand is an excellent one.

12/12/33
ACIDITY & ALKALINITY: DEBILITATION **F. 22 yrs.**
TUBERCULOSIS **418-2**

Mornings—Grapefruit juice. Do not take it when cereals are taken that milk is eaten with, though they may be altered.

3/1/41
F. Adult
ARTHRITIS: NEURITIS: TENDENCIES **838-3**

Starches and roughages should not be so much a part of the diet. Have rather those things that are alkalin-reacting even though they may be acid in themselves; such as plenty of citrus fruit juices. With the grapefruit use a little salt rather than sugar. Do not ever take these at the same meal with cereals, however, or even during the same day while such properties are working through the system.

This does not mean, of course, that these are to be the ONLY foods taken. We merely give a list of the DO'S and the DON'TS.

3/21/39
F. 49 yrs.
RELAXATION **1158-21**

Q. Grapefruit juice?

A. This may be taken each day if so desired; half a grapefruit or the juice thereof.

1/24/35
M. Child
738-2

COLD: CONGESTION

With the cold and congestion in the present, almost an entire liquid diet would be the better. Grapefruit juice, these are well for the body, and keeping the strength and vitality without the use of cane sugar, and ridding the system of the cold.

5/1/35
M. 1-1/2 yrs.
786-2

WORMS: PINWORMS: AFTEREFFECTS

Be very mindful that the diets are body and blood building. Citrus fruit juices of all kinds. Grapefruit juice, with a little salt rather than sugar in same. They may be taken two or three times a day, provided the body can be induced to take same.

5/29/34
F. 57 yrs.
1309-4

OBESITY

Q. Should I take grapefruit juice? If so, at what time of day and how much?

A. As we find, if taken occasionally—a small quantity at various times through the day, as the activities of the body are carried on—they should be helpful to the body.

8/15/38
F. 48 yrs.
1468-5

ASSIMILATIONS: POOR
NERVOUS TENSION

Grapefruit juice is most excellent for the body. As often as possible have it FRESH, and we will find it much improved.

Q. What can I do for my nerves and to overcome tenseness?

A. Take those things as we have indicated. For as outlined, when we supply the food values that with their assimilation supply the necessary—we would say—elasticity to the nerve reactions, we will find these conditions materially improved.

1/6/44
F. 44 yrs.
3525-1

OBESITY

Q. Am I allergic to citrus fruits?

A. These under the present conditions are not good. After there has been a good irrigation and the vibrations have been used for some ten days, we find that the effect of citrus fruits will be entirely different. Then don't overdo it, but these are well in the diet. It will be much better if you will add a little lemon with grapefruit—not too much, but a little. It will be much better and act much better with the body. For, many of these are hybrids, you see.

3/14/32
M. Adult
5672-1

TOXEMIA

Mornings—Coddled egg and toast; dry toast or milk toast. There may be taken fresh fruits with the toast, as grapefruit. They would be better taken as the juice than with the pulp of the fruit itself.

5/20/38
F. 68 yrs.
TOXEMIA 1593-1

Do not add lemon or lime to grapefruit . . .

2)—Lemon Juice

8/1/34
M. 36 yrs.
BRONCHITIS 555-4

Let the diet be only fruit juices, principally lemons. A little orange juice may be taken, but mix it rather with the lemon. And the other periods of diet would consist of vegetable juices.

3/21/39
F. 49 yrs.
RELAXATION 1158-21

Q. Lemon juice?
A. About once in TWO weeks; teaspoonful.

10/31/31
ANEMIA F. 60 yrs.
ASSIMILATIONS: POOR 501-2

Mornings—Citrus fruit, *principally* lemons in this diet. Lemon juices—this may be changed by the addition of water in greater or lesser quantities to suit the tastes of the body, but not with too much sugar. We would also include in this meal figs and prunes, and such—these not taken at the same period as the lemons, to be sure, but altering them from day to day.

1/4/36
BLOOD-BUILDING F. 22 yrs.
MINERALS: CALCIUM DEFICIENCY 578-5

Q. Please give in full a blood-building diet for my body.
A. Those as indicated that have a quantity or an excess of the calcium, and those that will make for a balance in the iodines with the potassiums of the system itself.

Quantities, then, of the lemon. These should form a portion of the diet at most *all* times. *Do not* combine cereals or starches of a great nature with the citrus fruit juices.

12/12/33
ACIDITY & ALKALINITY: DEBILITATION F. 22 yrs.
TUBERCULOSIS 418-2

Mornings—Lemon juice. Do not take it when cereals are taken that milk is eaten with, though they may be altered.

6/21/43
F. 24 yrs.
ACIDITY: TENDENCIES 1709-10

Q. Is lemon juice, as being taken now, helpful?
A. It is a good alkalizer. Squeeze a little lime in with it also, just two or three

drops in a full glass of the lemon juice taken. Best to mix the lemon juice with water, of course. Use half a lemon, or a full lemon to a glass of water, depending upon how soon the lemon is used after it is fully ripened or prepared for the body.

3/14/32
M. Adult
5672-1

TOXEMIA

Mornings—Coddled egg and toast; dry toast or milk toast. There may be taken fresh fruits with the toast, as lemon. They would be better taken as the juice than with the pulp of the fruit itself.

3)—Lime Juice

6/17/37
F. 29 yrs.
528-9

ACIDITY & ALKALINITY: TUBERCULOSIS

Drink plenty of citrus fruit juices of all natures. Lime with a little syrup and carbonated water would be very good, just so it is alive.

1/4/36
F. 22 yrs.
578-5

BLOOD-BUILDING
MINERALS: CALCIUM DEFICIENCY

Q. What is the cause of the wearing away of the front tooth and the crumbling of the jaw tooth? What can be done to save these teeth?

A. Drink more of lime juice, and make correction locally of those conditions existent there. Lack of proper amount of calcium in the system.

Q. Please give in full a blood-building diet for my body.

A. Those as indicated that have a quantity or an excess of the calcium, and those that will make for a balance in the iodines with the potassiums of the system itself.

Quantities, then, of the lime, these should form a portion of the diet at most *all* times. *Do not* combine cereals or starches of a great nature with the citrus fruit juices.

4)—Orange Juice

6/3/28
F. 2 yrs.
608-5

COLITIS

As for the diet—little orange juice occasionally will not be harmful. No apple or fruits of other characters, though, may be used as yet. These, as we find, would bring the normal forces—reducing the conditions in system.

8/23/43
F. 42 yrs.
3173-1

LOCOMOTION: IMPAIRED

We would also take into the system extra quantities of vitamins D—B and B-1. These may be had in orange juice.

11/8/35
F. Adult
1051-1

ANEMIA
ASSIMILATIONS: ELIMINATIONS: INCOORDINATION

Throughout the period be very mindful of the diets, that these are kept *tending* toward the alkaline-reaction. And we would have quantities at times of orange juice.

9/19/40
M. 33 yrs.
849-53

ARTHRITIS

In the matter of the diet—do not keep just ONE thing. It is necessary that each day there be plenty of liquids, both in the diet and in the quantity of water taken. Take the orange juices—AND if practical drink at least a pint or more each day!

1/4/36
F. 22 yrs.
578-5

BLOOD-BUILDING
MINERALS: CALCIUM DEFICIENCY

Q. What is the cause of the wearing away of the front tooth and the crumbling of the jaw tooth? What can be done to save these teeth?

A. Drink more of orange juice, and make correction locally of those conditions existent there. Lack of proper amount of calcium in the system.

Q. Please give in full a blood-building diet for my body.

A. Those as indicated that have a quantity or an excess of the calcium, and those that will make for a balance in the iodines with the potassiums of the system itself.

Quantities, then, of the orange. These should form a portion of the diet at most *all* times. *Do not* combine cereals or starches of a great nature with the citrus fruit juices.

12/10/36
F. 28 yrs.
1102-2

ANEMIA

Do not take this as the first or the morning meal, but during the day—*each* day for a week at a time, then leave off a week at a time—drink a *quart* (full quart) of orange juice! This may be taken two or three times during the day, but preferably *not* at a meal time, nor after or before cereals—rather after the vegetable meal, or preferably in the middle of the morning or afternoon, between the meals drink the orange juice—and preferably the Florida orange.

5/4/41
M. 14 yrs.
2488-2

ANEMIA

Give all the orange juice that the body will assimilate. These are best given from the fruit itself, that is, in the food, than by injections or the formations of vitamins that said to be of the same nature.

12/12/28
F. 48 yrs.
569-18

ACIDITY

Fruits that are non-acid producing as orange juice are good.

7/23/40
F. 37 yrs.
ACIDITY **2310-1**

Occasionally have orange juice for the morning meal, but this not oftener than once a week—and then not at the same meal with the cereal. This will not be found most advantageous (the orange juice) except occasionally.

10/14/35
M. 17 yrs.
GLANDS: INCOORDINATION: HYPOTHYROIDISM **1078-1**

Take sufficient amount of the carbohydrates or sugars, but these are more preferable to be taken in the quantities of orange juice (that is, supplied in that manner). For at least twice a day there should be a small glass of orange juice taken—before the morning meal and before retiring, a small glass of four to four and a half ounces. Take same for two to three weeks in straight succession each day. Then rest from same for a period, and then take again.

6/1/28
ASSIMILATIONS: ELIMINATIONS: LIVER **F. 23 yrs.**
ASTHENIA: LIVER, CHOKED **288-22**

The juices of oranges are well to bring about the more normal conditions. Be consistent, persistent, and *act*. There is as much of the necessity of filling the system, of the weight in the same and its activity, as of any activity for the body, see? Just keep 'em well balanced!

5/1/38
F. Adult
ARTHRITIS **932-1**

Mornings—All the orange juice that the body may take; or a large tumber full of either of these each morning.

8/27/32
F. 72 yrs.
CIRRHOSIS OF LIVER **2092-1**

Mornings—Citrus fruit juices (oranges). These will be well to be taken, even though they are used from the canned—just so they carry little of the preservatives. Libby's brand is an excellent one.

11/16/36
BLOOD: COAGULATION: POOR **F. 41 yrs.**
BODY-BUILDING **1100-8**

In the diet include those foods that are blood- and body-building, that carry iron in such manners as may be assimilated by the body. Plenty of orange juice, citrus fruit juices of all kinds. Preferably the orange juice would be with one-third lemon, but this taken for this body in the afternoon would be preferable.

Q. How can the bodily resistance be kept up, especially during the winter months?

A. By following those suggestions that have just been indicated, we find we may build resistances for this body, through the periods of sudden changes or distresses that may come from sudden changes to the bodily temperature.

2/25/41
F. 51 yrs.
DIABETES: TENDENCIES **454-8**

Q. What foods should she eat daily?

A. Those that are easily assimilated; less acid-producing, though plenty of orange juices and FRUITS of all kinds.

6/14/35
F. Adult
GLANDS: INCOORDINATION **935-1**

As to the DIET: We would have quantities each day of *orange* juice. There should be at least two full glasses of same taken each day; mornings the first thing, and in the evenings just before retiring. Do not *gulp* same but drink very slowly, so that this may be assimilated by the system without upsetting the body too much. Take five to ten minutes or more to drink same.

12/12/33
ACIDITY & ALKALINITY: DEBILITATION **F. 22 yrs**
TUBERCULOSIS **418-2**

Mornings—Orange juice. Do not take it when cereals are taken that milk is eaten with, though they may be altered.

10/17/27
M. 8 mos.
BABY CARE **5520-2**

Q. Can he take orange juice? If so, how diluted?

A. Diluted nearly half and half. Use boiled water, however.

8/15/25
COLITIS **F. 6 yrs.**
MALARIA: TENDENCIES **4281-6**

Orange juice may be given in small quantities as tonic.

3/10/41
M. 18 yrs.
LEUKEMIA **2456-2**

Each day include as much orange juice as may be easily assimilated by the body; preferably the Florida grown and tree-ripened fruit. These elements will—in assimilation—induce or produce red blood.

2/18/25
F. 33 yrs.
ANEMIA **2457-1**

Quantities of the juices of beef may be taken, *should* be taken, provided small quantities of stimulant in fruit juices are taken with same, such as orange taken with the meat juice or beef juice.

6/27/41
F. 18 yrs.
ANEMIA **1207-2**

Have the regular foods; those that carry quantities, or an excess, of vitamin B-1, especially such as would be found in all foods that are yellow in nature or color. Have plenty of orange juices, then, throughout the day. There should be excesses of these in the diet, though—to be sure—other foods would be taken normally.

2/10/38
F. 25 yrs.
SPIRITUAL **275-45**

Q. What kind of fruit juice is best upon rising?

A. When orange juice is taken, always take a little lemon juice with same. Change these, but not too many combinations. These are well, and the changing occasionally is preferable.

6/18/37
F. 22 yrs.
ASSIMILATIONS: POOR: ANEMIA **667-8**

Oranges should be used. However, do not take the orange juice *and* the cereal at the same meal or even the same day! A whole quart of orange juice taken at once (not swallowed at once but taken at the one sitting) would be well. This, of course, for the body would be impractical, but a whole glassful, at least, should be taken for a meal.

5/29/34
F. 57 yrs.
OBESITY **1309-4**

Q. Should I take orange juice? If so, at what time of day and how much?

A. As we find, if taken occasionally—a small quantity at various times—through the day, as the activities of the body are carried on—they should be helpful to the body.

3/14/32
M. Adult
TOXEMIA **5672-1**

Mornings—Coddled egg and toast; dry toast or milk toast. There may be taken fresh fruits with the toast, as oranges. They would be better taken as the juice than with the pulp of the fruit itself.

7/16/40
BABY CARE **M. 8 mos.**
COLD: CONGESTION **2299-2**

Orange juice *weakened* may be given once a day. Do not give same at the same feedings with the oatmeal! This should be tested for the quantity and as to how often given.

6/6/38
COLD: CONGESTION **F. 41 yrs.**
TEMPERATURE: FEVER **459-9**

Now as we find, there needs to be precautions taken as to the overtaxation and the UNBALANCING of the diet as related to the weaknesses produced by the temperature and the infectious forces through the system.

Take plenty of those things that are body and blood building. Plenty of citrus fruit juices, especially orange juice. If a pint is taken EVERY day it will be MOST beneficial for the body; though the same amount might be taken morning and evening and still not be too much. However, do not take cereals within several hours of any citrus fruit juices.

VII

Fruit Juice Diets

1)—Grapefruit Juice & Grapes

7/9/34
F. 54 yrs.
RHEUMATISM **133-3**

Then, in meeting the needs in the present we would find that we would first give an outline to prepare the body; for later—as we will find—it will be necessary to change the order of those things that would be applied for the corrections to be *permanent;* for the effects, as well as some portion of the causes, must be attended to first. First, then:

For at least three to five days, let the diet be only grapefruit juice and grapes.

Q. Should the grapefruit juice and grapes be taken at the same time?

A. No! One at one time, one at the other. But eat quantities of grapes—whether two, three, four, five or ten *pounds,* even!

Q. Any special kind?

A. Those that may be obtained at any place at present.

2)—Grapefruit & Grape Juice

8/28/41
M. 56 yrs.
OBESITY: TENDENCIES **619-10**

Also for this body we find that the grape juice and grapefruit diets would be beneficial.

Take two ounces of grape juice (Welch's preferably, unless fresh grapes are used) stirred in one ounce of plain water (not carbonated water), half an hour before each meal and at bedtime.

The grapefruit juice should be a drink taken once or twice each day, about two or three ounces.

5/4/41
BURSITIS: TENDENCIES **M. 52 yrs.**
KATABOLISM: METABOLISM: INCOORDINATION **1151-28**

If there is the desire to keep the weight normal, take grapefruit juice and grape juice combined—rather than just the grape juice in water, see? To two ounces and a half of pure grape juice add half an ounce of grapefruit juice. Take this four times each day (before meals and at bedtime) for five days, leave off five days, take again for five days, and so on. This should keep a normal balance.

3)—Orange & Grape Juice

9/28/35
F. 18 yrs.
PERITONITIS: AFTEREFFECTS **852-8**

We would continue at times to give orange juice with the *fresh* grape juice. This will be nourishing.

4)—Orange Juice & Grapefruit, Lemon or Lime Juice

9/27/37
F. Adult
DEBILITATION: GENERAL **1419-5**

Mornings—Alternate between these various things; not all of them at once but one day one, and another day the next, dependent upon the tastes of the body and their reaction with the body: Orange juice about a glassful, with half a lemon in same at one time and at another time half a lime; at another time half of the orange juice and half of the grapefruit juice. The fresh fruit of all of these is preferable.

1/26/35
F. 59 yrs.
INJURIES **3823-2**

Hence we would use those foods that carry in a soluble manner that which may be absorbed and become replenishing or rebuilding for the blood; or the calciums, irons, glutens that make for the urea. We would use principally an alkaline-reacting diet.

Mornings—Citrus fruit juices; orange juice and lemon juice combined.

4/19/41
F. 51 yrs.
ASSIMILATIONS **1158-30**

Q. Shall I supplement with additional vitamin B tablets?

A. We find that if this vitamin is supplied in the diet it will be better than taking an overquantity of vitamin B, which would be the case if the tablets were taken as a supplement. With the Adiron taken, that is to aid in assimilation, it would be better to supplement the vitamin B in the diet, with such as: Orange juice with a little lemon in it, these taken, as we find, with beef and fowl, should carry sufficient vitamins.

5/25/39
M. 5 mos.
BABY CARE **1788-6**

There are indicated those inclinations for regurgitation, as has been seen; that is, the body spits up its food—and the citrus fruit—as we have indicated—does not at all times agree.

As we find, do not attempt to give too much of the citrus fruits even yet. Do not give these on days that cereals are prepared for the body, which as we find are necessary.

And when the orange juice is given, preferably use the Florida rather than the California oranges; and mix a little lemon with same. This should not be any large quantity, but just—as it were—a few drops—say ten drops, from a quarter of a lemon, squeezed into half a glass of orange juice. At other times try it with the lime. These in their activity one with another, when well stirred together, will be found to be most beneficial in aiding the body not only to retain same but to gain from same. Don't give him too much at once. On the days that it is given, give it rather often than too much at a time.

5/6/40
F. 27 yrs.
COLD: COMMON: SUSCEPTIBILITY **2186-1**

Here we find that citrus fruit juices in quantities, regularly, will be helpful. Drink at least a pint of orange juice, with the juice of half a lemon squeezed into same, each day; for periods of ten days—then leave off for a period of ten days, and then take again for another ten days, and so on.

1/6/44
F. 44 yrs.
OBESITY **3585-1**

Q. Am I allergic to citrus fruits?

A. These under the present conditions are not good. After there has been a good irrigation and the vibrations have been used for some ten days, we find that the effect of citrus fruits will be entirely different. Then don't overdo it, but these are well in the diet. It will be much better if you will add a little lime with the orange juice. It will be much better and act much better with the body. For, many of these are hybrids, you see.

3/21/39
F. 49 yrs.
RELAXATION **1158-21**

Q. Orange juice?

A. This is better mixed with the lemon, or the lemon mixed with the orange juice—and this taken once or twice a week. But do not take ANY of these so they become routine! Let the appetite call for them, rather than expecting these to fill the appetite.

5/1/35
M. 1-1/2 yrs.
WORMS: PINWORMS: AFTEREFFECTS **786-2**

Be very mindful that the diets are body and blood building. Citrus fruit juices of all kinds. Orange juice with a little lemon in same, four or five parts orange juice to one part lemon or lime juice. These are very, very good for the body. They may be taken two or three times a day, provided the body can be induced to take same.

1/24/35
M. Child
COLD: CONGESTION **738-2**

Mr. Cayce: Yes, we have the body; this we have had before. As we find, there are decided changes for the better in the physical functioning of this body. We find that there are disorders as related to the cold and congestion. If there will be kept a more alkaline condition in the body, the better will be the general conditions and welfare. With the cold and congestion in the present, almost an entire liquid diet would be the better—and the greater portion of it orange juice and lemon juice combined, three parts of the orange juice to one part of the lemon.

Q. What should be done for the fever?

A. It may be reduced by the use of the fluids, or the non-acid fluids in the food.

3/15/40
M. 45 yrs.
BODY-BUILDING **2146-1**

This has much to do with the general building up of the body. Have plenty of citrus fruit juices, but do not attempt to take orange juice alone—always put a little lemon in same. These are preferable with a little lemon in same.

8/31/41
ARTHRITIS: PREVENTIVE **F. 51 yrs.**
BODY: GENERAL **1158-31**

Q. Orange juice with lemon?

A. Once to twice to three times a week.

3/1/41
F. Adult
ARTHRITIS: NEURITIS: TENDENCIES **838-3**

Starches and roughages should not be so much a part of the diet. Have rather those things that are alkaline-reacting, even though they may be acid in themselves; such as plenty of citrus fruit juices. With the orange juice put a little lemon. We would combine these in this manner. Do not ever take any of these at the same meal with cereals, however, or even during the same day while such properties are working through the system.

This does not mean, of course, that these are to be the ONLY foods taken. We merely give a list of the DO'S and the DON'TS.

4/27/35
F. 39 yrs.
908-1

ASSIMILATIONS: ELIMINATIONS: INCOORDINATION
NEURITIS

Now, these things are just the beginning, you see; they will have to be changed. For we must get the poisons *out* of the system—that have been infected into the system—or that have grown in the system from the bad activity of the circulation, before we can *begin* to build the body up!

As to the diet during this period, let it be on this order!

Mornings—Citrus fruit juices; combining lime or lemon with the orange juice—four parts orange juice to one part lime or lemon. At the same meal there may be taken whole wheat or brown toast, with a little butter if so desired, but only brown bread—and this doesn't mean white bread just browned!

3/8/35
F. 37 yrs.
631-6

ARTHRITIS

Mornings—Citrus fruit juices, or cereals. When the fruit juices or citrus fruit juices are taken, mix lemon *with* the orange juice—a teaspoonful of lemon juice to a glass of orange juice for this body. Any of these with brown bread, whole wheat or rye, or the combination of these but all toasted. A little butter may be taken with the brown bread.

4/2/39
F. 38 yrs.
1857-1

CHOLECYSTITIS

With orange juice always add a little lemon with same; this will act much better with the system.

11/19/43
F. 66 yrs.
3412-1

ELIMINATIONS: POOR

Do not take orange juice without lemon or lime juice in same, and this will keep down those tendencies for the formations of gas through the alimentary canal.

11/3/43
F. 54 yrs.
3337-1

MULTIPLE SCLEROSIS

Do add as much as may possibly be assimilated of the B vitamins, A and D vitamins. We find that these may be best supplied by quantities of citrus fruit juice—especially oranges with a little lemon juice squeezed in same. Take these often.

2/18/35
M. 29 yrs.
831-1

ASSIMILATIONS: POOR
GLANDS: INCOORDINATION

Mornings—Citrus fruit juices, including orange juice with lemon juice in same; this should be fresh fruit.

5)—Orange Juice Diet

2/15/39
ACIDITY **F. 41 yrs.**
ASSIMILATIONS: ELIMINATIONS: INCOORDINATION **1713-21**

There may be the use of citrus fruit juices in quantities; but this would necessitate, then, that there be not too great an activity, and that nothing else be taken but the citrus fruit for five days. This would include only oranges, or oranges with lemons—no other foods—for five days. Just how many? As many as the body wants to take!

On the evening of the last day of such a diet—take half a teacup of olive oil. This would cleanse the system from the impurities, preventing the inclinations for gas formation and for this regurgitation that is taking place in the lower portion of the duodenum.

VIII

GRAINS

1)—Breads, Cakes & Crackers

1)—Bread: General

7/16/35
F. 64 yrs.
ARTHRITIS **950-1**

In the middle of the afternoon we would take half a wine glass of *red* wine, with black or rye bread—preferably the very heavy or sour bread. (Yes, the entity's family used to make bread—not in this country, though.)

7/22/31
ACIDITY **F. 28 yrs.**
ASSIMILATIONS: ELIMINATIONS: INCOORDINATION **2261-1**

Those of bread—keep those that are of the whole wheat or those of the rye, or those of the nature that are easily assimilated, and we will find in two to three months a normal body, with the proper weight, proper adjustments, and feeling better, and a removal of those pains that come at times through the stomach as well as those under the shoulder blades.

4/2/38
F. 54 yrs.
ACIDITY & ALKALINITY **1563-1**

No fried foods at any time, not even fried cakes—though corn bread and whole wheat bread may be taken.

2/18/35
ASSIMILATIONS: POOR **M. 29 yrs.**
GLANDS: INCOORDINATION **831-1**

Evenings—Never too much starches. All breads taken at all of the meals should preferably be browned whole wheat or rye or of such natures.

12/22/42
ARTHRITIS **M. 34 yrs.**
VITAMINS: B-1: GENERAL **849-62**

DO keep up ALL foods that carry B-1 especially, the exercise or energy vitamin. These are found in the breads, of course, and especially sunshine—which may be just as valuable as a means or manner of obtaining same, when practical. Even eat IN the sunshine when practical—all foods.

Q. Is the diet all right?

A. As indicated, hold closer to the B-1 products and vitamins. Don't take them separate. For these are not as well assimilated and DO cause disturbances in other directions at times.

10/11/38
CYSTITIS: TENDENCIES **F. 35 yrs.**
ACIDITY & ALKALINITY **540-11**

Not great quantities ever of white bread, but rather use rye or whole wheat or the like—these are the more preferable.

2/24/32
M. 44 yrs.
ELIMINATIONS: INCOORDINATION **437-4**

Little or no bread, unless it is of the whole wheat, or such as the rye—or a combination of same as of the Swedish or that that is blessed in the making—of the Jewish whole wheat (Kosher bread).

6/17/41
NERVOUS TENSION **F. 26 yrs.**
RHEUMATISM **2517-1**

As to the diet throughout the period—keep close to those foods that will supply the greater quantity of B-1 vitamin.

The bread should be made with the reconditioned or revitalized flour, so that the phosphorus, iron and vitamins are all in same.

12/6/43
COLD: CONGESTION: PELVIC DISORDERS **F. 15 yrs.**
BODY-BUILDING **2084-15**

Q. Any changes in her diet other than these vitamins?

A. No great changes in diet, except don't get too much fats for the body. Don't have too much starches. Brown bread, and such foods are better for the body.

8/11/44
M. 55 yrs.
HEART: ENGORGED **1151-32**

Q. What starches?

A. Brown bread, not any white bread ever, nor any macaroni. The rest we would find in moderation would be very good.

1/6/42
HEMORRHOIDS M. 57 yrs.
INTESTINES: COLON: PROLAPSUS 462-14

Q. Please give me the foods I should eat at breakfast.

A. Crisp bacon, toast—or the salt or whole wheat bread.

10/30/37
M. 48 yrs.
DIABETES: TENDENCIES 470-19

But in the breads, of course the whole wheat, rye or the sour breads are preferable.

7/21/44
F. 60 yrs.
CANCER: LUNGS 5374-1

Not too large a quantity of starches; then, no white bread. The dark breads or what may be called pumpernickel or rye or whole wheat are well for the body.

1/7/37
CIRCULATION: POOR F. 44 yrs.
ELIMINATIONS: POOR 1315-6

Q. Does pumpernickel bread contain starch or anything that is bad for me?

A. Pumpernickel is of many varied characters or kinds. That which is properly made pumpernickel is *very* good for the body. But we would find rye bread or Ry-Krisp as a better bread than too much pumpernickel—as has been mostly used by the body.

7/8/44
F. 32 yrs.
ARTHRITIS 5331-1

Then, these are the don'ts: Don't have too much starches, don't have too great quantity of the combinations of sweets and starches together; thus cake, pastries or that nature eliminate while honey or corn syrup or Karo syrup would be very well in its proper proportions and at the right periods. These may be taken with corn bread or the like, but not white bread. Whole wheat bread might be very well.

i)—Corn Bread

4/30/40
ASSIMILATIONS: POOR M. 49 yrs.
CIRCULATION: LYMPH 2183-1

Each day throughout the afternoon, for instance, we would have vegetable juices with corn bread put in same.

4/28/43
F. 36 yrs.
ELIMINATIONS: POOR 2977-1

Corn cakes, corn bread would be good; provided sweets are not eaten with same.

8/11/36
M. 68 yrs.
ACIDITY **1245-1**

Do not eat white bread but corn bread—this preferably made with either plain hot water or with egg.

Not too much of sugars, but honey as sweets is very good and will be found to agree with the body—especially honey in the honeycomb, with corn bread.

11/20/25
M. Adult
ASSIMILATIONS: ELIMINATIONS: INCOORDINATION **4891-1**

No corn cakes or corn bread of any kind.

10/21/36
COLD: COMMON: SUSCEPTIBILITY **F. 41 yrs.**
BODY-BUILDING **1100-7**

Be mindful that in the rest of the diet it is kept close to the alkaline or twenty percent acid-producing to eighty percent alkaline-producing food values.

Plenty of corn bread, in whatever way prepared. The scalded or the egg bread. This with the meal cakes even of a morning. Honey as a carrier with same or to eat with same is very good.

ii)—Whole Wheat Bread

9/18/37
M. 17 yrs.
ASSIMILATIONS: ELIMINATIONS: INCOORDINATION **984-2**

Q. Will you please give a recipe for a perfect loaf of whole wheat bread made with the flour ground by local farmers, some of which I hold in my hand. Is this flour better than the commercial kind?

A. This as we find is better combined somewhat with the white flour. The proportions would be three-fourths of the whole wheat to one-fourth of the white; and the shortening or the activities of the seasoning to suit the taste.

7/30/36
ATTITUDES & EMOTIONS: WORRY: GENERAL **M. 30 yrs.**
COMBINATIONS **416-9**

Then, do not combine also the reacting acid fruits with starches, other than *whole wheat bread!* that is, citrus fruits.

7/16/35
F. 64 yrs.
ARTHRITIS **950-1**

Evenings—Always the breads should be toasted, and of the whole wheat variety.

12/29/41
M. 40 yrs.
ASSIMILATIONS: POOR **826-14**

The administering of the active forces through or in the body, by the chemical lack, rather than through the proper assimilation of the vitamins necessary, has tended—with the activities of the mind over same—to clog the system, rather than being assimilated by the system.

Thus the lacking elements of B-1 (or thiamine), and the acids that are a combination of B-1, G and D, have NOT been assimilated from the chemical standpoint. And the diet not being balanced caused the tiredness, the upsetting in the vital energies of the body; headaches, eyes tired, the trembly feelings through the body. All of these have come from this CONFUSION in the assimilating system.

As we find, the diets that bring a normal amount of the vitamins especially A, D, B-1, G and K may be had in the *proper* consideration of foods, rather than chemicals.

Hence, quantities of bread—as the whole wheat—is not sufficient in its supply. Though supplying B-1 sufficiently, it overclogs the system and causes a lack of reaction in the colon area; thus forming gases when this is attempted to be supplied by this means alone.

With this combine citrus fruits, though not at the same time.

8/23/37
SCLERODERMA **F. 29 yrs.**
TUBERCULOSIS **528-11**

Do not eat white bread, white potatoes and spaghetti during the same day; any one of these may be used—but preferably the whole wheat bread.

iii)—White Bread

2/27/35
M. 26 yrs.
EPILEPSY **567-7**

Never include any white bread . . . or any of the starchy elements for these tend to make for a slowing up of the conditions in the system.

5/30/36
ASSIMILATIONS: ELIMINATIONS: INCOORDINATION **M. 47 yrs.**
CIRCULATION: IMPAIRED **1151-2**

An eighty percent alkaline-reacting to a twenty percent acid-reacting diet would be preferable. The variations of same under the activities of the body at times makes this rather disturbing. But these are those things to be warned against, then otherwise there may be kept a near normal diet:

Not white bread and potatoes at the same meal. Not quantities of sweets *with* white bread. The meats and sweets should be preferably taken at the same meal. It isn't so much *what* the body eats as it is the *combinations* that are taken at times. Beware then of those things.

7/19/43
F. 33 yrs.
ARTHRITIS **3134-1**

The body should not take white bread. These should be barred from the diet.

8/25/39
F. 39 yrs.
TOXEMIA **1985-1**

Refrain from those foods that produce alcohol. We do not mean so much the combinations of the alcohol, but those things that produce an alcohol reaction in the system; such as those combinations of white bread with spaghetti or potatoes or macaroni or cheeses—no two of these at the same meal.

4/18/32
F. 61 yrs.
VITAMINS: D **658-11**

Q. How much bread is it necessary for a child four years old to eat a day to obtain the correct amount of vitamin D?

A. This, to be sure, depends upon the activities of the body, that which is lacking in its system, and what character of foods other than bread, if any, are taken. Ordinarily, six ounces is sufficient.

Q. What highest authorities absolutely guarantee to my family that every sunshine vitamin D claim made for Bond Bread is absolutely true?

A. Scientific research; notably Pediatric Foundation, supplemented by Steenbock patents.

Q. What changes in civilization cause us to be unlikely to get enough sunshine vitamin D as nature originally intended?

A. The tendency to have less sunshine activity, or less activity in the sunshine, and the taking of more foods that are not close to nature.

Q. Why does my table provide plenty of all other vitamins, yet fail to provide enough vitamin D unless Bond Bread is used?

A. Sufficient vitamins are found in the green vegetables that may be easily procured, but these lack that necessary sunshine vitamin D in their preparation or make-up; that is provided more safely, more certainly, in Bond Bread.

Q. Why do the members of my family absolutely need a constant and plentiful supply of sunshine vitamin D, especially right now?

A. The lack of sunshine at the present season, the necessity for the structural portions or frame portions of the body. These add, or this vitamin adds, to that necessary element in the structural building of the body, that is lacking when sunshine is not as plentiful, as at the present season.

Q. How does sunshine vitamin D help to insure better teeth, stronger bones, and the general well-being of my family?

A. Adding those necessary elements for the building, especially, of those structural portions of the body.

11/8/34
DEBILITATION: GENERAL **F. 12 yrs.**
BODY-BUILDING **632-6**

In the diet, beware of too much starches of *any* kind—that is do *not* include white bread or anything of this nature.

2)—Cakes

i)—Buckwheat Cakes

7/10/30
M. 65 yrs.
BLOOD-BUILDING: ASSIMILATIONS **4806-1**

We would be mindful of the diet, that there are those of the full rebuilding—especially of those that build for the blood supply.

Plenty of the citrus fruits—especially mornings. Alter these occasionally with buckwheat cakes, with a very *nominal* amount of syrup—but the syrup should be of the pure character, or *preferably* that of the honey in the honeycomb, of the fresh variety.

10/4/33
DERMATITIS: TOXEMIA **M. Adult**
ASSIMILATIONS: ELIMINATIONS: INCOORDINATION **463-1**

Be mindful that the diet contains little or no meats of any character. A diet easily assimilated, and that is nerve and blood building; hence carrying iron and silicon would be the better, and the foods carrying phosphorus and iodine would be the more helpful for the body. Not too much proteins or starch, but those that are more of the mineralized reactions.

Mornings—At times there may be taken buckwheat cakes or the like, but these should not be taken with any great quantity of syrup; though butter and honey may be used.

12/30/42
M. 21 yrs.
BODY-BUILDING: LOCOMOTION: IMPAIRED **2873-1**

The food values should be those well balanced with calcium, iron, and especially the vitamins B-1 and the B-Complex. These are much preferable for the body.

At least three times each week, then, supply these from the foods rather than the reinforced vitamins (though these reinforcements may be desirable if there is the inability of the body to assimilate foods that carry excesses of the full quantity of such vital forces).

These should include then such foods as these as an outline; though, to be sure, these are not all the foods that are to be taken:

Mornings—Buckwheat cakes, or the like, or cereals that are reinforced.

ACIDITY
ANEMIA **10/3/40**
COLD: COMMON: SUSCEPTIBILITY **F. 19 yrs.**
BODY-BUILDING **2374-1**

Mornings—Either cooked or dry cereal. Follow these at times with such as buckwheat cakes and honey (not syrup), milk, and plenty of butter.

Do these, and as we find we will bring bettered conditions for this body; not only making for the corrections but improving the vitality, the strength, and increasing the weight.

4/29/38
F. 77 yrs.
TOXEMIA **1586-1**

Do not eat fried foods of any kinds, nor cakes—though buckwheat cakes may be taken if they are fried in butter and then NOT any butter used on same, but these should not be eaten with syrup. Honey—a little may be taken if so desired.

8/12/40
F. 33 yrs.
ANEMIA: DIGESTION: INDIGESTION **2320-1**

If there is the desire for sweets, use only honey—and preferably in the honeycomb. This may be taken a little with buckwheat cakes.

7/8/44
F. 32 yrs.
ARTHRITIS **5331-1**

Then, these are the don'ts: Don't have too much starches, don't have too great quantity of the combinations of sweets and starches together; thus cake, pastries or that nature eliminate while honey or corn syrup or Karo syrup would be very well in its proper proportions and at the right periods. These may be taken with buckwheat cakes.

9/28/41
CONSTIPATION **M. 8 yrs.**
ASSIMILATIONS: POOR **2595-1**

Mornings—Take all the citrus fruit juices the body may assimilate. These may be varied. If possible take buckwheat cakes, that may be taken with Karo—and milk if desired. Occasionally have with these some bacon, very crisp. A little of these should be taken, but they may be altered or changed about.

ii)—Corn Cakes

12/11/38
F. 13 yrs.
GLANDS: INCOORDINATION **1206.-9**

Little or no fried foods should be in the diet, though of course cakes—as buckwheat, may be a part of the diet.

12/11/38
F. 13 yrs.
GLANDS: INCOORDINATION **1206-9**

Little or no fried foods should be in the diet, though of course cakes—as corn cakes may be a part of the diet.

7/30/40
F. Adult
OBESITY **2315-1**

Each meal should be preceeded by the grape juice—thirty minutes before eating.

Mornings—Corn cakes may be taken with a little honey or the like.

8/12/40
F. 33 yrs.
ANEMIA: DIGESTION: INDIGESTION **2320-1**

If there is the desire for sweets, use only honey—and preferably in the honeycomb. This may be taken a little with corn cakes.

iii)—Rice Cakes

12/6/43
COLD: CONGESTION: PELVIC DISORDERS **F. 15 yrs.**
BODY-BUILDING **2084-15**

Q. Any changes in her diet other than these vitamins?

A. No great changes in diet, except don't get too much fats for the body. Don't have too much starches. Rice bread, rice cakes, and such foods as have been indicated are better for the body.

12/30/42
M. 21 yrs.
BODY-BUILDING: LOCOMOTIVE: IMPAIRED **2873-1**

The food values should be those fully well balanced with calcium, iron, and especially the vitamins B-1 and the B-Complex. These are much preferable for the body.

At least three times each week, then, supply these from the foods rather than the reinforced vitamins (though these reinforcements may be desirable if there is the inability of the body to assimilate foods that carry excesses or the full quantity of such vital forces).

These should include, then, such foods as these as an outline; though, to be sure, these are not all the foods that are to be taken:

Mornings—Rice cakes or the like.

2/10/30
M. 41 yrs.
LACERATIONS: STOMACH **5545-1**

Occasionally there may be taken rice cakes, with honey—but the honey should *not* be other than that *with* the honeycomb. Not strained honey.

iv)—Rice Flour Cakes

9/28/41
CONSTIPATION **M. 8 yrs.**
ASSIMILATIONS: POOR **2595-1**

Mornings—Take all the citrus fruit juices the body may assimilate. These may be varied. If possible take rice flour cakes, that may be taken with Karo; and milk if desired. Occasionally have with these some bacon, very crisp. A little of these should be taken, but they may be altered or changed about.

v)—Whole Wheat Cakes

7/10/30
M. 65 yrs.
BLOOD-BUILDING: MENU: ASSIMILATIONS **4806-1**

We would be mindful of the diet, that there are those of the full rebuilding—especially of those that build for the blood supply.

Plenty of the citrus fruits—especially mornings. Alter those occasionally with whole wheat cakes, with a very *nominal* amount of syrup—but the syrup should be of the pure character, or *preferably* that of the honey in the honey-comb, of the fresh variety.

12/11/38
F. 13 yrs.
GLANDS: INCOORDINATION **1206-9**

Little or no fried foods should be in the diet, though of course cakes—as whole wheat may be a part of the diet.

7/30/40
F. Adult
OBESITY **2315-1**

Each meal should be preceeded by the grape juice—thirty minutes before eating.

Mornings—Wheat cakes may be taken with a little honey or the like.

8/13/30
M. 42 yrs.
DEBILITATION: GENERAL **2335-1**

Whole wheat glutens, or whole wheat flour, whole wheat muffins or cakes. These also should be a portion of the diet.

3)—Crackers

i)—Ry-Krisp

DEBILITATION: GENERAL **10/5/38**
TOXEMIA **F. 40 yrs.**
OBESITY: TENDENCIES **1657-2**

It is indicated that there are not the best eliminations; that there is too much of acid foods taken, or the "breaking over" owing to the demands of the appetite because of the glandular activities—and these should be noticed, or precautions taken as to same.

As we find, then:

We would use only such as Ry-Krisp as bread or ALWAYS using toasted whole wheat bread. Preferably the Ry-Krisp, though.

11/23/37
M. 13 yrs.
PSORIASIS **1484-1**

Evenings—only use brown bread, or preferably for this body, as much as possible of only Ry-Krisp.

2/13/37
F. 17 yrs.
OBESITY **1339-1**

Abstain from great quantities of starches. Most of the breads (if any are taken) should be of the rye bread or Ry-Krisp.

ii)—Whole Wheat Crackers

3/18/32
F. 38 yrs.
ADHESIONS: BLOOD-BUILDING **5515-1**

Noons—Preferably the entirely green vegetable diet, those cut together and used with some sauce or mayonnaise, with graham or whole wheat wafer or cracker.

iii)—Zwieback Crackers

8/15/25
COLITIS **F. 6 yrs.**
MALARIA: TENDENCIES **4281-6**

Q. What kind of bread or crackers?

A. Graham crackers and whole wheat bread. Zwieback very good, see?

4/27/35
ASSIMILATIONS: ELIMINATIONS: INCOORDINATION **F. 39 yrs.**
NEURITIS **908-1**

Mornings—Citrus fruit juices. At the same meal there may be taken Zwieback, or the like; with a little butter if so desired, but only brown bread—and this doesn't mean white bread just browned! Use whole wheat, rye, Zwieback or the like. Of course, Zwieback is of white, but the mixtures are of rye, wheat, barley and malt.

2)—Cereals

1)—Cereals: General

7/26/32
ANEMIA **M. 25 yrs.**
ASSIMILATIONS: POOR **481-1**

Mornings—If cereals are taken, do not mix these with the citrus fruits—for this *changes* the acidity in the stomach to a detrimental condition; for citrus fruits will act *as* an eliminant when taken alone, but when taken with cereals it becomes as weight—rather than as an active force in the gastric forces of the stomach itself. It requires a different element for the digesting of citrus fruits with cereals of any nature that are taken with milk; for curds with acids of fruits are as pouring milk in tea that has lemon in it. It produces a curd.

8/8/32
M. Adult

HERNIAS **246-1**

Mornings—Preferably citrus fruits, though it may be altered with fresh fruits that are used with the various cereals carrying an extraordinary amount of vitamins—as vitamin E, vitamin D. Vitamin E, especially, will act with the *regenerative* forces of the system.

5/12/44
F. 16 yrs.

DERMATITIS **2084-16**

Q. What foods would be best for her when she comes home from school so hungry?

A. Whole grain cereals if not too much sugar is used. Put in a little honey instead.

Cut down on the amount of sweets taken, not even using sugar on cereals or things of that nature.

1/12/40
F. 27 yrs.

NEURASTHENIA **2076-1**

Throughout this period the diet should consist more of the forces as in vitamin B-1; such as in whole wheat cereal (crushed wheat, cooked a long time); as in the combination of wheat and barley; as in steel cut oats.

8/17/38
M. 61 yrs.

LIFE: BALANCED **1662-1**

Not such a diet as to be contrary to natural laws, but that which is in keeping with the manner in which the body exerts itself—so that there may be brought the better resuscitating influences and forces.

Upon the natural things, then, that replenish and supply energies—as in these; not as the only things eaten, but this as an outline for the activities of the body to preserve and maintain a balance:

Mornings—The natural answer to the call for the foods that supply the body; such as whole wheat, whole rye—either in their combinations or separately, but in their natural state or natural sources. Not combining cereals at the same meal with fruits—for these defeat then their purposes.

4/23/42
F. 34 yrs.

VITAMINS: B **457-8**

Q. What foods carry most of the vitamin B?

A. All those that are of the yellow variety, especially whole grain cereals . . .

Q. Is it part of this vitamin which can prevent the hair from growing gray?

A. Not necessarily. This only supplies energy. Energy is not the activity, especially for the thyroid. It is from the thyroid that the activity is produced for hair upon the body.

5/2/44
M. 33 yrs.
PARKINSON'S DISEASE **3491-2**

Q. Please suggest foods to stress and foods to avoid in the diet.
A. Do stress B-1 and E. Do leave off too much starches. Have plenty of whole grains.

7/29/29
M. 50 yrs.
ULCERS **5641-2**

Q. What should be a sample of the diet for one day, for the three meals?
A. Morning—Should be of *gruels,* with those of oaten or corn or rice, or such. Little of the citrus fruits may be taken.

In the evening may be taken any of those that carry the iodine with the still whole wheat or those of the properties that carry the gruels with same.

6/13/23
F. Adult
ANEMIA **4102-1**

The diet shall be, not meats, but vegetables and vegetable matter, especially, gruels and coarser foods, see? that that carries vitamins and iron in the system to give more vital forces to the body to resist in the system.

12/1/30
COLD: COMMON: SUSCEPTIBILITY: WORMS **M. Child**
WORMS **203-1**

Beware of sweets for some time. Preferably would be as this: Mornings—Gruels, especially with citrus fruit juices.

11/18/30
F. 60 yrs.
ELIMINATIONS: POOR **505-1**

In the matter of diet—these, as we find, will be more of the well balanced that carry more of the irons in their reaction—as will be found in those of all the vegetable forces, as of those of the wheat or oaten, preferably in the *whole* grain rolled—not soured before rolled, but rolled—and made in a gruel. *These* would be well for the body, but should be *well* cooked; should be cooked at least three to four hours—in double boilers, *preferably not* aluminum.

11/4/25
COLITIS **F. 70 yrs.**
DEBILITATION: GENERAL **3776-10**

Whole wheat gruels and such. These will assist the body in gaining its normal equilibrium. Do that.

1/17/43
CIRCULATION: IMPAIRED **F. 6 yrs.**
BODY-BUILDING **2883-1**

In the diet—have plenty of calcium, the foods that carry plenty of calcium; as the whole grain cereals. These should be a part of the diet for the body.

12/30/42
M. 21 yrs.
BODY-BUILDING: LOCOMOTION: IMPAIRED **2873-1**

The food values should be those fully well balanced with calcium, iron and especially the vitamins B-1 and the B-Complex. These are much preferable for the body.

At least three times each week, then, supply these from the foods rather than the reinforced vitamins (though these reinforcements may be desirable if there is the inability of the body to assimilate foods that carry excesses or the full quantity of such vital forces).

These should include, then, such foods as these as an outline; though, to be sure, these are not all the foods that are to be taken.

Mornings—Cereals that are reinforced; that is, whole grain cereals, either cooked or those ready prepared.

7/30/41
M. 26 yrs.
ANESTHESIA: BODY-BUILDING **1710-6**

The general diet should be for body-building. Be sure that most of the foods carry especially vitamin B. These are best found in reinforced cereals.

9/3/41
GLANDS: THYROID **F. 33 yrs.**
BODY-BUILDING **2582-1**

Be mindful that there are the diets that carry full quantities of the vitamins that aid in the strength and body-building. These will be found in cereals. These should be a considerable part of the body's diet.

ACIDITY
CIRCULATION: INCOORDINATION **5/11/42**
COLD: CONGESTION **F. 74 yrs.**
BODY-BUILDING **2074-2**

Give foods that are very stimulating. Every form of better stimulant that is for building strength. And give plenty of the whole grain cereals.

9/16/41
ELIMINATIONS: INCOORDINATION **F. 2 yrs.**
VITAMINS **2015-8**

Be mindful as to the diets; keeping plenty of the vitamins, especially B-1, A and G. These will be found principally in cereals.

7/30/36
M. 30 yrs.
ATTITUDES & EMOTIONS: WORRY: GENERAL **416-9**

For the activities of the gastric flow of the digestive system are the requirements of one reaction in the gastric flow for starch and another for proteins, or for the activities of the carbohydrates as combined with starches of this nature—especially in the manner in which they are prepared. Then, in the combinations, do not eat great quantities of starch with the proteins or meats.

And do not have cereals (which contain the greater quantity of starch than most) at the same meal with the citrus fruits. These we will find will make for quite a variation in the *feelings* and in the activity of the body, if these suggestions are adhered to.

7/20/25
F. 20s
INJURIES: SPINE: LUMBAR **49-1**

Keep the diet free from meats as much as possible, save fish or seafoods, and keep vegetable forces more of the cereals than of the tuberous nature.

10/29/36
M. Adult
ANEMIA **1131-2**

Mornings—Principally cereals. May be balanced with a small amount of crisp bacon, or coddled eggs—using principally or altogether the yolk. These will carry with them an abundant amount of resisting forces in the system, and aid in the elimination; also add to the blood-building forces of the body.

The cereals should carry an overamount of vitamins E, D, A and B; E and D especially, for these are the life-resisting—or carry an overabundance of elements that add to the vitale of the body.

Q. Please give the foods that would supply these.

A. We have given them; cereals that carry the heart of the grain.

3/2/43
M. 10 yrs.
INJURIES: BIRTH: AFTEREFFECTS **2780-2**

Q. Would it be helpful to take some preparation such as cod-liver oil, iron or vitamins, to aid further development?

A. These are best taken in the regular diet, if there is supplied sufficient of those foods needed. If some good whole grain cereal is taken each day, or any such activity, it should supply sufficient. This, combined with the yolk of an egg each day, should supply sufficient, and be much better assimilated by the body than being reinforced from vitamins.

4/14/43
M. 5 yrs.
CHILDREN: ABNORMAL **2963-1**

As to the foods—keep a normal, balanced diet; not an oversupply of any particular vitamins, but plenty of the whole grains.

7/30/41
M. 26 yrs.
ANESTHESIA: AFTEREFFECTS **1710-6**

The general diet should be for body-building. Be sure that most of the foods carry especially vitamin B. These are best found in reinforced cereals.

12/22/42
ARTHRITIS **M. 34 yrs.**
VITAMINS: B-1: GENERAL **849-62**

Do keep up ALL foods that carry B-1 especially, the exercise or energy vitamin. These are found in the reinforced cereals.

Q. Is the diet all right?

A. As indicated, hold closer to the B-1 products and vitamins. Don't take them separate. For these are not as well assimilated and DO cause disturbances in other directions at times.

1/4/40
M. 32 yrs.
ATROPHY: NERVES **849-47**

With the taking of the wheat oil in the manner indicated, supply vitamins B-1, as well as A, B and G—through the cereals. We do not mean dried cereals! These should be cooked cereals! The cracked whole wheat at one time, the steel cut oats at another time, and wheat and barley at another time! These should be taken with cream or milk, and NOT TOO MUCH SUGAR! Put barely sufficient for making same palatable!

3/22/41
M. 62 yrs.
DEBILITATION: GENERAL **556-18**

As we find, there should be the more efficient supply and more quantities of the vitamins B and B-1 and D. These, through the food supply, would be the better means for obtaining helpful directions for the body forces.

We would have plenty of steel cut oats, well cooked, or cracked wheat and such forms.

12/9/41
F. 26 yrs.
RHEUMATISM **2517-3**

It is better, as we find that the B-1 vitamins that make for resistance be assimilated in the foods, so far as possible, and as much as practical—such as in reinforced cereals . . .

8/23/39
ASTHMA **F. 46 yrs.**
BODY-BUILDING: LOCOMOTION: IMPAIRED **1794-3**

Q. What should patient eat or do to regain her lost appetite and lost weight?

A. Eat whole wheat crushed, and this combined with fruit; and cereals of other natures, especially the steel cut oats—not rolled oats. These with plenty of liver, liver extract, will tend to help gain weight.

2)—Corn Cereal

7/18/40
F. 39 yrs.
ASSIMILATIONS: ELIMINATIONS: INCOORDINATION **2309-I**

Take plenty of food values that carry vitamin B-1 and G. These are found in cereals—especially corn. These should be in the diet almost daily.

3)—Oat Cereal

12/12/33
ACIDITY & ALKALINITY **F. 22 yrs.**
DEBILITATION: GENERAL: TUBERCULOSIS **418-2**

Noons—Stewed fruits and oaten cereals may be taken at the noon meal. The oaten cereals tend to be acid in their reaction unless there is plenty of fruit juices taken in the evening meal or period.

5/21/42
CONCEPTION **F. 34 yrs.**
VITAMINS **457-9**

Q. Are there any whole grain cereals containing vitamin B which are not too much starch for this body?

A. Oats are the better sources—oats and barley.

1/6/42
M. 57 yrs.
GENERAL **462-14**

Q. Please give me the foods I should eat at breakfast.

A. Citrus fruits, and especially once or twice or three times a week the reinforced cereals—but mostly the whole grain, especially oats—these well cooked, with little sugar, but with milk or cream.

1/10/41
APPENDICITIS: TENDENCIES **M. 33 yrs.**
ULCERS: DUODENAL **481-4**

Cereals—steel cut oats well cooked, and dry cereals that carry the vitamins in same, with plenty of milk, and malted milks.

4/27/42
F. 33 yrs.
ASSIMILATIONS: ELIMINATIONS: INCOORDINATION **2737-1**

Have citrus fruits AND plenty of whole grain cereals. Whole oats—these carry those elements that have been lacking and that will be stored or energized to activity in the system by the balance created in the chemical forces.

3/14/32
M. Adult
TOXEMIA **5672-1**

Mornings—Cooked cereals, preferably of rolled oats, but the oats should be the steel cut oats rather than those already heated, for they lose some of the necessary vitamins in such. Those that are cooked for a long period of time.

Do not mix cereals and fruit juices, though cereals with fresh fruits may be taken.

11/29/39
F. 40 yrs.
ANEMIA **2050-1**

In the matter of the diets through these periods—we will find that those foods combining a greater quantity of vitamin B-1 (thiamine) would be especially most beneficial to the body, as they will aid in eliminating those disturbances through the whole of the system, especially as related to the conditions carried in the bloodstream itself.

Eat especially a great deal of steel cut oats—not rolled oats so much, though these, to be sure, carry SOME, but a greater quantity will be found in the steel cut oats—these, of course, cooked a long time.

7/18/40
F. 39 yrs.
ASSIMILATIONS: ELIMINATIONS: INCOORDINATION **2309-1**

Take plenty of food values that carry vitamin B-1 and G. These are found in cereals—especially oats. These should be in the diet almost daily. Plenty of orange juice for the body, but do not take with cereals.

5/15/41
F. Adult
ANEMIA: DEBILITATION: GENERAL **2500-1**

We would add B-1 in the foods. Steel cut oats—cooked a long while. Cook these in a double boiler and keep covered throughout the cooking, so as to preserve the real value.

7/21/39
M. 24 yrs.
STREPTOCOCCUS **568-3**

Q. Any special diet?

A. Those foods that are easily assimilated, and that are strengthening, and that carry such vitamins as in plenty of steel cut oats, as well as those foods of every nature that carry the plasms of better blood supply. Vitamin B-1, vitamin A, B, C and G—these are those needed.

5/25/39
M. 5 mos.
BABY CARE **1788-6**

Also we would give the strained oatmeal, but use the steel cut oats, not rolled oats; and cook a LONG time, in a double boiler, of course. When it is strained the husks of course will be out, but it will retain much of the vitamin B and thiamine that will be most helpful in the developing of the nerves, as well as resistance against cold. Give this at least twice each week.

4/2/32
F. Child
ASTHMA **5682-2**

Mornings—There may be given cereal, and preferably such as carries more of the necessary elements in the vitamins; as in oatmeal use the steel cut, and as is cooked for a long period of time and altogether cooked with its own steam, *not* cooked in open pan or boiler. As double boilers, for three to five hours this should be cooked.

2/5/42
F. 24 yrs.
INJURIES **2679-1**

In the diets, also much may be accomplished. Have especially those foods that carry more of the calcium and of the vitamins A, D, B-1 and other B complexes.

Use plenty of crushed or steel cut oats and plenty of citrus fruits. However, DO NOT use citrus fruits AND cereals at the same meal. Rather alternate, having one on one day, the other the next.

5/4/39
M. 31 yrs.
LIVER: KIDNEY: INCOORDINATION **1885-1**

Not too much, yet, of those foods that are too heavy in the contents as from cereals. But oats, especially cut oats, are desirable—these, of course, in moderation.

2/5/42
F. 55 yrs.
ANEMIA **2067-9**

Keep up good eliminations—this by exercises as well as by eating plenty of oatmeal, this taken of evening before retiring as well as for the morning meal; though alter the morning meal at times with citrus fruits.

Q. Will I be able to overcome this condition and keep my job?

A. If you'll do as has been indicated! If you half do it and then are still pessimistic about it, no! Remember the word of the psalmist, "That which I hated has come upon me."

6/9/27
F. 20 mos.
TOXEMIA **608-3**

For the diet: do not give any water that is not first boiled, see? Do not give any milk unless it is first heated—not necessarily boiled, but heated, see? Give then those properties in dried milk gruels, especially oatmeal—let this be strained.

The water, the milk—in its precaution—is to meet those conditions as are seen produced in the assimilating system of the body. Hence when the conditions are *normal* again, this is not necessarily to be kept up.

9/27/37
F. Adult
DEBILITATION: GENERAL **1419-5**

Mornings—Use oatmeal, but the steel cut oats—Not the rolled oats. The rolled oats make for too much acidity. The steel cut oats would be well.

12/30/40
APPLES: ELIMINATIONS: ASSIMILATIONS: POOR **M. 52 yrs.**
UTENSILS: ALUMINUM: NOT RECOMMENDED **2423-1**

As to the diet after the first cleansing with the apples—we would have plenty of oatmeal—but preferably the steel cut oats and these cooked a long time, but in enamel or glassware, NOT in aluminum at all—for this body. For this body, do not eat foods prepared in aluminum at all; for, from the natural conditions and the supercharges of acids, the body will be allergic to the effects from aluminum on foods.

9/5/42
F. 27 yrs.
TUBERCULOSIS 2806-I

Do give other pre-digested foods; as the strained oatmeal, but not heavy foods nor fat foods.

4)—Rice Cereal

8/4/34
M. 36 yrs.
BODY-BUILDING 555-5

There are only those precautions necessary now in adding to the system those things that will gently build up the resistances and gain the bodily strength.

Begin with the semi-solid foods and gradually the solid foods; and we will find the general conditions will be *greatly* improved.

Rice. Things that are of the starch nature, yes, but *with* those combined for the body-building; which means green vegetables of fresh raw vegetables taken along with same. Not too much at the time, but satisfy the cravings of the body; not wholly, but so that the assimilating system may take same on properly.

And we will find conditions will continue to improve.

3/4/35
F. Adult
KATABOLISM: METABOLISM 844-I

This (diet) would be the outline, though it may be altered at times:

Mornings—Alter at times for the morning meal to rice, provided it is of the browned rice or the uncut rice or unpolished rice.

2/24/35
ASSIMILATIONS: ELIMINATIONS: INCOORDINATION M. 53 yrs.
ACIDITY & ALKALINITY 843-1

Noons—Only a gluten, as of rice boiled clear (and this preferably the brown rice, or cut rice). This may be used with a gravy, provided it is not too heavy or with too much grease; or, more preferably, use with butter alone. Fruits should be preferably taken at this meal, with the gluten, which may be of the rice or of the cracked wheat that might be cooked and used for same. These are adding the strength and the vitality.

5)—Whole Wheat Cereal

2/18/35
ASSIMILATIONS: POOR M. 29 yrs.
GLANDS: INCOORDINATION 831-1

Mornings—Citrus fruit juices. Whole wheat bread, preferably toasted. At least three times each week—only crushed wheat, whole wheat; not cooked so as to destroy any of the vitamins that carry the iron, the silicon and those influences that build with body and nerve and blood-building forces, but in such measures that these are retained—which would be as cooked in preferably steam cooker of such nature that will only break up the elements but release for the body the proper nutriments from same. These may be combined at times with the cereal known as Maltex, which is a combination of barley with wheat, which breaks up the activities of some influences.

3/22/41
M. 62 yrs.
DEBILITATION: GENERAL **556-18**

As we find, there should be the more efficient supply and more quantities of the vitamins B and B-1 and D. These, through the food supply, would be the better means for obtaining helpful directions for the body forces.

We wouid have plenty of cracked wheat and such forms.

10/4/35
M. 41 yrs.
DEBILITATION: GENERAL **1014-1**

Then, we would be very mindful of the DIET for the body. For this should be the greater healing influence that will aid in building up the body. This would be as an outline, though these are not the only foods to be taken—but let these be the greater portion of the foods as taken for the body:

Mornings—Citrus fruit juices; *or* whole wheat, that is crushed or rolled, that is not cooked too much but cooked sufficient that it may be active with the digestive forces of the system itself. About three or four times each week the whole wheat would be used, and at other times the citrus fruit juices—but do not have these both together.

7/3/35
ABRASIONS **M. 56 yrs.**
DEBILITATION: GENERAL **556-8**

The lacking for the system, then, is the *body*—or the weight, to make for the activities through the gastric flow of the digestive system: for these having been the first basis of disturbances, we must be precautious as to increasing this too fast or overbalancing in elements that would make for an infection—or a centralizing of poisons in the organs of assimilation.

Hence we would begin with what may be termed some of the predigested foods, or whole wheat that is rolled and then cooked for two or two and a half hours—only, though, in enamel or glassware. While this carries a great deal of starch, it would be very strengthening and helpful if taken in moderation; that is, in small quantities at the time and given the more often—every hour or the like, you see, not more than a half to a teaspoonful at the time, and this taken slowly, with milk and a little *brown* sugar for the seasoning. This carries those balances of iron and the vitamin elements in phosphorus, the forces in silicon, and the activities necessary to make for a complete balance in the body.

So the beef juices and the whole wheat (this rolled or crushed, not ground) should be sufficient for the next eight days, with—of course—the fruit and vegetable juices that have been indicated.

2/23/35
DERMATITIS **M. Adult**
BLOOD: HUMOR: PSORIASIS **840-1**

At least three mornings each week we would have the rolled or crushed or cracked whole wheat, that is not cooked too long so as to destroy the whole vitamin force in same, but this will add to the body the proper proportions of iron, silicon and the vitamins necessary to build up the blood supply that makes for resistance in the system.

2/5/42
F. 24 yrs.
INJURIES **2679-1**

In the diets, also, much may be accomplished. Have especially those foods that carry more of the calcium and of the vitamins A, D; B-1 and other B Complexes.

Use plenty of whole wheat grain—as cracked wheat.

5/4/39
M. 31 yrs.
LIVER: KIDNEYS: INCOORDINATION **1885-1**

Not too much, yet, of those foods that are too heavy in the contents as from cereals. Crushed wheat, especially, is desirable—these, of course, in moderation.

5/9/38
F. 51 yrs.
RHEUMATISM **920-12**

Mornings—About twice a week have the whole wheat—this crushed or cut WHOLE WHEAT, you see; bran and all; cooked very thoroughly—for this carries more of the vitamins that are necessary for the revivifying of the glandular system in all directions than may be had from most any other source. Hence there would be taken a nice bowl full for a meal, you see: thoroughly cooked, however. This may be taken with a little sugar or saccharine, and cream. Do not have the cereal AND juice at the same meal! or do not take them within several hours of one another, even!

5/23/35
M. 33 yrs.
GLANDS: INCOORDINATION **412-8**

We would keep nearer toward an alkalinity in the diet. Little or no food values carrying quantities of grease. Less of the breads or those things that make for the accumulation of elements that are clogging to the system, in the form of starches that have been and are indicated as a portion of the diet. So, a diet according to this outline would be well:

Mornings—The citrus fruit juices or cereals that have a great deal of all the elements; especially vitamins A, B, C, D, such as would be found in whole wheat or the cereals that are dry and the Maltex preparation (barley and wheat) for the cooked cereals.

And take time to masticate the food well!

12/12/33
ACIDITY & ALKALINITY **F. 22 yrs.**
DEBILITATION GENERAL: TUBERCULOSIS **418-2**

Mornings—Cereals of the whole wheat character, cooked cereals and plenty of milk eaten with same.

12/12/33
ACIDITY & ALKALINITY **F. 22 yrs.**
DEBILITATION: GENERAL: TUBERCULOSIS **418-2**

Noons—The whole wheat cooked cereals—any of those that employ or use the whole of the wheat, including the bran—may be used and are alkaline in their reaction.

10/8/36
ANEMIA **F. 54 yrs.**
ARTHRITIS: TOXEMIA **1269-1**

Mornings—Citrus fruits may be taken, or whole wheat, crushed wheat . . . or the combinations as in barley and wheat and the like for cooked cereal. Alternate these. These should be the morning meals, with a little breakfast bacon occasionally; and egg.

9/10/23
M. Adult
ELIMINATIONS: INCOORDINATION **4232-1**

Let the diet be not of meats, or of sweets but of gruels, whole wheat.

1/8/37
F. Adult
DEBILITATION: GENERAL **1278-7**

We would find it well to use every character of food that is body and blood building; as whole wheat cereal, or if preferred the combination of wheat and barley. These as we find should be the main or chief diet.

3/14/35
M. Adult
DEBILITATION: GENERAL **856-1**

At least twice each week, or three times each week, we would have a whole wheat cereal; that is, cracked wheat or rolled wheat; not cooked *too* done but sufficient to break up the cellular forces that the vitamins may be released for the activity of the body, see? (This may be used when citrus fruits are not.)

2/16/35
M. 45 yrs.
ACIDITY **829-1**

Mornings—At least twice to three times each week there should be taken the cracked wheat cereal or whole wheat; not oats, but that which is cooked in such a manner that the whole evaluation of the vitamins of the iron, silicon, the roughage as necessary for the creating of the proper balance in the blood supply, is effective to the body. There may be periods when fresh fruits may be taken in preference to either of these.

10/17/27
M. 8 mos.
BABY CARE **5520-2**

Well, too, that those of the glutens be used, which will be found by rolling wheat—raw wheat, see? or mashing same and this cooked as a gruel, and strained, seasoned—a little salt and little butter, and a very *small* quantity of sugar. This in small quantities will be well for this individual.

12/31/37
DEBILITATION: GENERAL M. 41 yrs.
ACIDITY & ALKALINITY 1476-1

Mornings—Whole wheat cereals—as Maltex (barley and wheat) or crushed wheat, that are well, WELL cooked (but do not combine cereals AND citrus fruits at the same meal!). These may be altered at times also with stewed fruits. But these should be taken at one time or another.

9/29/24
ULCERS: STOMACH M. 45 yrs.
ELIMINATIONS 4709-5

Take no foods save those that carry the incentive for the proper producing condition in the system. Namely these:

Whole wheat, pressed, cleansed and pressed, and this formed into a well-prepared gruel, with the milk as would be used, with this only beet sugar, and sufficient milk to make such palatable to the body. Do not take large quantities of this, but take it more often.

10/8/38
F. 51 yrs.
DEBILITATION: GENERAL 1703-1

Mornings—Citrus fruit juices, in their combinations, OR cereals. When cooked cereal is used, preferably use only the whole wheat. This may be merely rolled, crushed or ground—but the WHOLE of the grain is to be taken; because of the influence and vitamins, as well as the iron, as well as the very natures of the life of the wheat itself that are needed. Crushed or ground, then—whole; and cook for at least three hours—but do not cook same in an OPEN kettle nor in an aluminum kettle. Use either glass OR enamel ware with the top on at all times. This would be found to be MOST satisfying, most helpful for creating a proper balance. Do not eat overmuch of such in the beginning, until it becomes WELL-balanced in the system. Use same with a little sugar or honey to sweeten, and half milk and half cream. The milk should be preferably that which has been properly prepared for keeping.

Citrus fruit juice and cereal should never be taken at the same meal, or on the same day. Use one one morning, the other the next, or in that ratio. A little crisp bacon with whole wheat toast or fruit after these may be taken, if so desired.

2/5/36
F. 38 yrs.
TUBERCULOSIS 1045-6

Occasionally the *whole wheat* cereal, cooked for at least three to four hours, will be strengthening; but give only a tiny bit. This carries those vitamins necessary for combating the distressed conditions produced by strains upon the system.

4/18/40
F. 25 yrs.
VITAMINS: GLANDS 2171-1

At least once or twice each week have the whole wheat (crushed or rolled) as the cereal—this cooked a long time—that there may be more of the iron, sulphur, and the vitamins arising from this; especially B-1, as an aid in the circulatory forces of the body.

5/15/41
F. Adult
ANEMIA: DEBILITATION: GENERAL **2500-1**

We would add B-1 in the foods. Cracked wheat cereal occasionally—cooked a long while. Cook these in a double boiler and keep covered throughout the cooking, so as to preserve the real value.

3/11/36
NERVOUS SYSTEMS: INCOORDINATION **F. 18 yrs**
BODY-BUILDING **852-13**

Q. Am I keeping an equal balance in my diet now?

A. Very good. We would only add the salts or vitamins that come from crushed whole wheat as a portion of the diet occasionally for the morning meal, and these would be more helpful. For the iron, silicon, vitality combined in these elements as a portion of the diet will be most helpful.

5/20/38
F. 68 yrs.
TOXEMIA **1593-1**

Have at least two breakfast meals each week consisting of a whole cereal; as crushed wheat cooked WELL—or for at least two or two and a half to three hours. Have this crushed but the whole wheat, see? This may be taken either with dry milk or Carnation milk, but not with cow's milk that is RAW, see?

2/6/35
M. 31 yrs.
NERVES: TOXEMIA **815-1**

As we find, in bringing the better conditions for this body in the present (for, to be sure, the mental attitudes of the body, the worriment about the conditions of the physical forces, the indecisions as to the proper mental and material attitude towards those conditions that have surrounded the body, are contributory causes—but) there needs to be these applications that would *rid* the body of the disturbing forces, adding the necessary character of vibrations and of activity to the replenishing forces of the system as to overcome those conditions.

Then, we would find these to be the more helpful in the present:

We would not change a great deal, first, from the diet that has been given; save we would have at least four or five meals each week (preferably morning) that would be principally of the whole wheat or cracked wheat, prepared as a cereal; not cooked for long, but sufficient that there may be only the breaking up of the cellular forces for the vitamins to be supplied that are necessary for the creation of the necessary forces for the activity to the digestive forces, through the liver, the pancreas, the spleen, and through the gall duct area. We find these would be most helpful (but do not ever use citrus fruits *and* cereals at the same meal!).

CIRCULATION: LYMPH **2/21/35**
ELIMINATIONS: POOR **F. Adult**
DROPSY: TENDENCIES **838-1**

We would find it well to take at least twice or three times a week for breakfast the cracked or rolled *whole wheat;* this not cooked too much, but cooked rather in steam, that there may be preserved all of the vitamins. And *do not* cook in *aluminum!*

1/26/35
F. 59 yrs.
INJURIES 3823-2

Hence we would use those foods that carry in a soluble manner that which may be absorbed and become replenishing or rebuilding for the blood; or the calciums, irons, glutens that make for the urea. We would use principally an alkaline-reacting diet.

Mornings—The cereals that have more of the whole wheat with raisins in same—though do not use citrus fruit *and* cereal at the same meal. Whole wheat bread or cracked wheat bread toasted, with a little butter.

3/14/32
M. Adult
TOXEMIA 5672-1

Mornings—Cooked cereals, preferably of Wheatena cooked for a long period of time.

i)—Wheat & Barley Cereal

3/23/35
F. 47 yrs.
BLOOD-BUILDING 865-1

In the diet, keep to those foods of an alkaline-reaction, but more of the whole wheat or the whole wheat and barley as body and blood building of the nature with those vitamins necessary for maintaining the ironization in the bloodstream itself from that which is assimilated by the body.

Q. Would you recommend any specific diet?

A. As given, we would keep an alkaline-reacting diet; only using the whole wheat and barley at times as a body-building, you see. This should be at least one of the meals once or three times a week.

1/9/35
M. 1 yr.
WORMS 786-1

We would begin with a body-*building* diet for the body.

Mornings—A cooked cereal that is rich with vitamins A, B and D, which is preferably found in the Maltex—a combination of wheat or barley combined together.

3/8/35
F. 37 yrs.
ARTHRITIS 631-6

Mornings—Citrus fruit juices, or cereals. *Specifically,* at least two to three times a week, have the combination of the whole wheat with barley.

3/7/35
F. 43 yrs.
COLITIS: TENDENCIES **846-1**

Mornings—Cereals. At least once or twice a week it would be well to have cereals of the whole wheat with barley, or that combined in Maltex is well provided it is well prepared. *Do not* have cereals at the same meal with citrus fruits or citrus fruit juices; though they may be taken an hour or more apart, for their combination with the gastric juices of the stomach produces rather an acid than an alkaline.

5/25/42
M. 58 yrs.
NEURASTHENIA **816-13**

Have the reinforced cereals that carry B-1. Use as cooked cereals the combination of wheat and barley. These will aid in stimulating. Not that these should be the things alone taken, but these should form portions of the diet daily.

4/27/42
F. 33 yrs.
ASSIMILATIONS: ELIMINATIONS: INCOORDINATION **2737-1**

Have citrus fruits AND plenty of whole grain cereals, though do not take these at the same meal. The combinations of wheat and barley cereals, dry or cooked—these carry those elements that have been lacking and that will be stored or energized to activity in the system by the balance created in the chemical forces.

11/23/37
M. 13 yrs.
PSORIASIS **1484-1**

Mornings—A cooked cereal is preferable—when a cereal is to be taken; such as a combination of wheat and barley as in Maltex—this is the preferable of the cooked cereals for this body. This carries activities that when taken do not ferment easily as oats OR whole wheat rolled or preparations in other forms.

5/1/35
M. 1-1/2 yrs.
WORMS: PINWORMS: AFTEREFFECTS **786-2**

We would suggest that occasionally, once or twice a week, there be given the body a cooked cereal with a little milk (but not at the same meal with citrus fruit juices); and in this we would use either Carnation or Eagle Brand milk as the cream for same—or mixed with same. Maltex (wheat and barley) is preferable for growing children.

ii)—Whole Wheat & Malt Cereal

11/13/36
CHILD TRAINING **F. 11 yrs.**
BODY-BUILDING **1206-2**

Q. Should [1188] start taking chocolate calcium tablets such as he took last winter?

A. There's better resistance here than there was in the previous winter, as indicated. This is not a combination we would use in this time, unless changes come about.

Rather we would use the cereal combinations as of malt and the whole wheat, that would be better. These will supply a malt in the digestive forces, with the weight, with the activity for all—especially with those properties as indicated that produce a cleansing that is hard to surpass.

iii)—Whole Wheat & Oatmeal Cereal

7/26/43
M. 2 yrs.
ELIMINATIONS: INCOORDINATION 3109-1

Combinations of cereals are at times bad for the body, though oatmeal and whole wheat and the wheat germ with the oatmeal will be very good for the body.

iv)—Wheat Germ Cereal

5/1/44
M. 20 yrs.
COLITIS: ULCERATIVE: CHRONIC 5000-2

Q. What should be added to or taken from the present diet, if anything?

A. We wouldn't change anything, we would only add wheat germ. This preferably prepared from whole grain cereals, and taken in the morning, whether these are cooked or dry cereals, taken with milk or cream.

6)—Cereals: Dry—General

1/25/33
F. 44 yrs.
GLANDS: INCOORDINATION 757-3

If the citrus fruit is not taken there may be used the dry cereal—and do not use sugar on same, although the milk may be used—but preferably use that which is well balanced in the vitamin forces, or the pasteurized milk, or dry milk that is made for such usages.

10/24/34
CHILDBIRTH: AFTEREFFECTS F. 35 yrs.
DEBILITATION: GENERAL 637-2

Mornings—Citrus fruit juices, with a small *quantity* of *any* of the dry cereals afterward or with same—will be helpful for the body *in* its *existent* condition (very few (but what this would form acid for!); this should not be used with milk, but with the cereal itself. If milk is to be used, use rather the dry milk—not the regular formations, you see.

2/21/34
M. 20 yrs.
EPILEPSY **521-1**

Mornings—Dry cereals.

Do not take cereal with citrus fruit, though there may be taken at times cereals with fresh fruits. See?

2/23/28
F. 21 mos.
TOXEMIA **608-4**

Again we would change the diet into more of the gruels that give rebuilding forces in the system, as is seen in grapenuts . . .

1/10/41
APPENDICITIS: TENDENCIES **M. 33 yrs.**
ULCERS: DUODENAL **481-4**

Cereals—dry cereals that carry the vitamins in same such as Post Toasties, with plenty of milk, and malted milks.

8/15/25
COLITIS **F. 6 yrs.**
MALARIA: TENDENCIES **4281-6**

Those of the cereal—corn flakes or of nut flakes (that is, the brown nut flakes, see?) and cream that is sterilized rather than of the pure rich cream, see? More milk than cream, see? and that sterilized before used.

5/25/42
M. 58 yrs.
NEURASTHENIA **816-13**

Have the reinforced cereals that carry B-1. For the dry cereals use oats or corn and tapioca or corn flakes. These with yellow peaches or bananas or the like should be parts of the diet. These will aid in stimulating. Not that these should be the things alone taken, but all those should form portions of the diet daily.

3)—Flours

1)—Popcorn Flour

8/29/35
F. 45 yrs.
COLITIS **404-4**

In the matter of the diet, be mindful that this is not *over*alkaline; nor that there is taken too great a quantity of that ordinarily termed roughage. For with these tendencies for the inflammation that arises, as we have indicated, from changes in the activities in the system and the changes in the system caused by the congestion in the lymph circulation through the intestinal tract, these produce irritations.

As we find, a portion of the diet as nominally taken should be from popcorn flour, or the flour that is not wholly bolted—rather a combination of that bolted, or that bolted *without* the husks and brans left in same.

2)—White Flour

3/28/44
M. 41 yrs.
ACIDITY & ALKALINITY 4008-1

Do not use white flour except in pastries, and eat pastries not more than once a month.

9/30/40
F. 74 yrs.
ARTHRITIS 1224-6

Q. Should white flour be excluded?

A. This is better, as we find, to be excluded.

4)—Meals

1)—Corn Meal

11/16/36
BLOOD: COAGULATION: POOR F. 41 yrs.
BODY-BUILDING 1100-8

In the diet include those foods that are blood- and body-building, that carry iron in such manners as may be assimilated by the body.

Q. For what reason was corn meal suggested for my diet?

A. Because there are those elements from same—as of silicon, and the activities from those elements that produce a character of iron—that are helpful for the body.

Q. How can the bodily resistance be kept up, especially during the winter months?

A. By following those suggestions that have just been indicated, we find we may build resistances for this body, through the periods of sudden changes or distresses that may come from sudden changes to the bodily temperature.

10/7/40
F. 23 yrs.
ANEMIA 2376-1

Use yellow meal for the corn bread, and have this at least three to four times each week.

5/25/42
M. 58 yrs.
NEURASTHENIA 816-13

Corn meal wafers, or corn pones, made of yellow corn meal—all of these will aid in stimulating. Not that these should be the things alone taken, but those should form portions of the diet daily.

ARTHRITIS **10/11/43 F. 26 yrs. 3285-1**

We should have easily assimilated foods, but those very high in the adding of B-Complex, or the vitamin B. And also yellow corn meal—made in corn bread with egg or in batter cakes or in mush. Throughout the period do eat these.

5)—Oat and Wheat Germ Oil

VITAMINS: DEFICIENT **8/27/40 M. 39 yrs. 826-13**

It is only necessary that there be the consideration of the proper foods; especially such as the germ oils of wheat or oats. These in the varied forms or manners as may be prepared would be most helpful.

ANEMIA **6/5/44 F. 65 yrs. 5170-l**

As we find, we would use oft in the diet the supplementary vitamins especially of the E or the wheat germ oil, see? These as prepared by Squibb would be well for this body. Take one of those a day, one of the wheat germ oil, see?

Q. What can be done to strengthen eyes?

A. The same as is indicated, for the general treatments, see? The assimilations must carry more vital energies and thus suggestions for wheat germ oil and B-1 vitamin complex. These should be in addition to the regular diet.

PRURITUS
VITAMINS: E **3/17/42 F. 52 yrs. 1158-36**

Q. Shall I take vitamin E wheat oil capsules?

A. These are very satisfactory; though, as we find, if the wheat germ oil would be taken two drops daily it would be more effective than that prepared in the gelatin capsules; though, to be sure, this may be more convenient to some in the pellets or capsules—but it is not always as fresh, and neither does it act as effectively with the body as being assimilated first with the upper gastric flow.

Q. Any other capsules, pills or tonics I should take? If so, how much?

A. Others as we find are not necessary, if the eliminations are kept and especially if the normal vitamins, A & D and B-1 are taken in the daily diet.

NERVOUS SYSTEMS: INCOORDINATION **11/12/41 F. 74 yrs. 1553-26**

Q. What wheat germ oil would be the best to use?

A. That most easily absorbed in the system, as we find, is that prepared in the solution, NOT encased in other ingredients for the taking of same.

9/19/40
M. 33 yrs.
ARTHRITIS **849-53**

Again we would add, now, the wheat germ oil; not more than the system can stand, but that which aids the natural sources of supplying those energies builded in the system; aiding same through the rubs, the massage, the adjustments mechanically (osteopathically); and—by all means—keep up the exercise!

As we find, begin with about two drops of the wheat germ oil once each day. If this is assimilated, and does not cause an upset, after ten days increase it a drop; and after ten days increase it again—until it is possible to assimilate or handle at least five drops each day.

We would leave off the gelatin with the wheat germ oil.

Do these and, as we find, we will continue to see improvements in the GENERAL health, as well as the removal of causes in the disturbances in the system; and we will overcome those conditions that hinder in locomotion and activity.

5/9/44
M. 28 yrs.
MULTIPLE SCLEROSIS **5073-1**

In the diet, do not take any quantity of salt.

Also, at least once each day take wheat germ. This may be taken with foods or cereals, but preferably with cereals. If it is impractical to get wheat germ oil that is prepared, take one tablet, or if gotten in the bulk, take 5 drops of same once each day.

6/5/44
COLD: CONGESTION: DEAFNESS **F. 35 yrs.**
VITAMINS **5203-1**

Q. Are vitamins helpful in any way?

A. Vitamins are very helpful, especially the B-Complex and for this body especially "E" or use on the cereals the kernel or heart of wheat. B-1 Complex would be very good for the body also.

4/18/40
F. 25 yrs.
VITAMINS: GLANDS **2171-1**

Also we would take small quantities, about two minims every other day, of whole wheat oil. The Squibb's Germ Wheat Oil will be satisfactory, and if this is used, the quantity in one of the pellets is about correct—but this taken only every other day. Take it for two weeks, leave off a week; then take it for another two weeks, leave off a week; then take for another two weeks, and so on. This activity will be as an aid to the stimulating of the glands as they are aided by the purifying of same through the massage and the sweats.

1/4/40
ATROPHY: NERVES **M. 32 yrs.**
NERVES: REBUILDING **849-47**

Take three to four drops of the wheat oil about three times each week; not oftener, BUT DO NOT MISS TAKING IT AT THESE PERIODS! Its active principle is upon the stimulated glandular system, for not only reproduction of the red blood supply but of the genital reaction in the system; for, as "germ" indicates, this is the activity in the system.

IX

Meat and Game

1)—Meat: General

1/8/36
ELIMINATIONS: POOR **M. Adult**
ACIDITY **1095-1**

No red meats. These are too severe upon the system.

12/18/30
M. 24 yrs.
BACILLOSIS: POLIOMYELITIS **135-1**

In the evenings—flesh may be taken in moderation, but none that does not have the hoof divided and that does not chew the cud. In these, these should not be rendered in other than their *own* fat, and should *not* be in any grease other than their own—whether boiled, fried, or roasted. This will, of course, include breads also. Rye, whole wheat, or it may be mixed. At this meal light wines or malt extracts may be also taken as drinks.

11/10/36
F. Adult
ACIDITY **1288-1**

In the diet be mindful that there is not too great a combination of starches, as to form for the circulatory forces and the digestive area too great an acidity which not only produces the conditions that disturb through the poor elimination and the toxic forces through the alimentary canal, but produces in the bloodstream itself the inability—with the activities of the properties indicated—for proper coordination. Twenty percent acid to eighty percent alkaline-reacting should be the proper balance, or as these:

Do *not* combine ever any red meats with the starches, as of white bread or white potatoes, at the same meal. The meats should consist principally of fowl, fish or lamb. Not *any* fried foods at any time.

10/25/22
F. Adult
ANEMIA **2219-1**

This will assist the conditions that arise at times through the sciatic nerve force and give a better supply of blood force to the whole system, and make more capillary circulation and more Iymphatic action to all the Iymphatic glands in this body; both internal and external action of these glands need to be excited, so we will have more secretions from the food that is taken. The food should be that of wild game or fish, no meat should be eaten by this body. See?

7/30/36
M. 30 yrs.
ATTITUDES & EMOTIONS: WORRY: GENERAL **416-9**

Q. What foods should I avoid?

A. Rather is it the combination of foods that makes for disturbance with most physical bodies, as it would with this.

In the activities of the body in its present surroundings, those tending toward the greater alkaline reaction are preferable. Hence avoid combinations where corn, potatoes, rice, spaghetti or the like are taken all at the same meal. Some combinations of these at the meal are very good, but all of these tend to make for too great a quantity of starch—especially if any meat is taken at such a meal. If no meat is taken, these make quite a difference. For the activities of the gastric flow of the digestive system are the requirements of one reaction in the gastric flow for starch and another for proteins, or for the activities of the carbohydrates as combined with starches of this nature—especially in the manner in which they are prepared. Then, in the combinations, do not eat great quantities of starch with the proteins or meats. If sweets and meats are taken at the same meal, these are preferable to starches.

8/29/40
M. 27 yrs.
PSORIASIS: TENDENCIES **641-5**

Eat rather regularly, and not spasmodically. Be very consistent in the diets as much as practical; keeping away from sweets, keeping away from meats that are of red or rare meats—though meats are not harmful that are WELL cooked, save hog meat.

1/15/31
M. 47 yrs.
ACIDITY & ALKALINITY: TOXEMIA **5544-1**

Beware of too much meats, and especially of condiments during this period.

12/28/43
F. 56 yrs.
CANCER **3515-1**

Keep away from all meats for at least three to six months. Meat substitutes may be used, but use a great deal of herbs, soups in which even the timothy hay is put for the cleansing of the system.

5/7/35
F. 33 yrs.
ELIMINATIONS: INCOORDINATION **919-1**

Do not make too much of a diet of meat, but when meats are to be eaten eat little else at the same meal—except a little sweet, and let that sweet be honey.

12/12/28
F. 48 yrs.
ACIDITY **569-18**

Q. What should the diet be?

A. Those that are of non-acid producing conditions in the system, as has been outlined. Much of this, as is seen, in most conditions where the body is exceedingly acid and eliminations necessarily are kept at a high point or above normal in eliminations—the body, as it were, *feels* its way with what it may eat—but meats and acid-*producing* foods should be barred by the body, unless conditions are much bettered. *Do* that.

5/8/35
M. 29 yrs.
ASSIMILATIONS: ELIMINATIONS: INCOORDINATION **416-6**

In the diet, be mindful that we do not have too great a quantity of meats; but those that are boiled, roasted or broiled are much better than any fried meats of *any* kind. Not too great a quantity, or *little* of the fats should be taken with same.

ASSIMILATIONS: ELIMINATIONS: INCOORDINATION **5/30/36**
CIRCULATION: IMPAIRED **M. 47 yrs.**
ACIDITY & ALKALINITY **1151-2**

Q. Any suggestions as to diet?

A. As has been indicated, the elements or salts through the system are necessary for the maintaining as well as resuscitating the portions where disturbances have been brought about by high temperature or burning of tissue. An eighty percent alkaline-reacting to a twenty percent acid-reacting diet would be preferable. The variations of same under the activities of the body at times makes this rather disturbing. But these are those things to be warned against, then otherwise there may be kept a near normal diet:

The meats and sweets should be preferably taken at the same meal. It isn't so much *what* the body eats as it is the combinations that are taken at times. No *red* meats; that is, rare meats.

5/12/28
M. 33 yrs.
LIVER: KIDNEYS: INCOORDINATION **900-383**

Q. Is the albumin on the decrease or increase in the urine?

A. On the decrease. Beware of meats.

8/23/34
CYSTS **M. Adult**
ASSIMILATIONS: ELIMINATIONS: INCOORDINATION **643-1**

In the diet, beware of very much meat; and *no* fried meat or fried food of *any* kind. Rather eat those foods that are blood and nerve building.

7/7/30
M. 39 yrs.
ACIDITY: ALKALINITY: RHEUMATISM **99-5**

In the diet, beware of meats—especially of red meats. Those of the vegetable—those of even more starches may be better taken than too much of that, that must form acid—and which produce pressure.

10/23/36
BLOOD: HUMOR **F. 35 yrs.**
OBESITY **1276-1**

Do not combine potatoes with rice or spaghetti or white bread, or if either or any one of these is taken *do not* eat meat at that meal!

3/27/35
F. 52 yrs.
ACIDITY & ALKALINITY **805-2**

Q. What can I do to avoid losing so much weight? Outline the proper diet.

A. Those foods, now, that are the body-building; as starches and proteins, if these are taken without other food values that make for the combinations that produce distress or disorder; that is, not quantities of starches and proteins combined, you see, but these taken one at one meal and one at another will be most helpful. As potatoes, whether white or the yam activity with butter, should not be taken with fats or meats; but using these as a portion of one meal with *fruits* or vegetables is well. When meats are taken, use mutton, fowl or the like, and do not have heavy starches with same—but preferably fruits or vegetables.

7/22/31
ACIDITY **F. 28 yrs.**
ASSIMILATIONS: ELIMINATIONS: INCOORDINATION **2261-1**

But no fried meats—nothing *fried* should be taken by the body—see?

8/14/26
MEAT: AFTEREFFECTS **M. Adult**
ELIMINATIONS **3896-1**

Now, we find there are many abnormal conditions, and to give the cause of existing conditions would be first to give much of the histology of those conditions as have existed in times back that now bring about the existent conditions. Then, we find these conditions existent in this body:

The condition at present produced in the blood supply by the poor eliminations as have long existed in the body, and through same has produced a combination, and complication, of distressing conditions to the functioning of organs. Hence the depression, and the dis-ease, as has existed in the organs from time to time. Much of this produced in times back by too much meat not well cooked for the body . . .

During this time no meats of any character are to be taken.

12/11/38
M. 49 yrs.
COLD: CONGESTION: SUSCEPTIBILITY 1151-19

Q. Should he cut down on his red meats?

A. This is desirable, especially under the condition where congestion affects the circulation to the heart and liver.

1/11/37
ACIDITY & ALKALINITY: GENERAL M. 61 yrs.
ELIMINATIONS: POOR 1217-2

But do not make bad combinations; that is, fried meats with starches or potatoes. Leave off any fried foods altogether. Let the meats be rather fish, fowl or lamb. And the combinations of sweets—do not have too great a quantity of sweets with vegetables, but at times when meats are taken a little sweets may be taken.

5/13/44
F. 35 yrs.
CYSTS: CANCER: TENDENCIES 5113-1

Keep a normal diet, not too much of any kind of meats, and never any "red meats" of any character.

8/29/44
F. 62 yrs.
ARTHRITIS 5402-1

Do these and in the diet keep away from animal matter. For this body there should be little or no animal fat or animal matter. For the form of the activity of the infection is that which is created by, or lives upon, the animal matter.

1/3/23
ASSIMILATIONS: ELIMINATIONS: TOXEMIA M. 50 yrs.
DEBILITATION: GENERAL 4189-1

Q. Should this body eat meats?

A. Not good for body; very little, if any.

2/17/41
M. Adult
COLD: COMMON: PREVENTIVE 902-1

Q. Is the absence of meat in the diet an important factor in avoiding colds?

A. Not necessarily. It depends upon the combinations, rather than any one element that may be singled out as producing destructive forces. If rare meats are taken, or those that have the life in same, in such measures as to set up a weakening of some portion of the digestive forces, in the attempt of the body to assimilate, it may produce a condition of susceptibility. In that case meats should be avoided by that particular body, or in such quantities at least.

5/18/43
M. 63 yrs.
ARTHRITIS 3009-1

Keep away from meats, especially such as beef or hog meat or the like; though fish, fowl and lamb may be taken in moderation, but NO FRIED FOODS OF ANY KIND!

4/29/38
F. 77 yrs.
TOXEMIA **1586-1**

Evenings—Do not take fried foods morning, noon OR evening! nor fried ham, nor fried meats—even fried chicken! But the meats—if any are taken—should be preferably fish, fowl or lamb; and these boiled, broiled or baked.

11/20/25
M. Adult
ASSIMILATIONS: ELIMINATIONS: INCOORDINATION **4891-1**

Meats in moderation, and the principal meats should be as much wild game or fowl, or fish, see? with a moderate amount of vegetable matter that grows *above* the ground, not using that below the ground. No tuberous vegetable of *any* character.

4/29/37
ASSIMILATIONS: ELIMINATIONS: INCOORDINATION **M. 45 yrs.**
BLOOD: HUMOR **877-16**

In the diet—of these things beware. Others may be taken very well. Do not have red meats; that is, raw meats—unless it is steak or venison or the like; though any that are highly seasoned or barbecued might be taken. But as pot roast or roast beef that is rare, no—these are tabu for the body.

3/28/44
M. 41 yrs.
ACIDITY & ALKALINITY **4008-1**

Q. Is there any combination of foods that could be truthfully called Brain Foods, Nerve Foods, Muscle Foods?

A. Those that are body-building; those that are nerve-building and those that supply certain elements. For, as indicated, those foods suggested are to be taken by the body. Fish, fowl and lamb are those that supply elements needed for brain, muscle and nerve-building.

1)—Fat Meat

12/17/31
F. Adult
ACIDITY & ALKALINITY: PSORIASIS **5557-1**

In the matter of meats, beware of those that are much of the fats of same, and never have any that is cooked in its own fat, nor seasoned with the products of its own kind.

3/26/25
ASTHMA **F. Adult**
ELIMINATIONS **85-1**

As much of the rough foods as possible, taking fats of meats rather than of the lean or fleshy portions. Not in large quantities, but that the assimilations may be better corrected in the system.

9/2/41
ARTHRITIS **F. 50 yrs.**
ELIMINATIONS: INCOORDINATION **2581-1**

Keep away from a great deal of fat. Not that the body is to become diet conscious, but keep away from fats. Not that no meats should be taken, but no fat meat.

Q. Why does using my right hand in writing especially cause a general crippling?

A. Because of the effect it has upon the very things as indicated that are to be eliminated. Fats are not assimilated as other conditions in the system, but pass into the activities upon which the gall duct has acted, and then are emptied into the circulation through the right side. Hence the use of this then causes distress, or stress.

7/3/36
ASSIMILATIONS: ELIMINATIONS: INCOORDINATION **F. Adult**
COMBINATIONS **1197-1**

Be mindful of the diet, that there are not the combinations of fat meats with starches. These make for the use of the varied activities and cause a superacidity.

6/26/36
F. 61 yrs.
COMBINATIONS: CHOLECYSTITIS **760-21**

Q. Any other advice at this time?

A. In the rest of the diet keep near to those things as has been indicated. It's the combinations rather than the food values, as has been indicated, that cause upsets. No fat meats. And when beans or things of such natures are cooked, do not cook them in too much fat meat. Butter, or cooked in the straight water and then with butter and seasoning is preferable to fat meats.

7/1/44
F. 44 yrs.
ARTHRITIS: TENDENCIES **5298-1**

Keep away from too much fats, especially pork or beef. Fish, fowl and lamb are preferable.

2)—Roasts

10/30/37
M. 48 yrs.
DIABETES: TENDENCIES **470-19**

The leafy vegetables, of course, should be the main—though this should not exclude meats, but preferably not those that are fried, but roasts, these are very well—though these should be very well done.

10/26/34
F. Adult
ACIDITY **710-1**

We would keep those foods that are the more alkaline; that is, do not take red meats—such as roast beef or heavy roasts that carry a great deal of grease and fats. No fried meats.

7/26/32
M. 25 yrs.
481-1

ANEMIA
ASSIMILATIONS: POOR

We would be mindful of the diet, that those foods are taken that are easily assimilated. Do not take quantities of grease of any nature. When meats *are* taken, they should be those of roast beef or roast mutton.

Evenings—Cooked vegetables, and the meats *when* these are taken. Do not eat meat more than three times each week, and don't gorge self when this is done!

9/29/34
M. Adult
675-1

ABRASIONS: TOXEMIA

Evenings—Well-cooked vegetables. Do not have very fat roasts—they are detrimental to the better eliminations from the system.

2)—Beef: General

4/6/44
F. 62 yrs.
4033-1

NERVE-BUILDING

Q. Please suggest foods to stress and foods to avoid in the diet.

A. In the diet there should be the stressing of those that are nerve-building; such as beef . . .

8/11/25
F. 27 yrs.
4618-1

BLOOD-BUILDING

Diet should be of the nature of rebuilding red blood. Meats, beef especially. Not of the rough character, rather the lean, not too well cooked, but of the nature that will digest in the system, using pepsins in its preparation.

7/23/41
F. 45 yrs.
811-7

ANEMIA

Q. Does the body get the proper kinds of food elements, or is there a deficiency?

A. If so, we wouldn't give the special food values. Those that carry vitamins A and B and B-1 especially should be taken by the body. These are found most, of course, in the fruits and vegetables of the yellow variety as well as especially in beef.

7/1/26
M. Adult
43-1

BLOOD: HUMOR

Not meats, especially not fat meats. Lean meat of beef may be eaten. No hog meat or any fish for this body.

2/23/25
M. 20 yrs.
BODY: BUILDING **77-2**

Q. What special foods should be given the body that would give to the mind and body strength, endurance and activity?

A. Beef, raw or the blood of beef would be the meat taken. Not large quantities, but that which would assimilate with the system.

5/18/43
M. 63 yrs.
ARTHRITIS **3009-1**

Keep away from meats, especially such as beef; though fish, fowl and lamb may be taken in moderation, but NO FRIED FOODS OF ANY KIND!

2/6/31
F. 22 yrs.
EPILEPSY **543-7**

Q. Would eating beef occasionally be detrimental to body?

A. If well prepared, and not too *much* taken, it may be taken in moderation—well cooked.

11/29/37
M. 42 yrs.
GENERAL: RHEUMATISM **1334-2**

As to meats, we find beef may be taken if it is PREPARED well in it OWN juices—not so much as a roast, but rather as broiled—but cooking same.

4/15/38
ASTHENIA: TENDENCIES **M. 20 yrs.**
BODY-BUILDING **487-22**

In the diet, keep to those foods that are body-building. When there IS the taxation through the physical exercise, have plenty of meats—beef; but let these be WELL DONE. Preferably not the fried foods.

5/21/42
CONCEPTION **F. 34 yrs.**
VITAMIN **457-9**

Q. Among the meat foods that may be taken, can well done beef be included?

A. Beef may be included at times but not too often.

8/31/41
ARTHRITIS: PREVENTIVE **F. 51 yrs.**
BODY: GENERAL **1158-31**

Q. For balanced diet, what quantities should I take per week of beef?

A. This should be a part of the diet about once a week—about three or four ounces of this, well prepared, but in its own juices.

5/7/40
ARTHRITIS **M. 33 yrs.**
BODY-BUILDING **849-50**

Then, fowl, fish, lamb—and once each week the beef. This should not be hard, but cooked well done, and more of the juice of same taken into the body than the flesh itself.

7/22/31
F. 28 yrs.
2261-1

ACIDITY
ASSIMILATIONS: ELIMINATIONS: INCOORDINATION

Meats—only those that are of the beef.

8/31/40
F. 12 yrs.
2153-4

EPILEPSY

Q. Should she be allowed to have a lamb chop, steak or other meat occasionally besides the fish and fowl?

A. Fish, fowl or lamb—but NOT fried foods! As to beef, this is not so well—unless it is very, VERY thoroughly cooked; and then well, WELL masticated!

12/18/36
F. 50 yrs.
1259-2

ARTHRITIS: ANEMIA

Q. What should I do about taking the hydrochloric acid internally? I seem to be much better when taking it.

A. If that is the desire of the body, that these be added in this form, then take it! For the mental outlook has as much to do with the results as the material applications! But this acidity and this unbalanced condition is what prevents the effluvia of the blood from producing resistances in the body. And if the balances for the diet are kept, these as we find are much preferable to the synthetic reactions that the body itself *should* produce within itself! If these are taken then occasionally, it may be very well. But the body should know that if the system depends upon that to be supplied that it does not have to use, it is just as in any other condition, the body depends upon same and it is as habit forming as any drug.

Q. Would it be wise for me to include in my diet any other body-building foods such as red meats or fattening foods?

A. Know that if there is to be taken, to be sure, beef and it is *required* that there be taken the acids to digest same—and they are not taken, this will be hard upon the system! But if the food values are taken in combinations and in manners that the system will assimilate same, this is much preferable.

Q. Please explain the reaction of foods on my system.

A. It's just been given! Those that required the bodily foods—there are foods that require (as meats) acids for their proper fermentation, while most of the foods as of the vegetable forces, especially of the leafy nature, require more of the slow combination of the lacteals' reaction or the greater quantity of the combination of acid and alkaline. Then if foods are taken in quantities that require an alkaline for their digestion and an acid is in the system—this produces improper fermentation. If foods are taken where acid is necessary and it is not being produced by the system, or not taken into the system in synthetic state, then these produce the disturbances, see? See how the combinations of these, then, make for the necessity of watching, experimenting as it were with that which is good today and may be bad tomorrow. For what would be poison for someone, to another may be a cure. This is true in every physical organism. And unless these balances are being cared for properly, they produce disturbances.

9/30/40
F. 74 yrs.
ARTHRITIS 1224-6

Q. Should beef be excluded from diet?

A. This is not a matter of excluding so much as to how often and the manner of preparation! As we find, it is best that it not be taken too often, though it may be taken at times; that is, once a week, twice a month or the like.

6/10/38
F. 13 yrs.
ASSIMILATIONS: ELIMINATIONS: INCOORDINATION 1206-8

Q. Is it well to eliminate beef?

A. As to the use of beef: this is very well to be discontinued.

ANEMIA 10/31/31
ASSIMILATIONS: POOR F. 60 yrs.
INJURIES: ACCIDENTS: AFTEREFFECTS: FRACTURES 501-2

In the evening, then, may be those of the whole vegetables—with the meat juices, or those that will supply more gluten will be taken at this time . . . as the *joints* of beef, and the marrow of same—these are well for the body.

1)—Roast Beef

10/5/36
CIRCULATION: POOR F. 42 yrs.
UREMIA 1016-1

Beware of roast beef that is rare, or the fats of same.

2)—Steaks

4/18/35
ANEMIA M. Adult
MENU: ASSIMILATIONS: POOR 898-1

Evening meal—About once a week a good raw steak, not oftener. Not other red meats. No hog meats of any kind should ever be taken unless it is very crisp bacon.

Keep these consistently, persistently; we will gain weight, we will put off this dullness, this tendency for catching cold, this weakness throughout the whole system; and bring the body—in six to eight months—to its normal weight of about a hundred and fifty pounds.

9/29/34
M. Adult
ABRASIONS: TOXEMIA 675-1

Evenings—Well-cooked vegetables. Do not have fried food such as steak—they are detrimental to the better eliminations from the system.

MENU: INTESTINES: CATARRH

4/30/35
F. 42 yrs.
913-1

Evenings—Occasionally there may be taken a steak, *provided* this is *well* done. And never eat any *fried* foods!

ANEMIA
DEBILITATION: GENERAL

3/16/36
F. 38 yrs.
954-2

Evenings—Occasionally a steak that is broiled rather than fried, and rather scrape same than eating *all* of same—see?

CIRCULATION: POOR
ACIDITY & ALKALINITY

2/11/37
F. 40 yrs.
1337-1

Do not have any fried foods, especially as of steak or things of that nature—but broiled, boiled or the like.

ATROPHY: NERVES

1/4/40
M. 32 yrs.
849-47

Occasionally, about once a week, give the body a good stiff steak, SMOTHERED IN ONIONS! and mushrooms may be added if so desired.

ELIMINATIONS: INCOORDINATION
VITAMINS

9/16/41
F. 2 yrs.
2015-8

Be mindful as to the diets; keeping plenty of the vitamins, especially B-1, A and G. These will be found principally in scraped beef or steak.

3)—Goat Meat

ANEMIA
BLOOD-BUILDING

11/24/24
F. Adult
2221-1

Take care that the system is supplied with those properties of iron and the food values that dilate the system in its course through the system. Little meats, save that or goat meat. These carry the necessary properties. This should all be roasted, not with much fat. Lean portions carrying the juices of the meats proper.

ACIDITY & ALKALINITY: ANEMIA

6/3/17
M. Adult
4834-1

Q. Would mutton be good?

A. No, goat would be better. Nothing that is actively acid should be taken.

4)—Lamb & Mutton

ANEMIA: TENDENCIES **10/2/43**
ASSIMILATIONS: ELIMINATIONS: INCOORDINATION **F. 37 yrs.**
KIDNEYS **1695-2**

Then take at least once each day the vitamins B-1. Do not take A.

Do take D and G, but these more in the foods than supplementing in the combinations. These will bring better forces to the body; that is, in the food values take a little lamb; not other meats.

12/9/36
ARTHRITIS: TENDENCIES **F. 63 yrs.**
BODY-BUILDING **1302-1**

In the matter of the diets: here we need body-building foods but those that tend to be more alkaline-producing than acid. For the natural inclinations of disturbed conditions in a body are to produce acidity through the bloodstream. Hence we need to revivify same by the use of much of those that produce more of the enzymes, more of the hormones for the blood supply; yet not overburdening the body with those unless the balance in the vitamin forces is carried.

Hence as we will find, not heavy foods or fried foods ever, nor combinations where there are quantities of starches with sweets taken at the same time. But lamb preferably as the meats.

8/25/39
F. 39 yrs.
TOXEMIA **1985-1**

The activities of red meats would become more disturbing to the body. Lamb should be a portion of the diet as the meats, if there is any of these taken.

7/30/40
F. Adult
OBESITY **2315-1**

Each meal should be preceeded by the grape juice—thirty minutes before eating.

Evenings—Take a little of one or the other of the raw vegetables as a salad; with baked, broiled lamb, but NOT any fried. All cooked vegetables should be cooked in their own juices (as in Patapar Paper), rather than with meats or fats.

6/25/40
M. Adult
ARTHRITIS **228-1**

As to the diet, refrain from any foods carrying any elements as of silicon, lime or the like. Hence not much meats unless lamb. No fried foods of ANY character.

2/5/36
M. 28 yrs.
ARTHRITIS **849-13**

Be most careful that there are not shell fish. Not too great a quantity of meats, and when meats are taken let same be roast lamb. These, we find, with *quantities* of the green vegetables, would supply greater quantities of those elements to create this balance in *conjunction* with the indicated manipulative and electrical treatments and the baths.

5/22/44
F. 56 yrs.
1895-2

ARTHRITIS: TENDENCIES

Do decrease any red meats. Lamb we would take but none of any heavy foods, none of these fried.

4/18/35
M. Adult
898-1

ANEMIA
ASSIMILATIONS: POOR

Evening meal—In the meats have those especially, whenever possible, of lamb.

Keep these consistently, persistently; we will gain weight, we will put off this dullness, this tendency for catching cold, this weakness throughout the whole system; and bring the body—in six to eight months—to its normal weight of about a hundred and fifty pounds.

3/31/43
F. 18 yrs.
2947-1

ASSIMILATIONS: ELIMINATIONS: INCOORDINATION
BODY-BUILDING

Keep the diet body-building. Plenty of vitamins A and D; plenty of B-1 and the B-Complex.

No hog meat of ANY character. Let there be occasionally lamb.

This is not to be all the diet, of course, but these should form a great part of the diet—just so often as not to become obnoxious to the body; altering in the manner of preparation.

Q. What causes pain in arms, shoulders and back, and what can be done for relief?

A. The lack of sufficient energies being supplied to the nerve forces and the stimulation of the nerve plexus calling for more activity. AND at times a pressure in the assimilating system.

Thus the needs of keeping good eliminations.

Q. How can she best overcome constipation?

A. By the diet; and, as indicated, these are taken into consideration.

8/27/40
F. 40 yrs.
2332-I

ATHLETE'S FOOT: ECZEMA

If meats are taken, only take such as lamb, broiled, baked, stewed or the like.

4/15/38
M. 20 yrs.
487-22

ASTHENIA: TENDENCIES
BODY-BUILDING

In the diet, keep to those foods that are body-building. When there IS the taxation through the physical exercise, have plenty of meats—as lamb; but let these be WELL DONE. Preferably not the fried foods.

3/21/39
F. 49 yrs.
RELAXATION **1158-21**

Lamb about three times a week—this about three and a half ounces.

2/11/37
F. 40 yrs.
CIRCULATION: POOR
ACIDITY & ALKALINITY **1337-1**

Do not have any fried foods, especially as of steak or things of that nature—but broiled, boiled or the like; and especially lamb should be used if meats at all are taken.

2/5/42
F. 24 yrs.
INJURIES **2679-1**

In the diets, also, much may be accomplished. Necessarily, there must be plenty of those properties that aid in keeping a correct balance in the production of Iymph, leucocyte AND the red blood supply.

Then, have especially those foods that carry more of the calcium and the vitamins A, D, B-1 and other B Complexes.

Hence we would have plenty of lamb; these alternated as parts of the diet.

3/28/44
M. 41 yrs.
ACIDITY & ALKALINITY **4008-1**

Q. Is there any combination of foods that could be truthfully called Brain Foods, Nerve Foods, Muscle Foods?

A. Those that are body-building; those that are nerve-building and those that supply certain elements. For, as indicated, those foods suggested are to be taken by the body. Lamb will supply elements needed for brain, muscle and nerve building.

INCOORDINATION **5/19/35**
GLANDS: SALIVARY: DIGESTION: GENERAL **F. 27 yrs.**
PREGNANCY **808-3**

The meats should be such as lamb. Occasionally the *broiled* steak, or liver, or tripe, would be well. A well balance between the starches and proteins is the more preferable, with sufficient of the carbohydrates. And especially keep a well balance (but not an excess) in the calciums necessary with the iodines, that produce the better body, especially through those periods of conception and gestation.

8/12/37
F. 36 yrs.
LACERATIONS: STOMACH **1422-1**

No food that makes for a quantity of alcohol in its activity in the system.

Meats—never rare meats. Rather use those that are broiled or roasted; preferably only lamb.

11/23/37
M. 13 yrs.
PSORIASIS **1484-1**

Evening—Lamb—these would be taken in moderation, with any of the vegetables that are grown UNDER the ground, with one or two of the green variety or nature that grow above the ground.

7/26/32
ANEMIA **M. 25 yrs.**
ASSIMILATIONS: POOR **481-1**

We would be mindful of the diet, that those foods are taken that are easily assimilated. Do not take quantities of grease of any nature. When meats *are* taken, they should be those of roast mutton.

Evenings—Cooked vegetables, and the meats *when* these are taken. Do not eat meat more than three times each week, and don't gorge self when this is done!

9/19/35
ASSIMILATIONS: POOR **F. 80 yrs.**
CANCER **975-1**

Evenings—When meats are taken let them be preferably either small quantities of mutton or the like. These should never be fried. These would only be those that were prepared very thoroughly, and in most instances after preparation be *chilled* almost, as it were, that they may be the easier assimilated by the gastric forces that have had so much disturbance; but these will be aided by the properties we have indicated in the compound for the body.

11/24/24
ANEMIA **F. Adult**
BLOOD-BUILDING **2221-1**

Take care that the system is supplied with those properties of iron and the food values that dilate the system in its course through the system. Little meats, save that of mutton. These carry the necessary properties. This should all be roasted, not with much fat. Lean portions, carrying the juices of the meats proper.

2/22/34
ASTHENIA **F. 65 yrs.**
ACIDITY & ALKALINITY **509-2**

Beware of too much starch and too much fat. But oils, as the olive oil or the fats of any that are taken in the foods—as mutton (provided the same is not the *gross* fat)—will be helpful. But no red meats, nor too much of those foods that will make for sugar reaction in the system.

7/1/26
M. Adult
BLOOD: HUMOR **43-1**

Not meats, especially not fat meats. Lean meat of mutton may be eaten. No hog meat or any fish for this body.

1/6/42
M. 57 yrs.
GENERAL **462-14**

Noons—Juices, but with such as mutton. These with plenty of vegetables should supply sufficient needs for the body.

3/27/35
F. 52 yrs.
ACIDITY & ALKALINITY **805-2**

Q. What can I do to avoid losing so much weight? Outline the proper diet.

A. Those foods, now, that are the body-building; as starches and proteins, if these are taken without other food values that make for the combinations that produce distress or disorder; that is, not quantities of starches and proteins combined, you see, but these taken one at one meal and one at another will be most helpful. When meats are taken, use mutton, or the like, and do not have heavy starches with same—but preferably fruits or vegetables.

7/22/31
ACIDITY **F. 28 yrs.**
ASSIMILATIONS: ELIMINATIONS: INCOORDINATION **2261-1**

Meats—only those that are of the mutton.

5)—Pork: General

5/17/28
M. 55 yrs.
COLITIS: MEAT: HOG: NOT RECOMMENDED **4874-3**

To be sure, there must be kept for the body properties that will continue to act as an antiseptic for the lungs, throat, bronchials, and the constant building up of the blood supply; but no hog meat should *ever* be taken by the body—not even hog liver!

11/4/40
M. 56 yrs.
ARTHRITIS **2392-1**

Keep away from any meats, especially hog meats. A little fish or fowl may be taken.

Q. Will this treatment if carefully carried out give permanent cure?

A. This will depend upon the body's returning to those things that would bring back the reaction. Keeping off of hog meat and fats, and these eliminated as indicated should be, we find that it should be a permanent cure.

12/18/36
F. 50 yrs.
ARTHRITIS: ANEMIA **1259-2**

Q. Would it be wise for me to include in my diet any other body-building foods such as red meats or fattening foods?

A Know that if there is to be taken, to be sure, pork ham, and it is required that there be taken the acids to digest same—and they are not taken, this will be hard upon the system! But if the food values are taken in combinations and in manners that the system will assimilate same, this is much preferable.

1)—Bacon

CIRCULATION: POOR **10/5/36**
UREMIA **F. 42 yrs.**
1016-1

Q. Any other advice as to diet?

A. As indicated from the slowed circulation, and the tendencies at times for the acidity, those things that pertain more to the alkaline-reacting diet would be the better. Rather would we give those things that the body should be warned against, and then most everything else may be taken if it is taken in moderation, and *when* there is the *desire!* As there is the desire for food, whether it is the regular meal time or at others, it would be best for *this* body to eat! If it desires to eat this or that, eat it! but do not mix it with other foods! Beware of hog meats, though, in every form save a little crisp bacon may be taken at times.

6/6/34
F. Adult
ANEMIA **574-1**

Q. Please give the diet I should follow.

A. Keep the diet rather alkaline. That means not too much meats nor too much starches, nor too much of *any* of those things that *produce* acidity. But don't make self as subject to a diet. Rather subject the diet to self, by self's activity; that is, keep a normal well-balanced diet, but no hog meats ever—unless a little crisp breakfast bacon at times.

4/9/43
ASSIMILATIONS: POOR **F. 33 yrs.**
BODY-BUILDING **2959-1**

Mornings—Citrus fruit with bacon and egg, and brown toast.

DO NOT eat hog meat, other than the crisp breakfast bacon.

9/12/37
BLOOD: COAGULATION: POOR **M. 62 yrs.**
ACIDITY & ALKALINITY **1411-2**

Noons—Preferably vegetables that are well cooked, preferably WITHOUT fat meats in same. DO NOT eat hog meat, save the bacon of morning.

7/26/37
DEBILITATION: GENERAL **F. 60 yrs.**
TEMPERATURE: FEVER: AFTEREFFECTS **1409-4**

Since the temperature has been allayed, there is the necessity, to be sure, that there are not foods used nor activities that would tend to make for the weakening of the digestive forces, nor the allowing of activities of the assimilating system—the liver, the kidneys or the whole hepatic circulation—to become so congested as to allow the temperature to arise again.

Hence we would keep rather a tendency to the alkaline-producing foods.

To be sure . . . crisp bacon may be gradually added; not all at once, to be sure, but just sufficient that the body gains the strength physically. And keep the eliminations well.

10/29/36
M. Adult
ANEMIA **1131-2**

Mornings—Principally cereals or citrus fruits, but these should *not* be taken at the same meal; either may be balanced with a small amount of crisp bacon.

4/28/43
F. 36 yrs.
ELIMINATIONS: POOR **2977-1**

Not too much of fats. Never hog meat, save crisp breakfast bacon.

6)—Game: General

4/7/23
NERVOUS SYSTEMS: INCOORDINATION **M. Adult**
NERVE-BUILDING **4730-1**

The diet—all those that lend energy to nerve-building forces and those that give the blood force the eliminating properties—vegetables, those that are green. Meats, very little. When used, only game or the sinew of any other force. Do that.

7)—Wild Game

1/20/24
F. Adult
BLOOD-BUILDING **4120-1**

The diet should be watched closely, taking those properties that will create stimulation to blood supply, especially nerve-building forces in blood. Meats only that of wild game.

9/13/43
M. 41 yrs.
ARTHRITIS **3077-1**

Liquids and semi-liquids for the present, but include in same a great deal of wild game—as much as practical . . .

4/18/35
ANEMIA **M. Adult**
ASSIMILATIONS: POOR **898-1**

Evening meal—In the meats have those especially, whenever possible, of wild game.

Keep these consistently, persistently; we will gain weight, we will put off this dullness, this tendency for catching cold, this weakness throughout the whole system; and bring the body—in six to eight months—to its normal weight of about a hundred and fifty pounds.

11/27/34
M. 32 yrs.
749-1

KATABOLISM: METABOLISM: INCOORDINATION

Q. Will you outline a diet for the body?

A. Wild game would be most preferable for the meats. No red meats. No fried foods of any kind. Keep a well-balanced diet that will make for the better assimilations; strengthening, of course, more in those things that carry phosphorus and iron . . .

6/9/44
M. 12 yrs.
5192-1

ASTHMA

Q. What causes the deep ridges in thumbnail and what treatments should be followed?

A. These are the activities of the glandular force, and the addition of those foods which carry large quantities of calcium will make for bettered conditions in this direction. Eat wild game of any kind, but chew the bones of same. These will be well for the body.

5/17/28
M. 55 yrs.
4874-3

ENVIRONMENT: ALTITUDE: TUBERCULOSIS COLITIS

As much wild game as may be obtained, or may be taken and assimilated by the body. Keep in the open as much as possible.

11/16/22
F. Adult
4810-1

BLOOD: OXIDIZATION BLOOD-BUILDING

Q. Should this body eat any meats, Mr. Cayce?

A. Very little meats. When meats are eaten, preferably those of wild game and those not in large quantity, but something of those that carry the sinew and vital forces—no hog meat.

6/3/17
M. Adult
4834-1

ACIDITY & ALKALINITY: ANEMIA

Meats should be wild game, nothing that has been killed with blood in it. Eat wild game which eats from nature, tame game eats what it is fed.

12/17/38
M. 45 yrs.
1564-3

TUBERCULOSIS

Beware of any fried foods.

Have wild game whenever practical.

5/5/44
F. 40 yrs.
5053-1

TUBERCULOSIS

In the diet take strengthening foods.

Have squirrels, rabbit, or any wild game. Any of these are good for the body. Chew the bones when masticating same, as this will add to the strength and blood-building and resistance of the body.

1/9/26
F. 7 yrs.
4281-10

COLD: CONGESTION: FLU: AFTEREFFECTS
BABY CARE

Q. Should she eat rabbit?

A. Any wild game good for the body—never fried though.

12/8/41
F. 23 yrs.
2514-4

SCLERODERMA

Q. Is it all right for me to eat rabbit and squirrel, baked or stewed?

A. Any wild game is preferable even to other meats, if these are prepared properly. Rabbit—be sure the tendon in both left legs is removed, or that as might cause a fever. It is what is called at times the wolf in the rabbit. While prepared in some ways this would be excellent for some disturbances in a body, it is never well for this to be eaten in a hare. Squirrel—of course, it is not in same. This stewed, or well cooked, is really more preferable for the body, of course—but rabbit is well if that part indicated is removed.

5/12/28
M. 33 yrs.
900-383

LIVER: KIDNEYS: INCOORDINATION

Q. Is the albumin on the decrease or increase in the urine?

A. On the decrease. Little fowl—preferably though game, as hare, squirrel.

3/14/32
M. Adult
5672-1

TOXEMIA

Noon—Broths of fresh meats, preferably of wild game—of the hare or of the squirrel—these would be well for the body; but little of the meats would we take—but thick broths.

11/11/38
F. 13 yrs.
1206-9

GLANDS: INCOORDINATION

As for meats . . . when practical the wild game would be desirable. Little or no fried foods should be in the diet.

10/30/37
M. 48 yrs.
470-19

DIABETES: TENDENCIES

The leafy vegetables, of course, should be the main—though this should not exclude meats; but preferably not those that are fried . . . WILD GAME of every nature—all of these are well for the body.

10/21/32
F. 18 yrs.
951-1

ELEPHANTIASIS: TENDENCIES
ARTHRITIS: GLANDS: INCOORDINATION

Supply an overabundant amount of those foods that carry iron, iodine and phosphorus in the system.

The meats should be preferably (when taken at all) of wild game.

8)—Meat Juices & Puddings

1)—Meat Juices: General

1/9/35
M. 1 yr.
WORMS **786-1**

We would begin with a body-*building* diet for the body. We would give every day (this is outside of the other meals, you see) at least two tablespoonsful of beef juice and liver juice; these *not* mixed, but given at different times. Give the juice *warm,* of course, but not a large quantity at a time; half to a teaspoonful, or half a teaspoonful given at a dose—first one and then the other, you see—and this may be done two, three or four times in the morning and in the afternoon. Graham or whole wheat crackers may be eaten with same.

8/17/34
F. 53 yrs.
ARTHRITIS **634-1**

Be very, *very* mindful of the diet; which should consist, of course, of more of those foods carrying more and more of the Iymph and white blood-*building* influences. Hence little of the proteins as *fats,* while proteins in the *juices* of *lean* meats are very good. These should be a portion of the diet, but not great quantities of fats.

3/25/30
ACIDITY & ALKALINITY **F. 45 yrs.**
DIGESTION: INDIGESTION **5625-1**

Little of the meats, though those that are taken should be principally of the juices of same; not of the flesh itself. This rather in the evening meal.

8/8/29
HEART **M. 61 yrs.**
BLOOD-BUILDING **2597-6**

Q. Does he require any special foods, and what food is most beneficial to him?

A. Those that have blood-building, and especially carrying iron. Those of meats—rather the juices than the fleshy portions.

4/18/35
ANEMIA **M. Adult**
ASSIMILATIONS: POOR **898-1**

Noons—Meat juices, but not that which carries great quantities of grease in same. Let the greases be taken in vegetable oils, as olive oil, as butter or the like; and this should be taken with the brown bread—but do not take the brown bread without it being toasted, at *any* time, for this particular body.

4/17/31
M. 19 yrs.
1225-1

DEBILITATION: GENERAL
CHOREA

Noon—We would give those that carry more of the silicon, lime, salts—*these,* as we find, will be in the *green* vegetables. Following same with broths or the *juices* of meats—see? not the meats.

2/24/32
M. 44 yrs.
437-4

ELIMINATIONS: INCOORDINATION

Noon—The *juices* of meats *with* vegetables—see? or the broth of meats. No meats!

i)-Beef Juice

6/5/34
M. 68 yrs.
570-1

CANCER

As to the matter of the diet; this should be nerve- and blood-building, a liquid diet through the greater part of the time; a great deal of beef juices. Not meat nor stews nor soups or the like, but rather the juice itself—very small quantities.

DIRECTIONS FOR MAKING PURE BEEF JUICE

Put small chunks raw beef in covered fruit jar. Put jar inside pan of water (water coming to about half the depth of jar). Boil until chunks of beef are thoroughly done. Strain. Keep juice in cool place. Dosage: usually, for an adult, a tablespoonful at meals, diluted with water as a broth—but very small quantities: must mean about a teaspoonful every two or three hours.

11/28/22
F. Adult
4439-1

ANEMIA

Juice of beef well seasoned prepared much in this manner of the clear, good roast, would be cut into small cubes or pieces, placed in a glass jar sealed without any water and then put on in water and let this water boil for an hour and a half, squeeze the juice from beef and season well with salt and as much of the hot pepper, not black, as the body can take.

2/18/25
F. 33 yrs.
2457-1

ANEMIA

No great amount of meats. None carrying much fat. Quantities of the juices of beef may be taken, *should* be taken, provided small quantities of stimulant in fruit juices are taken with same. Citrus fruit juices should be taken with the meat juice or beef juice.

11/3/43
F. 54 yrs.
3337-1

MULTIPLE SCLEROSIS

Do add as much as may possibly be assimilated of the B vitamins, A and D vitamins. We find that these may be best supplied by quantities of beef juice taken as medicine. Take often—but very small quantities at a time.

12/31/40
F. 58 yrs.
STOMACH: SPASMS **805-6**

Have prepared the beef tea to begin taking at least when the Castoria is begun; not stew or the like, but the beef JUICE—only the juice of the beef itself, you see. Take a teaspoonful about every two hours, and take three to five minutes to sip that quantity of the beef juice. This will give strength to the body, even with the natural strain through the taking of the eliminant for the system.

Then, rest; not too much of foods save those easily assimilated.

5/18/43
F. 56 yrs.
CANCER **2956-2**

Q. What should be avoided in the diet, other than fats?

A. That mainly to be avoided is fats.

DO give the body beef juice as a strengthening factor, but no fats in same—and this only in small quantities, and very little taken at a time. Give as medicine.

7/27/39
F. 27 yrs.
DEBILITATION: GENERAL **480-52**

Keep a general upbuilding in the diet, by the body-building influences. Have plenty of beef juice; not too much of roast beef.

These as we find should bring much better results and experiences for the body.

6/4/26
M. 54 yrs.
BLOOD-BUILDING **4769-2**

Let the diet be beef juice—not the meats, but the juice as extracted from pure fresh meats, see? seasoned well.

3/4/40
F. 53 yrs.
GLANDS: ADRENALS: BODY-BUILDING **2025-3**

But if there will be more of the beef juices, these will aid in BUILDING the body for better strength, better resistance, and less of this disturbance.

Q. As I cannot eat enough to keep my strength, is there anything I can do to increase my weight?

A. Keep those things that have been indicated, and these will GIVE the strength—the beef juice, not as a drink but as a medicine. And the beef juice would be sipped, and not taken as a drink, but sipped very slowly.

5/11/42
F. 74 yrs.
BODY-BUILDING **2074-2**

Give beef juices and semi-liquids and liquids, foods that are very stimulating. Every form of better stimulant that is for building strength, as the beef juices. These especially, with the fish foods.

1/5/44
DEBILITATION: GENERAL **M. 27 yrs.**
ANEMIA **3535-1**

Also as oft as possible take beef juice, or as regularly as you can obtain the beef. It is much preferable to use the juice in this manner than to take transfusions, though you might have to take transfusions if you don't do these things—and it wouldn't be very good for this body!

So take all the beef juice you can assimilate—don't let it become obnoxious, but at least every day take one or two slices of calf liver—with all the blood in it that you can keep, just to make it palatable by broiling in butter.

Take a teaspoonful of the beef juice at a time—don't swallow it down, but let it mix with the juices of the mouth and be assimilated in that manner, by sipping it. Take at least a minute in sipping a teaspoonful. Do this two or three times a day, if it is possible to obtain the beef. Prepare the juice in the manner we have suggested—no fat at all in it.

Don't try to eat fats.

9/23/43
F. 49 yrs.
ANEMIA: MULTIPLE SCLEROSIS **3232-1**

Q. Is it necessary to take as much liver as prescribed?

A. As we find, beef juice taken instead of the liver would be more effective and better. Take this as medicine, a tablespoonful during the day but divided—half in the morning, half in the afternoon. Let the body be at least a minute in sipping a teaspoonful. Eat a whole whet cracker with it when it is being sipped.

12/5/43
F. 6 yrs.
EPILEPSY **3398-1**

Do give the body beef juice. Give a teaspoonful of this each day, or two teaspoonsful—not more than that. This should be given more as drops than as spoonful, though, so that proper assimilation may take place. A teaspoonful of this taken during a day will be more strengthening than a glassful of the eggnog. A teaspoonful may be taken during the morning and a teaspoonful in the afternoon, if it is sipped slowly so as to be properly assimilated.

7/6/44
F. 62 yrs.
ASTHENIA **5327-1**

In the diets, those which are easily assimilated, beef juice, liver extract, not necessary for this to be given by injection but beef juice taken often will give strength and will not be adverse to the condition of the heart or of the eliminations. All foods which are strengthening and body-building.

6/5/34
M. Adult
TUBERCULOSIS **572-1**

We find that the beef juice would be well.

Q. Why does weakness continue?

A. The poor circulation. The lack of the resistances in the body, and especially those things as indicated. If four to six ounces of the beef juice were taken during the day, it would not be too much—if the body assimilates it. But it should never be more than two or three teaspoonsful at a time, and *sipped*—rather than taking gobs or spoonsful at the time, you see. Taken often, every twenty to thirty minutes, would be better.

6/3/41
DEBILITATION: GENERAL **M. 25 yrs.**
APPENDICITIS **1970-1**

Then, after these have been followed out for the week or ten days—we would THEN begin to live more or less on the milk and cheese diet; with, of course, the beef juices—taken in small quantities often. No meats except the beef juices, you see. (Do not begin this diet, of course, until after the period of the grape poultices and the grape diet.)

7/3/35
M. 56 yrs.
DEBILITATION: GENERAL **556-8**

For the building up of the body's strength, we would *gradually*—as the assimilations are able to be carried on—increase the properties that would be given for strengthening.

If the beef juice is prepared properly, a tablespoonful of this carries *all* of the elements that are most worthwhile for the system—as much as from as large a steak as an ordinary person might eat.

10/27/43
ANEMIA: TENDENCIES **F. 53 yrs.**
ARTHRITIS: RHEUMATOID **3316-1**

When there is weakness indicated (as the body tends towards anemia, even from the character of swellings that occur), give the body plenty of beef juice. This should be taken as medicine. Give a teaspoonful at the time, but let the body be at least two minutes in sipping that quantity. Let it rather be absorbed than swallowed. Let it just flow with the salivary glands and be absorbed through the body-force by the gentle swallowing. There will be little or none to digest, but will be absorbed.

CHILDBIRTH: AFTEREFFECTS **8/3/26**
DEBILITATION: GENERAL **F. 34 yrs.**
ASSIMILATIONS: ELIMINATIONS: INCOORDINATION **583-4**

Take at least the juice of two to three pounds of steak, or beef (fresh), each day. None of the meat, but the juice. This, in itself, would apparently be heavy for the kidneys, under strain, yet the system is in that condition as is needed for this condition to produce some counter-irritation, as would be brought by this condition. Adding, then, as this: to each three tablespoonsful of such solution (that is, the beef juice), add syrup of pepsin one minim, oil of sassafras one minim. See? This, as we see, will meet the needs of the condition in the assimilation as created by this condition.

Then, as much green vegetable matter as the system will assimilate. Eat only graham crackers with the juice or tea.

2/23/34
F. 22 yrs.
TUBERCULOSIS 418-4

As to the matter of diet, prepare all the *beef* juice (not broth, but beef *juice*) that the body may take, and do not have any fats in the meat when the juice is prepared—and cook it *done,* the meat, you see, for an hour and a half to two or three hours; then strain off, but don't eat the meat—it isn't good for a dog even! Take the juice in very small quantities. If it is given every thirty minutes, a teaspoonful or so, so much the better.

And if there are the proper amounts of the beef juices taken, and the liver juices, and the foods that are blood-building, we will build up resistances to this body. Do not use too much sugar, but stick to the blood-building foods.

9/18/43
M. 22 yrs.
TUBERCULOSIS 3222-1

Do take daily two teaspoonsful of beef juice, one in the morning—or between breakfast and the noon meal, and one in the afternoon just after the body has rested and slept for at least a few minutes. Let the body be a minute or two minutes in sipping the teaspoonful.

1/22/36
F. 38 yrs.
TUBERCULOSIS 1045-5

For the assimilations, we find that beef juices sipped every few minutes (not drunk, but sipped), with whole wheat wafers, would be helpful; as also would the arrowroot biscuit, or popcorn wafers.

3/20/36
F. 38 yrs.
TUBERCULOSIS 1045-9

While the strength and the vitality and the resistances are low, if the diet is followed that will be the more easily assimilated, we find that building influences will be created—as we have indicated. *None* of the foods should be in great quantities, but the liquid and semi-liquid diet—the beef juice formed in the manner indicated; and these sipped a little now and then, three, four, five times a day, is much preferable to giving quantities at a stipulated time.

6/22/39
F. 83 yrs.
DEBILITATION: GENERAL 1907-2

The strengthening forces from the use of the beef juice are very well. This should not be taken in too large quantities, but may be sipped often; and as conditions progress it is well that the graham or whole wheat crackers be crumbled in the small quantity taken—or grated in same.

6/5/37
M. 45 yrs.
CANCER 1382-1

Give the body only liquids or semi-liquids in the beginning: beef juice (made from the lean beef, no fats nor fatty portions in same) . . . Not soups—these carry too much greases.

4/30/40
M. 49 yrs.
ASSIMILATIONS: POOR **2183-1**

In the diet—give small quantities of beef juice often; at least a tablespoonful each day, but not more than that, and this taken in several doses—that is, take a teaspoonful at the time only, and take about ten minutes to sip this amount, letting it mix thoroughly with the saliva of the mouth. Even half a teaspoonful at the time would be better, and this taken often during the day. Use only the lean beef, no fats whatever in same, and use only the juice.

4/12/35
F. Adult
TUMORS: LYMPH **889-I**

Q. Will the disturbance in the lungs clear up?

A. This will clear up, for we will make for the building of resistances that have been low—as indicated in the conditions that arise from the activities of the circulation.

Beef juices . . . should be the more of the meats for the body.

6/29/42
F. 25 yrs.
ANEMIA **2376-2**

Fish, fowl and lamb may be taken. Do not eat beef, for this body; though beef juice may be taken if it is desirable—not a stew, but beef juice.

11/28/33
M. Adult
ANEMIA **461-1**

Before retiring each evening take at least a tablespoonful of beef juice, but never the beef! Not juice extract, but *beef* juices and take it very *slowly.*

Q. How should the beef juices be prepared?

A. Take a pound to a pound and a half of beef—*lean* beef, not fat! Dice it into small pieces, about the size of a good sized marble—or the thumb. Put in a glass jar. Seal the jar, no water in same. Put this in water, with a cloth or something in to prevent from breaking or cracking the jar. Let it boil for two to three hours. Extract the juice. Throw the meat away. Season the juice and take it as directed. There will be enough in a pound to last for two or three days. Keep in a cool place. Not beef broth, but beef *juice!*

6/18/37
F. 22 yrs.
ASSIMILATIONS: POOR: ANEMIA **667-8**

Take beef juice. Make quantities of it, but be sure it is kept rather fresh; or make it fresh each day. Sip it two, three, four, five, six times a day. A teaspoonful of this is worth much more than a quarter pound steak. This is worth much more than five pounds of potatoes. It is worth much more than a whole head of cabbage, unless the cabbage is eaten raw—and this wouldn't be very well for this body. Take, then, at least a teaspoonful four, five, six times a day. Do not gulp it when this is taken, but make at least five or six swallows of same. A salty cracker or whole wheat cracker or the like may be taken with same, but keep this *consistently* for at least three to four weeks and we will see a vast difference!

1/23/39
M. 32 yrs.
ASSIMILATIONS: POOR **1798-1**

Prepare first the beef juice, not a broth—none of the fats with same at all. A little of this may be given every twenty minutes if it is so desired, but do not EVER take more than a teaspoonful—and this taken in three, four, five sips.

Do not ever take so much as to overcrowd the stomach and cause greater regurgitation than occurs at times even now.

Malted milk with apple brandy may be alternated with beef juice.

6/27/41
F. 18 yrs.
ANEMIA **1207-2**

Twice each day take a tablespoonful of beef juice; spending at least ten to twenty minutes in sipping that quantity.

Soon after, or with the beef juice, take an ounce to two ounces of red wine—with brown bread or whole wheat crackers. Also take time to sip this—not gulping it nor taking it all at once.

Then have the regular foods; those that carry quantities, or an excess, of vitamin B-1, especially.

1/24/38
F. 37 yrs.
ANEMIA **1520-1**

We would be precautious as to the DIETS of the body. Make for self, or have made, quantities of beef juice. Not so much at the time but make it rather every day—BEEF JUICE! Not the broths, but JUST the beef juice! Do not take this in large quantities, but take it often—three to four times a day, so that there will be at least two or three tablespoonsful taken during the day. This sipped with whole wheat wafers would be the better—seasoned to the taste. This will give strength, this will produce blood supply.

Of course, there are to be other foods in the diet than the beef juice, but the beef juice is to be taken as a tonic, as a stimulant. DO NOT eat ANY fried foods at ANY time! Whether vegetables or meat or whatnot, let these be broiled or boiled. The principal meats should be mutton, fowl or fish—but not fried, *any* of these!

12/18/36
F. 50 yrs.
ARTHRITIS: ANEMIA **1259-2**

Q. Would it be wise for me to include in my diet any other body-building foods such as red meats or fattening foods?

A. This depends upon what is termed red meats. Juices of meats, as has been given—and there is more strength and body-building in one spoonful of beef juice than a pound of the raw meat or rare meat or cooked! and the system will build more from same if taken in that way and manner. Especially where those conditions in the system have been as they have been.

7/14/30
M. 19 yrs.
OBESITY **488-3**

Q. Does beef contain iron?

A. Depends upon how soon it is used after being slaughtered. Depends upon the characterization of the preparations. The *juices* contain iron. The meats contain little.

2/5/36
F. 38 yrs.

TUBERCULOSIS **1045-6**

More of the beef juice would be well. Do not put *any* fat, for this becomes hard upon the stomach. There has been allowed a little of this, through the tendons being left in same. Preferably use round steak or rump steak. This should be diced and put in a jar with *no* water, *no fats;* almost sealed, and put on in either a double boiler or in a boiler (in the glass jar, you see), with a cloth or something to prevent the cracking of same. And *only* use the *juices* that come from boiling this from two, three to four hours. The juice may be seasoned with a little salt to make it more palatable, but give in sips often—rather than in quantities. It will be very strengthening. It may be taken with the whole wheat crackers or toasted brown bread, or whole wheat bread.

3/2/38
M. 12 yrs.

BLOOD-BUILDING **1519-1**

Greater precaution needs to be taken in the diet that there are blood-building foods; as the whole wheat, beef juices. These carry the hormones and the gluten that supplies in the assimilating system the better body-building.

1/26/27
F. 22 yrs.

TUBERCULOSIS **4236-1**

Also use in the diet as much beef juice as the body can assimilate—a little at the time may be taken, see? even though a half a teaspoonful at the time—just so the body *assimilates* same.

Do not let this become old, but this will assimilate in the system.

3/30/38
F. 36 yrs.

TUBERCULOSIS **1560-1**

At least twice or three times a day take a tablespoonful of beef juice, but in *very* small sips. Not just swallowed; not as spoonful—but just sipped, so that the assimilation not only begins by digestive forces but—prepared properly—begins with the salivary glands, the throat, the esophagus, the cardiac portion or the assimilation of the stomach; and will give STRENGTH to the body. If there is the feeling of weakness even in the evenings or night, sip just a little of this: it will give strength.

1/24/35

CANCER: TENDENCIES **F. Adult**
DEBILITATION: GENERAL **799-1**

We would be very mindful of the diet; and while it should not be too rich, it should be particularly nourishing. So we find that beef juices would be well.

2/19/38
ASSIMILATIONS: ELIMINATIONS: INCOORDINATION **M. 60 yrs.**
ANEMIA **1539-1**

Beef juices occasionally; not the meats but the beef juices should be a portion of the diet. Not gobs of it, but small quantities taken often. Or have regular days when a tablespoonful to two tablespoonsful would be taken, but in small sips during an evening or during a rest period at some time.

6/30/41
F. 62 yrs.
ASTHENIA **2521-1**

Take at least a teaspoonful of beef juice during a day; not the beef, but the juice; not more than half or a third of a teaspoonful at a time, and this merely sipped—not taken all at once, but sipped, so that it is almost assimilated from the activity produced by the salivary glands—and this swallowed.

9/24/40
DEBILITATION: GENERAL **F. 16 yrs.**
ELIMINATIONS: INCONTINENCE **2367-1**

We would take small sips of pure beef juice several times during the day; never more than a teaspoonful at the time, and take at least three to four minutes in sipping that quantity, you see.

7/20/43
ARTHRITIS **M. 64 yrs.**
ASSIMILATIONS: POOR **3101-1**

Beef juice taken as medicine will be the most strengthening as food. This being already digested will make for better assimilation. During a day take at least a tablespoonful, but take only half to three-quarters of a teaspoonful at the time, letting several minutes elapse while sipping that amount, see? This may be taken with a whole wheat cracker, so it will be more palatable for the body.

8/24/35
F. Adult
ACIDITY & ALKALINITY: ANEMIA **978-1**

Be very mindful of the diet. Eat those foods that are alkaline in their reaction. *Do not* partake of the heavier meats. Beef *juice* (not beef extract) may be taken; this made fresh once or twice a week, and a teaspoonful two or three times a day will be very *strengthening* to the body.

Hold to those things that are alkaline in their reaction. Not too much of sweets, not too much of starches; but rather those things that are well-balanced and those special foods as indicated should be a portion of the diet from day to day. Keep a well-balance, knowing that the alkaline-reacting foods are *preferable* for the body; for they prevent acidity. And acidity is irritating to the blood flow.

12/12/33
ACIDITY & ALKALINITY: DEBILITATION: GENERAL **F. 22 yrs.**
TUBERCULOSIS **418-2**

Noons—Beef juices or broths, but do not take the broths of beef *and* beef juice—for they don't work very well together. Take the beef *juice* preferably.

2/5/42
F. 55 yrs.
ELIMINATIONS: ANEMIA **2067-9**

Now, we would take regularly—for the body—the combinations of vitamins A, B-1 and D.

Then DO have, or do take—to work with these, the pure beef juice. This may be prepared for two days at a time—that is, for taking it the day it is made AND the next day, but DO NOT keep it beyond that time—make it fresh. Take a tablespoonful of morning and a tablespoonful of evening; just before going to work and just after returning from work. But PLEASE don't gulp it! else it will be more harmful than beneficial! Take at least five minutes to sip that quantity, slowly. Season to taste. And keep this up for some time.

Q. For some time before this trouble, I have had splitting headaches—I awake with them. What is the cause?

A. These have come from the strain upon the system by the lack of vital energies, and the calling upon the whole system for the better energizing forces. As indicated, do these things; being persistent and consistent, and we will find we will overcome.

These are opportunities, don't balk at them!

Q. Any further advice?

A. Do these things, and live—in thy dealings with others—as ye would seek that the Creative Influence or Force deal with thee.

1/12/40
F. 27 yrs.
NEURASTHENIA **2076-1**

Little of meat, save fish, fowl or lamb. Occasionally, for the strengthening of the body, take pure beef juice as a medicine; not as a drink or as a soup. When taken, this would be taken in a small quantity—as a tablespoonful once or twice a week, but this sipped—taking five to ten minutes to sip that quantity, see? With it there may be taken a whole wheat wafer. This will prove very strengthening.

7/15/41
F. 61 yrs.
DEBILITATION: GENERAL **2535-1**

Once a day it will be most beneficial to take beef juice as a tonic; not so much the beef itself but beef juice; followed with red wine. Do not mix these, but take both about the same time. Take about a teaspoonful of the beef juice, but spend about five minutes in sipping that much. Then take an ounce of the red wine, with a whole wheat cracker.

5/15/41
F. Adult
ANEMIA: DEBILITATION: GENERAL **2500-1**

We would add B-1 in the foods. The beef juice is a source of same.

7/17/44
M. 51 yrs.
ANEMIA **5334-1**

Take at least a teaspoonful of beef juice four times each day and take at least a minute and a half in sipping this. That is, just sip it sufficiently that there is scarcely the need for even swallowing but let it be absorbed in the mouth as well as just trickle, as it were, to the throat and stomach, and then a swallow, but let it be with a whole wheat wafer which might be taken with same.

6/29/42
F. 25 yrs.
ANEMIA **2376-2**

Fish, fowl and lamb may be taken. Do not eat beef, for this body; though beef juice may be taken if it is desirable—not a stew, but beef juice.

10/26/40
ADHESIONS: LESIONS **M. 40 yrs.**
BODY-BUILDING **2276-3**

We need more VITAL strength. The properties being taken (the B injections) are beneficial in this direction. These are sufficient, provided there is kept plenty of those foods in the diet that carry the same properties also.

Beef juices here would be excellent, taken as a tonic. Prepare this, and take sips of it several times a day. Do not just take it as a drink of water, or milk, or just to be swallowed, but sip it very slowly—about a teaspoonful at the time.

5/9/29
F. 64 yrs.
ACIDITY: ASSIMILATIONS: BLOOD-BUILDING **1377-3**

Q. 1 am taking a half cup full of blood pressed from the beef. Would the blood from liver be better?

A. The juices of well-cooked beef, without water in same, more beneficial than blood. That of the *juices* from beef, without bulk, works directly with the duodenum and the active forces in the pancreas and spleen, giving new blood to the body.

Q. Am I making any good blood?

A. Were the body not making some good blood, it would wear out in about seven days. Sure, there is some good blood being made. The activities for the system, much in the manner given for blood-building, will make *more* blood—but *do not* make *more* than may be taken care of by the body. This *also must* produce acid.

8/6/34
F. 56 yrs.
DEBILITATION: GENERAL **626-1**

Begin with the activities in the diet that will make for the resuscitating of more vital forces. Do not overfeed, so that the body becomes a dross pit—as it were; but only take sufficient that the body does assimilate, does *use u*p those forces that are taken into the system.

Take at least during the day as much as an ounce and a half of *beef juice;* not broths, but beef juice! unless this disagrees with the body. Of course, there may be periods when it may burn the stomach, or should it do this then reduce the *quantity* but keep on taking. It would be better for this to be taken just as medicine, every two or three hours, you see, and keep assimilating it.

ii)—Liver Juice

9/7/34
CANCER: TENDENCIES **F. 12 yrs.**
BLOOD-BUILDING **632-3**

Should the weakness continue it would be necessary eventually for the blood transfusion; though, as we find, if we are rather patient we will find the blood itself being built up—with the *diets* that will make for blood-building juices. Not too much at the time, but plenty of liver juice made in the same way and manner as the beef juice—this will be strengthening to the body.

While these conditions as described may be found to be in adverse opinions of those that minister to the body, give time sufficient for at least the trying of these suggestions for a few days and see the results. Then, should the judgment constrain thee to follow those that would do different—decide in self.

7/21/32
NERVOUS SYSTEMS: INCOORDINATION: PRURITUS **F. 81 yrs.**
BLOOD: HUMOR **5431-4**

Q. Just exactly what proteins should she have to strengthen her?

A. Those that will give the greater amount of strength will be those juices from liver.

5/9/29
F. 64 yrs.
ACIDITY: ASSIMILATIONS: BLOOD-BUILDING **1377-3**

Q. I am taking a half cup full of blood pressed from the beef. Would the blood from liver be better?

A. The activities of juices from liver would be better, were these steamed and the juices as *well* as the flesh itself, in small quantities, be taken. Well that these be alternated, for their activities for the system are entirely different. That of the liver is, with the bulk, active directly with the changing of assimilations in the system, or with those glands where the assimilating takes place, working directly with the active forces of same.

Q. Am I making any good blood?

A. Were the body not making some good blood, it would wear out in about seven days. Sure, there is some good blood being made. The activities for the system, much in the manner given for blood-building, will make *more* blood—but *do not* make *more* than may be taken care of by the body. This *also must* produce acid.

10/21/36
COLD: COMMON: SUSCEPTIBILITY **F. 41 yrs.**
BODY-BUILDING **1100-7**

For the general building up of the system, we would take the juices of liver or liver extract.

And be mindful that in the rest of the diet it is kept close to the alkaline, or twenty percent acid-producing to eighty percent alkaline-producing food values.

8/29/35
F. 45 yrs.
COLITIS **404-4**

In the matter of the diet, be mindful that this is not *over* alkaline; nor that there is taken too great a quantity of that ordinarily termed roughage. For with these tendencies for the inflammation that arises, as we have indicated, from changes in the activities in the system and the changes in the system caused by the congestion in the lymph circulation through the intestinal tract, these produce irritations.

Liver juices; these are well for a portion of the diet for the body.

2)—Blood Pudding

3/22/32
F. 42 yrs.
COLITIS **404-2**

Evenings—Cooked vegetables, with those that make for more blood-building, as would be in those of . . . blood pudding or the like, as combined *with* a well-cooked and well-balanced vegetable diet.

10/23/42
M. 10 mos.
BABY CARE: HEMOPHILIA **2832-1**

As we find, there are conditions that are lacking in the structural or building properties in body, that cause those disturbances and anxieties to those about the body—the lack of those elements in the blood supply to build the walls, and resistances necessary in the walls of the arteries and the veins in the body.

So, with bruises or injuries to the body, there is the formation of blood spots, or clots.

That with the formation of such clots or blots there is lack of full coagulation is well, but that there is lack of coagulation AND also the lack of the elements as to build in the glandular forces or activities those elements that arise from what is called the active forces of the B-1 Complex AND G as vital energies, is not so well. And this is that which needs correction.

We find that the outlines which have been given for diet are very good; but we would add small quantities regularly of blood pudding.* Necessarily, from the age, this will require that very small quantities be given, about three times each week. If you get him to take a teaspoonful it'll be fine!

4/17/31
DEBILITATION: GENERAL **M. 19 yrs.**
CHOREA **1225-1**

Evenings—We would give those of blood pudding and any that carry with same the *digestive* food values—see?

These, as we find, will bring about a great *change* for the betterment in the physical forces of this body.

---

*To be prepared as follows:
1/2 pound ground calf's liver;
1/2 cup blood (which you can get butcher to save from grinding the liver). Butter a pan six inches across and two inches deep. Season the liver with salt to taste and piece of butter the size of a walnut. Melt and mix with liver, then pour blood over the liver. Run in hot oven about ten minutes.

i)—Liver Pudding

2/21/43
F. 33 yrs.
CANCER **2918-1**

About two, three or four times a week it will be helpful to take the liver pudding. These will make for helpful forces, though not curative forces. Use as much blood in same as practical, though cook to some extent.

5/1/35
M. 1-1/2 yrs.
WORMS: PINWORMS: AFTEREFFECTS **786-2**

Be very mindful that the diets are body- and blood-building.

Especially the liver made as a liver pudding would be well. Calves' liver is preferable.

3/13/43
F. 81 yrs.
BLOOD-BUILDING: PURPURA **2935-1**

In the diet, give excess quantities of liver pudding and the like. These will be beneficial.

3/10/41
M. 18 yrs.
LEUKEMIA **2456-3**

It will be better for the liver pudding to be eaten and assimilated, to give activities for the body itself, rather than being administered wholly by the injections. For, this produces a different reaction. And, if there is to be helpful forces, there must be set up in the system itself an activity of the assimilating and distributing system.

The Iymph reaction and the red forces of the blood supply will be aided much better through taking it in the manner indicated, to be active enough through the assimilating system, as we find.

3/14/41
M. 18 yrs.
LEUKEMIA **2456-4**

Q. Is there any way to make the liver more palatable so he can eat it?

A. This we would grind and steam, keeping all the juices in same. We would grind and cook in Patapar paper, or heat in Patapar paper, saving the juices; and this then, of course seasoned, may be made more palatable.

Q. Is there any way we can disguise the liver so when he takes it he doesn't know it?

A. This, of course, may be mixed with bread or other things, but if prepared properly this should not be disturbing to the body.

Q. Why does liver make him so ill?

A. As has been first given, it's the natural reaction to those things that are abhorrent to the body-consciousness, see?

Q. Could it be given hypodermically?

A. It may be given by hypodermic, but—as we have indicated—not unless it is assimilated by the body through the eating of it in the manner outlined.

Q. Why is liver so hard to digest once it gets into the stomach?

A. This should not be hard to digest. With lactics it may be made to digest the easier, if it is desirable for same.

Q. What else can the doctors do to aid the body to help it take hold of itself to bring about a recovery?

A. Just the encouraging and stimulating to the mental self to fight back. Be more and more optimistic and creative, and not expressing that of fear.

ii)—Oxblood Pudding

2/21/43
F. 33 yrs.
CANCER **2918-1**

About two, three or four times a week it will be helpful to take oxblood pudding. These will make for helpful forces, though not curative forces. Use as much blood in same as practical, though cook to some extent.

9)—Stews & Broths

1)—Beef Stew

7/27/41
M. 45 yrs.
ASSIMILATIONS: ELIMINATIONS: INCOORDINATION **2546-1**

Beef juices should be taken; preferably not so much in steak but in stews. These are better.

4/17/41
DEBILITATION: GENERAL **M. 63 yrs.**
DIABETES **584-8**

Keep the better body-building foods—as not too much of the meat but the juices of beef if it is well cooked. CHEW same but do not swallow the meat so much. These prepared in stews or broths or the like are well.

2)—Wild Game Stew

11/4/25
COLITIS **F. 70 yrs.**
DEBILITATION: GENERAL **3776-10**

As much as the wild game as possible, see, for this body, in the form of stews, *not fried*—any kind of meats, see? Rather that of prepared in other manners than fried meats, or fried *any* character, see? These will assist the body in gaining its normal equilibrium. Do that.

3)—Meat Broths: General

9/29/34
M. Adult
ABRASIONS: TOXEMIA **675-1**

Noons—Preferably either a raw green vegetable salad—or meat juices—though it should never be a combination of meat juices together; either chicken broth, lamb broth or the like.

9/6/33
ASSIMILATIONS: POOR **F. 3 yrs.**
MALARIA: TENDENCIES **402-1**

Noons—There also may be taken at this time a little meat broth, see? Not any of the meats.

i)—Beef Broth

9/22/36
M. 75 yrs.
CANCER **1263-1**

In the matter of the diet, keep more to the liquids and semi-liquids. Beef broths . . . The broths are to supply nutriment as well as weight.

6/8/40
M. 55 yrs.
ANEMIA **2273-1**

Beef may be taken occasionally, but more of the broth with the cooked vegetables, rather than the roast or steak or the like.

8/27/32
F. 72 yrs.
CIRRHOSIS OF LIVER **2092-1**

Evenings—Well-cooked vegetables. Also there may be the strengthening foods such as broths of beef, with barley, but not with rice.

10/8/36
ANEMIA **F. 54 yrs.**
ARTHRITIS: TOXEMIA **1269-1**

Noons—There may be beef stock with combinations of vegetables; but *preferably* only vegetable juices *or* meat juices.

ii)—Lamb & Mutton Broth

3/14/32
M. Adult
TOXEMIA **5672-1**

Noon—Broths of fresh meats, as of lamb—these would be well for the body; but little of the meats would we take—but thick broths.

8/27/32
F. 72 yrs.
CIRRHOSIS OF LIVER **2092-1**

Evenings—Well-cooked vegetables. Also there may be the strengthening foods such as broths of mutton, with barley, but not with rice.

5/29/34
F. 19 yrs.
ANEMIA **562-1**

Noons—Preferably entirely green or raw vegetables, or the meal may be changed to only the juices of meats—but *not* the meats; as mutton broth or the like.

9/28/41
CONSTIPATION **M. 8 yrs.**
ASSIMILATIONS: POOR **2595-1**

Noons—Take small quantities of raw vegetables and meat juices—as mutton broth; any of such broths, but be sure they have a cereal in them—such as barley or rice or the like.

6/20/34
TUBERCULOSIS **M. Adult**
ELIMINATIONS: POOR **572-2**

Q. Any other advice for the body at this time that would be of benefit?

A. We would follow these, which we find will be the most helpful and we will find strength being gained. Take all the beef juice that may be assimilated. Broths may be taken at times of such as mutton—anything that is *strengthening* to the body and that doesn't strain some organ already involved.

X

Variety Meats (Offal)

1)—Brains

12/10/36
F. 28 yrs.
ANEMIA **1102-2**

In the rest of the diet—fish, fowl and lamb are preferable as the meats; though brains, any of those activities of such natures are well.

4/1/31
APOPLEXY **M. 52 yrs.**
NERVE-BUILDING **3747-1**

The diets will be along those lines that make for nerve-*building.* Little or no meats, to be sure though those that will add for nerve forces as brains, these will be beneficial to the body in small quantities.

ANEMIA **10/31/31**
ASSIMILATIONS: POOR **F. 60 yrs.**
INJURIES: ACCIDENTS: AFTEREFFECTS: FRACTURES **501-2**

In the evening, then, may be those of the whole vegetables—with the meat juices, or those that will supply more gluten will be taken at this time . . . Brains, and such—these are well for the body.

12/27/41
F. 19 yrs.
PREGNANCY **711-4**

Brains and the like should be the character of meats.

2)—Kidneys

4/1/31
APOPLEXY **M. 52 yrs.**
NERVE-BUILDING **3747-1**

The diets will be along those lines that make for nerve-*building*. Little or no meats, to be sure though those that will add for nerve forces as kidneys, these will be beneficial to the body in small quantities.

6/7/37
DEBILITATION: GENERAL **F. 65 yrs.**
ACIDITY & ALKALINITY **658-15**

No hog meat of *any* kind unless it is the kidneys—these are very good in keeping a balance and in producing that for the system to aid in keeping down anemia or uremic reaction from a taxed system.

7/27/41
M. 45 yrs.
ASSIMILATIONS: ELIMINATIONS: INCOORDINATION **2546-1**

Kidneys—kidney stew, all forms of the internal organs that are kosher killed, or prepared in a manner in which there is the inspection to be sure that there are no infections of any kind or character. Let all of these be taken often in the diet.

Keep away from fats.

3)—Liver: General

1/5/31
ANEMIA **F. 20 yrs.**
ASSIMILATIONS: ELIMINATIONS: INCOORDINATION **421-2**

In the evening—those of the liver, or such. These that carry the *glucose,* that make for a change in the blood supply, that aid to build up.

ACIDITY **9/21/34**
ANEMIA **F. 19 yrs.**
LACERATIONS: STOMACH **667-1**

Evenings (or one meal in the day)—Well-cooked vegetables, with quantities at certain given periods during a week's meals of liver, and those things that tend to make for the building up of the blood supply in the system; yet keep an even balance.

After each meal *rest* for at least ten to fifteen minutes, and while resting have your feet higher than your head; lying down in repose but feet higher than the head, that there may be the proper assimilations and proper positions for the stomach itself.

2/21/36
F. 38 yrs.
TUBERCULOSIS **1045-7**

Then, instead of so much of the fruit juices that tend to react so easily upon the system—we would use rather the ground liver, or goose liver or a mixture of pig's liver with calf's liver (not beef liver but calf liver). Any of these would be helpful, but *not* in large quantities.

7/21/39
M. 24 yrs.
STREPTOCOCCUS **568-3**

Q. Any special diet?

A. Those foods that are easily assimilated, and that are strengthening, and that carry such vitamins as in plenty of liver as well as those foods of every nature that carry the plasma of better blood supply. Vitamin B-l, vitamin A, B, C, G—these are those needed.

6/22/39
F. 31 yrs.
DEBILITATION: GENERAL **808-10**

We would take often the liver, or liver extract. If it is preferable to take the liver, take a little of it broiled, at least twice a week.

3/4/40
F. 53 yrs.
GLANDS: ADRENALS: BODY-BUILDING **2025-3**

But if there will be more of the liver extract or broiled liver itself and not too much cooked, these will aid in BUILDING the body for better strength, better resistance, and less of this disturbance.

Q. As I cannot eat enough to keep my strength, is there anything I can do to increase my weight?

A. Keep those things that have been indicated, and these will GIVE the strength. The broiled liver, of course, would be masticated very thoroughly.

ACIDITY
CIRCULATION: INCOORDINATION **5/11/42**
COLD: CONGESTION **F. 74 yrs.**
BODY-BUILDING **2074-2**

Mr. Cayce: Yes—this we have had before. This may become rather serious for the body, unless there is the ability to build some more resistance in the system. For, the complications of the disturbance from cold and congestion in the lymph circulation, which arises from superacidity, as combined with the low vitality AND the heart disturbance, may produce distressing disturbances unless this may be aided without overstimulating heart's activity.

Give foods that are very stimulating. Every form of better stimulant that is for building strength, as liver.

8/3/34
M. 56 yrs.
ANEMIA **556-4**

Q. Could any other tonic be substituted for the Ventriculin?

A. Could eat liver. These will be much slower; they will not carry as much of the iron, but *more* of those things in some forms that will be more easily assimilated. You see, these are the juices of these very portions of the animal fat (in the Ventriculin) that are assimilated by the system; and if these are used in their regular state, of course, this should supply then at least one meal each day from the liver or the like, see?

7/23/41
F. 45 yrs.
ANEMIA **811-7**

Q. Is there anything to do to increase the blood pressure?

A. All of these that we have given are for doing this, especially all the liver that may be taken.

Q. Does the body get the proper kinds of food elements, or is there a deficiency?

A. If so, we wouldn't give the special food values. Those that carry vitamins A and B and B-l especially should be taken by the body. These are found most, of course, in the fruits and vegetables of the yellow variety, as well as in liver.

5/4/41
M. 14 yrs.
ANEMIA **2488-2**

Give all the liver or liver extract that the body will assimilate. These are best given from the liver itself, that is, in the food, than by injections or the formations of vitamins that are said to be of the same nature.

9/5/29
SPINE: SUBLUXATIONS **M. 55 yrs.**
MEATLESS **5459-5**

Q. Will the elimination of meat from my diet have a weakening effect temporarily?

A. No. Only so far as the mental forces allow same, for there is as much *vitality* in the outline of those things the body *should* eat as would be with the meats, and when conditions are of the nature as has been given, *meats* aggravate, while vegetables, or characters of meats that build—that is, such as liver, these do not carry those vibrations that aid in accentuating such pressures as disturb this body—but rather give the tendency to give more strength and endurance to a physical body.

10/14/35
M. 17 yrs.
GLANDS: INCOORDINATION: HYPOTHYROIDISM **1078-1**

In the general diet have always those things for the meals that are in accord with body, blood and nerve-building. But not great quantities of meats. No red meats. No fried meats, nor fried foods of any kind. Let these when taken be roasted or broiled, or prepared in such a manner. Liver should be the principal food taken in place of meat. Also lamb, fowl and wild game may be included.

3/8/35
F. 48 yrs.
CONSTIPATION **848-1**

We would keep close to a body and nerve and blood-building, but as much towards an alkaline reaction as possible. Have at least three days each week or three meals each week of either juices of liver or liver broiled.

7/27/41
M. 45 yrs.
ASSIMILATIONS: ELIMINATIONS: INCOORDINATION **2546-1**

Keep away from fats, the mixing of too many starches. Liver, all forms of the internal organs that are kosher killed, or prepared in a manner in which there is the inspection to be sure that there are no infections of any kind or character. Let all of these be taken often in the diet.

6/3/41
M. 25 yrs.
DEBILITATION: GENERAL: APPENDICITIS **1970-1**

We would THEN begin to live more or less on the milk and cheese diet; with, of course, the beef juices—taken in small quantities often. No meats except the beef juices, you see. (Do not begin this diet, of course, until after the period of the grape poultices and the grape diet.) No meat save the beef juices, and liver and liver extract. It would be well if the liver were ground, and patties made, and save as much of the blood in same as is practical or possible—if it is perfect or good liver—not cow's but calf's liver; also hog liver would be very well.

4/17/31
DEBILITATION: GENERAL **M. 19 yrs.**
CHOREA **1225-1**

Evenings—We would give those of liver, and any that carry with same the *digestive* food values—see?

These, as we find, will bring about a great *change* for the betterment in the physical forces of this body.

3/16/43
ASSIMILATION: POOR **F. 21 yrs.**
BODY-BUILDING **2937-1**

Do give vitamin-rich foods; such as liver. Season with butter or the like, rather than with other forms of greases.

4/1/31
APOPLEXY **M. 52 yrs.**
NERVE-BUILDING **3747-1**

The diets will be along those lines that make for nerve-*building*. Little or no meats, to be sure though those that will add for nerve forces as liver, these will be beneficial to the body in small quantities.

4/18/35
ANEMIA **M. Adult**
ASSIMILATIONS: POOR **898-1**

Evening meal—Occasionally broiled liver may be taken in small quantities, but once a week should be sufficient for these.

Keep these consistently, persistently; we will gain weight, we will put off this dullness, this tendency for catching cold, this weakness throughout the whole system; and bring the body—in six to eight months—to its normal weight of about a hundred and fifty pounds.

4/8/38
M. 30 yrs.
849-26

ASSIMILATIONS: POOR

We would have quite often the broiled liver—not too done; only broiled sufficient so that it may be eaten by the body.

1/29/44
F. 37 yrs.
1695-3

CIRCULATION: INCOORDINATION

Q. Should I continue to leave off the red meats? If so, for how long a period?

A. You may begin to add red meats, if you don't add too much of them. Eat more liver.

7/16/35
F. 64 yrs.
950-1

ARTHRITIS

Noons—Either *broiled calf's* liver or vegetables that are of the leafy rather than bulbular nature. And drink about half a glass of the juice from *kraut.*

Evenings—The meats when taken should always consist of the broiled liver or the like (but not fried).

11/6/35
M. 24 yrs.
533-7

BODY-BUILDING

In the diets keep those things that will agree, yet we will find it will be necessary to change; but that are body-building. Liver is of the nature that will supply the effluvium in the blood.

2/5/42
F. 24 yrs.
2679-1

INJURIES

In the diets, also, much may be accomplished. Necessarily, there must be plenty of those properties that aid in keeping a correct balance in the production of Iymph, leucocyte AND the red blood supply.

Then, have especially those foods that carry more of the calcium and the vitamins A, D, B-1 and other B Complexes.

Hence we would have plenty of liver; these alternated as parts of the diet.

3/13/43
F. 81 yrs.
2935-1

BLOOD-BUILDING: PURPURA

In the diet, give excess quantities of liver, liver extract and the like. These will be beneficial.

3/30/38
F. 36 yrs.
1560-1

TUBERCULOSIS

Have liver often, and this the rarer the better, taken at least two or three times a week.

Then the foods for weight and that will aid in caring for the activities through the absorptions and through the digestive forces.

3/14/32
M. Adult

TOXEMIA **5672-1**

Evenings—Particularly blood-building foods, as of liver. This may be taken with some cereal drink, or coffee—but not coffee with milk in it.

2/16/35
M. 45 yrs.

ACIDITY **829-1**

Noons—Rather a sandwich of broiled liver. These are preferable for the noon meal, but *not* roast beef or any fried meats or any hog meats.

5/23/35
M. 45 yrs.

TUBERCULOSIS **929-1**

Take the food values that make for *body-building,* but let them be rather alkaline-reacting.

Noons—Broiled liver or things of such natures; not too much of same, but those that are body- and blood-building. These may be had either with the uncut (unpolished) rice or with the other cereals or grains that may be used with such; that is, in the soups or broths. Not too much grease, but plenty of those things that make for the body-building.

8/24/35
F. Adult

ACIDITY & ALKALINITY: ANEMIA **978-1**

Be very mindful of the diet. Eat those foods that are alkaline in their reaction. Let the body have at least two or three times each week the broiled liver. No *red* meat; no fried meat nor fried food of any kind; not even *boiled* fat meat. But fish, fowl, lamb may be taken. However, *do not* partake of the heavier meats.

Q. Please outline a specific diet.

A. As indicated, hold to those things that are alkaline in their reaction. Not too much of sweets, not too much of starches; but rather those things that are well-balanced and those special foods as indicated should be a portion of the diet from day to day. Keep a well-balance, knowing that the alkaline-reacting foods are *preferable* for the body; for they prevent acidity. And acidity is irritating to the blood flow.

3/2/38
M. 12 yrs.

BLOOD-BUILDING **1519-1**

Greater precaution needs to be taken in the diet that there are blood-building foods; as the broiled liver. These carry the hormones and the gluten that supplies in the assimilating system the better body-building.

4/24/34
M. 43 yrs.

ACIDITY & ALKALINITY **642-1**

Liver, all the enzymes—especially the Ventriculin character—these would be more helpful to the body, as we find, in building up through the food values.

3/22/41
M. 62 yrs.
DEBILITATION: GENERAL **556-18**

As we find, there should be the more efficient supply and more quantities of the vitamins B and B-l and D. These, through the food supply, would be the better means for obtaining helpful directions for the body forces.

These vitamins would be found in goose liver, chicken liver, calf's liver. These may be alternated, but these should be broiled—or ground and cakes lightly cooked with same—in the various forms.

7/22/31
ASSIMILATIONS: DEBILITATION: GENERAL: **F. 28 yrs.**
BLOOD-BUILDING **3842-1**

We would give a diet that is easily assimilated. Let the diet be that as is nerve- and blood-building. Let it be composed of liver—at least once each week—cod liver, fish liver, pig liver, calf liver—any of these.

6/7/37
DEBILITATION: GENERAL **F. 65 yrs.**
ACIDITY & ALKALINITY **658-15**

No hog meat of *any* kind unless it is the liver—these are very good in keeping a balance and in producing that for the system to aid in keeping down anemia or uremic reaction from a taxed system.

1)—Calf's Liver

9/11/31
M. 42 yrs.
CANCER **2097-1**

Beware of *any* element that carries too much alcohol in same. The foods would be those that are *nourishing*, as those of the calf's liver (not sodden, but not with grease), those of blood pudding *with* the liver would be well. This will give stimuli and active forces with those of the system. Do this for at least twenty days, then we may alter or change as to meet the needs of the condition.

6/21/32
F. 48 yrs.
ASSIMILATIONS: POOR **428-7**

Evenings—Two or three evenings each week have liver (calf's liver, not fried—but broiled in butter—not too rare, but such that the activities of same are for the replenishing of the blood supply in system), and well-cooked vegetables alternated. Do not stuff nor overeat, but eat—at all meals, slowly—all that may be well taken.

9/4/41
BABY CARE **F. 2-1/2 yrs.**
ELIMINATIONS **1521-5**

There needs to be those considerations for more of the foods carrying the vitamins B and D, rather than these taken separately.

We find that these would be obtained in the correct proportions, at least two or three times each week, of calf's liver.

Q. What is causing excessive growth of hair over entire body, particularly in back of neck and across shoulders, and what can be done to correct it? (especially noticeable for last six months).

A. This is a natural development, if we indicate the conditions of the body and its meeting itself. But these will not become unsightly if there is kept the normal balance in especially the B and D vitamins in the foods for the body.

4/18/32
DEBILITATION: GENERAL **F. Adult**
BLOOD-BUILDING **4164-1**

Evenings—A well-*balanced* diet, occasionally using the diet that is more blood-building in its nature. All those foods carrying the *blood*-building properties, as of calf's liver—especially. These should be a portion of the diet at most periods, though altered occasionally.

11/13/36
(F. 11 yrs. [1179])
BODY-BUILDING **1206-2**

Q. Should [1179] start taking her liver extract again? If so, how much and how often?

A. This as we find may he altered, in that the broiled liver itself if given would be much preferable to the body to the using of the extract. And this would be well for all, for this then supplies elements needed. Broiled; do not fry; do not have too hard, and only the calf's liver, see?

12/10/36
F. 28 yrs.
ANEMIA **1102-2**

In the rest of the diet—fish, fowl and lamb are preferable as the meats; though calf's liver, any of those activities of such natures are well.

7/16/35
F. Adult
ARTHRITIS: ASSIMILATIONS: POOR **946-1**

Also we would have a portion of the meals to consist of calf liver, broiled (not fried, but broiled); not too done, but sufficient that this may be taken in small quantities and will make for assimilation.

7/21/44
F. 60 yrs.
CANCER: LUNGS **5374-1**

Plenty of calf's liver, broiled, two or three times a week.

2/8/30
DEBILITATION: GENERAL: FLU: AFTEREFFECTS **F. 71 yrs.**
BLOOD-BUILDING **5604-1**

We would be mindful or careful of the diet, that it consists of those foods that, while easily digested, are blood- and nerve-building in their nature. Let the diet be of the calf's liver, at least twice a week.

1/8/30
F. 29 yrs.
BLOOD-BUILDING: VITAMINS: DEFICIENT 5615-1

Plenty of the vitamins as may be had in liver. Also the meat *juices,* but not too much of the body of the same. But much of the calf's liver, for these carry that *necessary* vital force to meet the needs of that that may be created in the blood as to *combat* the conditions existent, and *build* vital forces.

5/12/41
M. 72 yrs.
ANEMIA 2565-1

The administering of blood supply (through transfusions) has not aided, because there has been little or nothing accomplished in aiding the body to better assimilate that it HAS been able to retain as foods or diets.

Have liver—calf liver, especially—all that the body can absorb; this preferably broiled, not fried; never hard, but that which is the better and more easily assimilated.

8/13/30
M. 42 yrs.
DEBILITATION: GENERAL 2335-1

Eat liver—calf's liver—not fried—it may be broiled, or parboiled—at least three times each week.

4/1/43
POLIOMYELITIS F. 11 yrs.
KIDNEYS: BODY-BUILDING 2948-1

Have plenty of liver, calf's liver—this once or twice or three times a month.

5/1/35
M. 1-1/2 yrs.
WORMS: PINWORMS: AFTEREFFECTS 786-2

Be very mindful that the diets are body- and blood-building.

Especially the liver would be well-broiled liver; but never fried. Calf's liver is preferable.

2)—Goose Liver

ACIDITY
ANEMIA 10/3/40
COLD: COMMON: SUSCEPTIBILITY F. 19 yrs.
BODY-BUILDING 2374-1

Noons—A sandwich with green or raw vegetables—such as tomatoes and lettuce with mayonnaise (using brown bread, of course), and NOT ham or the like. Goose liver or the like is very well, if desired.

Do these, and as we find we will bring bettered conditions for this body; not only making for the corrections but improving the vitality, the strength, and increasing the weight.

4)—Marrow

1/9/40
F. 31 yrs.
CONCEPTION **1523-8**

None of those foods that are of themselves contraceptive in their nature, or in their reactions to the system.

Thus, have plenty of the stabilizing foods that are within themselves creative, rather than of the palliative nature.

Have the marrow of beef, or such, as a part of the diet; as the vegetable soups that are rich in the beef carrying the marrow of the bone, and the like—these as a part of the diet once or twice a week—and EAT THE MARROW!

7/23/41
F. 45 yrs.
ANEMIA **811-7**

Q. Does the body get the proper kinds of food elements, or is there a deficiency?

A. If so, we wouldn't give the special food values. Those that carry vitamins A and B and B-l especially should be taken by the body. These are found most, of course, in the fruits and vegetables of the yellow variety as well as especially in marrow.

6/17/41
NERVOUS TENSION **F. 26 yrs.**
RHEUMATISM **2517-1**

As to the diet throughout the period—keep close to those foods that will supply the greater quantity of B-l vitamins.

Evenings—Any marrow stews are well for the body; marrow fat or marrow bone prepared or broken and put in the soups or stews. These are well.

5)—Pig's Knuckles & Feet

8/31/41
ARTHRITIS: PREVENTIVE **F. 51 yrs.**
BODY: GENERAL **1158-31**

Q. What are the best sources of calcium in foods?

A. Gristle, pig's feet and the like.

1/5/31
ANEMIA **F. 20 yrs.**
ASSIMILATIONS: ELIMINATIONS: INCOORDINATION **421-2**

In the evening—those of pig knuckle, or such. These that carry the *glucose,* that make for a change in the blood supply, that aid to build up.

6/21/32
F. 48 yrs.
ASSIMILATIONS: POOR **428-7**

Evenings—Two or three evenings each week have pig knuckle, and well-cooked vegetables alternated. Do not stuff nor overeat, but eat—at all meals, slowly—all that may be well taken.

7/26/32
ANEMIA **M. 25 yrs.**
ASSIMILATIONS: POOR **481-1**

We would be mindful of the diet, that those foods are taken that are easily assimilated. Do not take quantities of grease of any nature. No hog meat of *any* kind, save that as may be taken in pig knuckle or the like. These would be prepared then without grease, rather with those that make for the easy assimilating in the system.

Evenings—Cooked vegetables, and the meats *when* these are taken. Do not eat meat more than three times each week, and don't gorge self when this is done!

ACIDITY **9/21/34**
ANEMIA **F. 19 yrs.**
LACERATIONS: STOMACH **667-1**

Evenings (or one meal in the day)—Well-cooked vegetables, with quantities at certain given periods during a week's meals of pig's feet, and those things that tend to make for the building up of the blood supply in the system; yet keep an even balance.

Q. Why have I lost so much weight, and how can I regain it?

A. The strain of the acidity in the system has made for the hardships upon the digestive system, as indicated, which has gradually eaten up not only the reserve supply but deficiency is created in the bloodstream that has made for the losing of weight, and as indicated when we have formed those positions and conditions in the system whereby we may rectify these conditions, so that digestion and assimilation takes place in the normal way, before there has been such an attack upon the organs themselves—or the glands of the body, we will find the body will return to its *normalcy* in weight—and it'll be very good!

3/22/41
M. 62 yrs.
DEBILITATION: GENERAL **556-18**

We find that these in the main, as related to the blood supply, may be met by change in the diet. For, the tendencies for the swelling in portions of the face, as we find, are from the lack of supply of the vital energies in the veins and the inability thus to prevent the drainages, or hemorrhages.

As we find, there should be the more efficient supply and more quantities of the vitamins B and B-1 and D. These, through the food supply, would be the better means for obtaining helpful directions for the body forces.

These vitamins would be found supplied best by having at least twice a week the pig's feet, well cooked and well jellied—using the gristle portions especially, or mostly.

In these may there be obtained those influences best for this body in the present.

4/18/32
DEBILITATION: GENERAL **F. Adult**
BLOOD-BUILDING **4164-1**

Evenings—A well-balanced diet, occasionally using the diet that is more blood-building in its nature. All those foods carrying the *blood*-building properties, as of pig knuckle. These should be a portion of the diet at most periods, though altered occasionally.

3/2/38
M. 12 yrs.
BLOOD-BUILDING **1519-1**

Greater precaution needs to be taken in the diet that there are blood-building foods; as pig's feet and the like. These carry the hormones and the gluten that supplies in the assimilating system the better body-building.

8/3/34
M. 56 yrs.
ANEMIA **556-4**

Q. Could any other tonic be substituted for the Ventriculin?

A. Pig's feet. These will be much slower; they will not carry as much of the iron, but *more* of those things in some forms that will be more easily assimilated. You see, these are the juices of these very portions of the animal fat (in the Ventriculin) that are assimilated by the system; and if these are used in their regular state, of course, this should supply then at least one meal each day from pig's feet or the like, see? and when the pig's feet, eat *only* the gristle force, not fat!

Q. How would they be prepared?

A. Roast.

12/10/36
F. 28 yrs.
ANEMIA **1102-2**

In the rest of the diet—fish, fowl and lamb are preferable as the meats; though pig's feet or pig's feet jelly is *well* to be taken occasionally, for this aids and adds with the very activity of the assimilating system that gluten necessary for this better coagulation.

4/18/35
M. Adult
ASSIMILATIONS: POOR **898-1**

Evening meal—Occasionally pig's feet may be taken in small quantities, but once a week should be sufficient for these.

Keep these consistently, persistently; we will gain weight, we will put off this dullness, this tendency for catching cold, this weakness throughout the whole system; and bring the body—in six to eight months—to its normal weight, of about a hundred and fifty pounds.

4/17/31
DEBILITATION: GENERAL **M. 19 yrs.**
CHOREA **1225-1**

Evenings—We would give those of pig knuckle and any that carry with same the *digestive* food values—see?

9/12/37
BLOOD: COAGULATION: POOR **M. 62 yrs.**
ACIDITY & ALKALINITY **1411-2**

Noons—DO NOT eat hog meat, save the pig's feet—these may be taken occasionally, but should be those that are roasted, NOT those that are EVER fried.

4/27/35
ASSIMILATIONS: ELIMINATIONS: INCOORDINATION **F. 39 yrs.**
NEURITIS **908-1**

Evenings—When a little meat is taken, let it be either of wild game, fish, fowl or lamb. No other kinds of meat; though at times there may be taken a little pig's feet or the like—this is only for the gelatin in same that is active in making for coagulations in the body-building.

6/20/39
M. 32 yrs.
ARTHRITIS **849-37**

Give the body, now, pig's feet (if he would eat same) would be very well, because of the needed activities for the muscular force and because of the gluten that forms from same.

8/11/31
ELIMINATIONS: POOR **F. 42 yrs.**
BLOOD-BUILDING **484-1**

In the matter of the diet, keep those things that are *blood*-building. Pig knuckle, or those that carry that that makes *for* the characterization of that glucose in the blood, that may aid in aiding and abetting, with that solvent force created by the use of the salts, rubs, and massage, and that will work *with* the *glands* of the system . . .

6)—Souse

4/17/31
DEBILITATION: GENERAL **M. 19 yrs.**
CHOREA **1225-1**

Evenings—We would give those of souse, and any that carry with same the *digestive* food values—see?

8/31/41
ARTHRITIS: PREVENTIVE **F. 51 yrs.**
BODY: GENERAL **1158-31**

Q. What are the best sources of calcium in foods?
A. Souse and the like.

7)—Spleen

4/1/31
APOPLEXY **M. 52 yrs.**
NERVE-BUILDING **3747-1**

The diets will be along those lines that make for nerve-*building*. Little or no meats, to be sure though those that will add for nerve forces as spleen, or such, these will be beneficial to the body in small quantities.

8)—Sweetbread

12/27/41
F. 19 yrs.
PREGNANCY **711-4**

Sweetbread and the like should be the character of meats.

9)—Tongue

ACIDITY
ANEMIA **10/3/40**
COLD: COMMON: SUSCEPTIBILITY **F. 19 yrs.**
BODY-BUILDING **2374-1**

Noons—A sandwich with green or raw vegetables—such as tomatoes and lettuce with mayonnaise (using brown bread, of course), and NOT ham or the like. Tongue is very well, if desired.

Do these, and as we find we will bring bettered conditions for this body; not only making for the corrections but improving the vitality, the strength, and increasing the weight.

10)—Tripe: General

9/11/31
M. 42 yrs.
CANCER **2097-1**

Beware of *any* element that carries too much alcohol in same. The foods would be those that are *nourishing,* as those of tripe. Do this for at least twenty-one days, then we may alter or change as to meet the needs of the condition.

4/24/34
M. 43 yrs.
ACIDITY & ALKALINITY **642-1**

Tripe, all the enzymes—especially the Ventriculin character—these would be more helpful to the body, as we find, in building up through the food values.

1/5/31
ANEMIA **F. 20 yrs.**
ASSIMILATIONS: ELIMINATIONS: INCOORDINATION **421-2**

In the evening—Those of the tripe. These that carry the *glucose,* that make for a change in the blood supply, that aid to build up.

7/26/32
ANEMIA **M. 25 yrs.**
ASSIMILATIONS: POOR **481-1**

We would be mindful of the diet, that those foods are taken that are easily assimilated. Do not take quantities of grease of any nature. No hog meat of *any* kind, save that as may be taken in tripe, or the like. These would be prepared then without grease, rather with those that make for the easy assimilating in the system.

6/7/37
DEBILITATION: GENERAL **F. 65 yrs.**
ACIDITY & ALKALINITY **658-15**

No hog meat of *any* kind unless it is the tripe—these are very good in keeping a balance and in producing that for the system to aid in keeping down anemia or uremic reaction from a taxed system.

ACIDITY **9/21/34**
ANEMIA **F. 19 yrs.**
LACERATIONS: STOMACH **667-1**

Evenings (or one meal in the day)—Well-cooked vegetables, with quantities at certain given periods during a week's meal of tripe, and those things that tend to make for the building up of the blood supply in the system; yet keep an even balance.

4/18/32
DEBILITATION: GENERAL **F. Adult**
BLOOD-BUILDING **4164-1**

Evenings—A well-*balanced* diet, occasionally using the diet that is more blood-building in its nature. All those foods carrying the *blood*-building properties, as of tripe. These should be a portion of the diet at most periods, though altered occasionally. Beware of too much sweets.

7/22/31
ASSIMILATIONS: DEBILITATION: GENERAL **F. 28 yrs.**
BLOOD-BUILDING **3842-1**

We would give a diet that is easily assimilated. Let the diet be that as is nerve and blood-building. Let it be composed of tripe—at least once each week.

8/3/34
M. 56 yrs.
ANEMIA **556-4**

Q. Could any other tonic be substituted for the Ventriculin?

A. Could eat tripe. These will be much slower; they will not carry as much of the iron, but *more* of those things in some forms that will be more easily assimilated. You see, these are the juices of these very portions of the animal fat (in the Ventriculin) that are assimilated by the system; and if these are used in their regular state, of course, this should supply then at least one meal each day from the tripe.

7/23/41
ANEMIA **F. 45 yrs.**
HYPOTENSION **811-7**

Q. Does the body get the proper kinds of food elements, or is there a deficiency?

A. If so, we wouldn't give the special food values. Those that carry vitamins A and B and B-1 especially should be taken by the body. These are found most, of course, in the fruits and vegetables of the yellow variety as well as especially in tripe and the like.

10/14/35
M. 17 yrs.
GLANDS: INCOORDINATION: HYPOTHYROIDISM **1078-1**

In the general diet have always those things for the meals that are in accord with body, blood and nerve-building. But not great quantities of meats. No red meats. No fried meats, nor fried foods of any kind. Let these when taken be roasted or broiled, or prepared in such a manner. Tripe should be the principal food taken in place of meat.

3/8/35
F. 48 yrs.
CONSTIPATION **848-1**

Tripe and the like should be a portion of the diet to make for the greater and better body-building and the better eliminations through the system.

7/21/32
NERVOUS SYSTEMS: INCOORDINATION: PRURITUS **F. 81 yrs.**
BLOOD: HUMOR **5431-4**

Q. Just exactly what proteins should she have to strengthen her?

A. Those that will give the greater amount of strength will be those juices from tripe (or this may be taken itself, provided it is not cooked in grease).

4/27/35
ASSIMILATIONS: ELIMINATIONS: INCOORDINATION **F. 39 yrs.**
NEURITIS **908-1**

Evenings—When a little meat is taken, let it be either of wild game, fish, fowl or lamb. No other kinds of meat; though at times there may be taken a little tripe or the like—this is only for the gelatin in same that is active in making for coagulations in the body-building.

9/12/37
BLOOD: COAGULATION: POOR **M. 62 yrs.**
ACIDITY & ALKALINITY **1411-2**

Noons—DO NOT eat hog meat, save the tripe—these may be taken occasionally, but should be those that are roasted, NOT those that are EVER fried.

4/1/31
APOPLEXY **M. 52 yrs.**
NERVE-BUILDING **3747-1**

The diets will be along those lines that make for nerve-*building*. Little or no meats, to be sure though those that will add for nerve forces as tripe, these will be beneficial to the body in small quantities.

4/18/35
ANEMIA **M. Adult**
ASSIMILATIONS: POOR **898-1**

Evening meal—Occasionally tripe may be taken in small quantities, but once a week should be sufficient for these.

4/12/35
F. Adult
TUMORS: LYMPH **889-1**

Q. Will the disturbance in the lungs clear up?

A. This will clear up, for we will make for the building of resistances that have been low—as indicated in the conditions that arise from the activities of the circulation.

Tripe should be the more of the meats for the body.

5/23/35
BODY-BUILDING **M. 45 yrs.**
TUBERCULOSIS **929-1**

Take the food values that make for *body-building,* but let them be rather alkaline-reacting.

Noons—Tripe, or things of such natures; not too much of same, but those that are body- and blood-building. These may be had either with the uncut (unpolished) rice or with the other cereals or grains that may be used with such; that is, in the soups or broths. Not too much grease, but plenty of those things that make for the body-building.

8/24/35
F. Adult
ACIDITY & ALKALINITY: ANEMIA **978-1**

Be very mindful of the diet. Eat those foods that are alkaline in their reaction. Let the body have at least two or three times each week tripe.

Hold to those things that are alkaline in their reaction. Not too much of sweets, not too much of starches; but rather those things that are well-balanced and those special foods as indicated should be a portion of the diet from day to day. Keep a well-balance, knowing that the alkaline-reacting foods are *preferable* for the body; for they prevent acidity. And acidity is irritating to the blood flow.

8/13/30
M. 42 yrs.
DEBILITATION: GENERAL **2335-1**

Also we will find, that at least *twice* a week, were beef tripe or hog tripe taken as a diet, this will be a real value in blood-building, but *do not* fry same.

1/8/30
F. 29 yrs.
BLOOD-BUILDING: VITAMINS: DEFICIENT **5615-1**

Plenty of the vitamins as may be had in tripe. Also the meat *juices,* but not too much of the body of the same. But much of the tripe—beef tripe, or mutton tripe, or hog tripe—for these carry that *necessary* vital force to meet the needs of that that may be created *in* the blood as to *combat* the conditions existent, and *build* vital forces.

1)—Pork Tripe

4/1/30
ANESTHESIA: AFTEREFFECTS **F. 64 yrs.**
ANEMIA **1377-5**

And *especially* would we take that of the hog tripe—not *pickled,* but that that is nicely prepared, and *not* fried. This will add and build *blood,* and build it quickly.

XI

Nuts

1)—Nuts: General

10/21/32
ELEPHANTIASIS: TENDENCIES **F. 18 yrs.**
ARTHRITIS: GLANDS: INCOORDINATION **951-1**

Supply an overabundant amount of those foods that carry iron, iodine and phosphorus in the system.

Then there should be one meal almost entirely of nuts, and the oils of nuts; so that the activities from these in the system are such as to produce a different character of fermentation with the gastric forces of the stomach and the duodenum itself; so that the type of the lactics that are formed in the assimilation become entirely changed, so that the hydrochlorics that are formed in the system—or that are necessary to supply to the non-acid forces as they enter the system, or acid that make for turning into lacteal fluids—cause the lacteals to throw off to those portions of the system that which will gradually build in the pancreas, the spleen, the kidneys, the duodenum, those various folds themselves, more of those forces that will lessen the tendency for the accumulation of those conditions in extremities, where carried by the circulation itself.

10/7/40
F. 23 yrs.
ANEMIA **2376-1**

To be sure, have plenty of nuts of all characters.

8/15/38
M. 54 yrs.
KIDNEYS: STONES **843-7**

Q. Will a substance known as "Mineral Food" be of value for my condition?

A. Not necessarily. While it is necessary for the vitamin activities through the system, these may be obtained by a better balance being kept in the vital forces as may be obtained from nuts than from concentrated forces such as those.

8/25/39
F. 39 yrs.
TOXEMIA **1985-1**

Refrain from those foods that produce alcohol. We do not mean so much the combinations of the alcohol, but those things that produce an alcohol reaction in the system; such as nuts.

3/15/29
M. 40 yrs.
ACIDITY & ALKALINITY **5567-1**

While acid may be taken in moderation, these would be better—that the sugars were created in system from nuts, as may be taken in their reaction with the other elements taken.

7/21/32
NERVOUS SYSTEMS: INCOORDINATION: PRURITUS **F. 81 yrs.**
BLOOD: HUMOR **5431-4**

Q. Just exactly what proteins should she have to strengthen her?

A. Those juices that come from nuts and from fruit. Nuts especially will be strengthening to the body. No other character of oils.

11/12/35
M. 50 yrs.
ADHESIONS: LESIONS **1055-1**

In the diets, be mindful that we keep those things that add iron, silicon, and gold in the system. It may be necessary later to change some of these, but in the present let the diet consist greatly of nuts, in salads.

6/17/44
ARTHRITIS **F. 63 yrs.**
ELIMINATIONS: POOR **3395-4**

Not too heavy a diet. Nuts may be included or a few of the nuts. Not too many through these periods because these would ferment easily in the intestinal tract.

12/4/22
F. Adult
TUBERCULOSIS **5703-1**

Let the diet be that that will give the vital forces to the body, principally of nuts or nut fats. Do that. We will bring the proper forces and incentives to this body.

7/12/35
BODY-BUILDING **F. 23 yrs.**
DIS-EASE: CONTAGION: PREVENTIVE **480-19**

The diet should be more body-building; that is, less acid foods and more of the alkaline-reacting will be the better in these directions. Those food values carrying an easy assimilation of iron, silicon, and those elements or chemicals. Nuts and the like, should form a greater part of the regular diet in the present—and in the preparations for those activities to come later, whether in relationships in the physical manner or those in the mental forces that are necessary in such activities.

8/28/28
F. 48 yrs.
CANCER **569-16**

Beware of meats. This has caused the greater distress at the present time.

Q. What would be a correct diet for the body at this time?

A. Vegetable diet, or pre-digested foods. Those that are not acid. Nuts in small quantities, or nut foods; but no meats.

4/11/35
ARTHRITIS: TENDENCIES **F. Adult**
BLOOD: HUMOR **888-1**

In the matter of the diet, be more mindful that there are less of the acid-producing foods; more of carbohydrates—that is, sweets—but sweets such as nuts.

9/15/35
F. 44 yrs.
TUMORS **683-3**

Let the general diet at other periods be body-building. Not meats; only fowl or fish along this line would be taken at all. Principally, nuts and the like. And, as we find, these would eliminate and make for a building of a near normal body.

Q. Is this growth in my breast cancerous?

A. No. Tumorous.

Q. It can be eliminated without an operation?

A. It can be eliminated *without* an operation. As indicated, the activities of the glands through all portions of the system have made for segregation of those conditions that have acted as a throw off from a catarrhal condition which has existed—and settled in the mammary glands.

Then, the application of those things indicated will create activities in the blood supply, *with* the keeping of the eliminations, that the condition may be absorbed and thrown off from the system.

ANEMIA **12/8/36**
ASSIMILATIONS: POOR **F. Adult**
TOXEMIA **1303-1**

Have plenty of nuts, as a portion of the meal; rather than so much meats—and *never* any fried meats.

11/9/38
ANEMIA: TENDENCIES **M. 7 yrs.**
BODY-BUILDING **773-16**

Q. Please outline diet for each of the three meals daily.

A. Keep these rather generally well-balanced.

Eat that which the bodily forces call for that supply the necessary building; though do not, of course, overbalance same with too much sweets. Keep the natural sweets—as with nuts.

11/4/35
F. 4 yrs.
GLANDS: INCOORDINATION **795-4**

At least once each day, even for the developing body, have nuts.

6/26/39
F. 21 yrs.
DIET: ENVIRONMENT: HAY FEVER **1771-3**

Use nuts, of all natures or characters that are grown in the environ of the body, especially.

9/2/29
CHILDREN: ABNORMAL **M. 7 yrs.**
NERVOUS SYSTEMS: INCOORDINATION **758-2**

No nuts that carry too much oils—unless these have been well grated and are mixed with other elements; though the oils of same are beneficial at times for these conditions.

10/17/34
F. 40 yrs.
HYPONCHONDRIA **1000-2**

In the matter of the diet . . . those of the phosphorus nature, and of those that carry these properties as are necessary—the creation with the chlorine foods carry the gold in its combination—follow these closely.

Q. What foods contain gold, silicon and phosphorus?

A. These are contained more in those of the vegetable. Those of the nuts—those should be the character of the diet.

10/26/34
ELIMINATIONS: INCOORDINATION **F. Adult**
NERVOUS SYSTEMS: INCOORDINATION **710-1**

Beware of *any* fried vegetables or cakes with syrup or any large quantities of the sweetmeats or very rich foods where too much of the nuts of certain natures are used. *Not* black walnuts, nor pecans nor of such natures. Not coconuts: Nuts such as almonds, peanuts, English walnuts, Brazilian nuts and filberts are very good.

10/7/39
M. 58 yrs.
GLANDS: INCOORDINATION **2020-1**

Not a great quantity ever of nuts, though filberts or almonds may be taken if combined with a salad or the like.

ASSIMILATIONS: ELIMINATIONS: INCOORDINATION **5/30/36**
CIRCULATION: IMPAIRED **M. 47 yrs.**
ACIDITY & ALKALINITY **1151-2**

Nuts are good, but do not combine same with meats. Let them take the place of same. Filberts and almonds are preferable in the nuts.

8/6/34
F. 56 yrs.
DEBILITATION: GENERAL **626-1**

Begin with the activities in the diet that will make for the resuscitating of more vital forces. Do not overfeed, so that the body becomes a dross pit—as it were; but only take sufficient that the body does assimilate, does *use up* those forces that are taken into the system.

We will also find that the eating of nuts will be the better diet, just so they are assimilated; especially almonds and peanuts—each one of these well masticated. All others may be included somewhat.

10/29/36
M. Adult
ANEMIA **1131-2**

Noons—Foods that will carry sufficient amount of the carbohydrates, and the sugars in quantities and qualities that are absorbed. If there are to be used desserts, or sweets, they should be taken at this period of the diet. Nuts; especially those that are of the fruit of trees—almonds, English walnuts, pecans, these especially. The walnuts known as Black Walnuts are not good for this particular body; neither are the Brazil nuts particularly good.

ASSIMILATIONS: ELIMINATIONS: INCOORDINATION **5/30/36**
CIRCULATION: IMPAIRED **M. 47 yrs.**
ACIDITY & ALKALINITY **1151-2**

Nuts are good, but do not combine same with meats. Let them take the place of same. Filberts and almonds are preferable in the nuts.

1/11/35
F. Adult
NERVE-BUILDING **787-1**

As to the building supply for the system through the diets, we would cling rather to that which makes for the reduction of acidity; the building of the white *and* red blood supply, through a consistent activity towards nerve-building foods and values.

Necessity demands that there be the proper amount of the activities through the digestion, that these do not cause or produce an overfermentation without sufficient of the gastric flows through the lacteal activity to produce overacidity.

Hence, there should be a reduction in sugars—only taking those sugars from the vegetables; with the fats that would be from nuts, preferably. Use rather almonds and filberts than black walnuts, English walnuts or even Brazilian nuts; though these will be helpful at times, but very small amounts of same.

Not meats, then, that are of the red nature; nor greases of meats. These elements should be supplied rather from the vegetables and nuts.

4/21/36
F. Adult
TUMORS: LYMPH: UTERUS: FIBROID 1140-2

Q. With lacteal area disturbed, shall I continue to drink so much sweet milk?

A. If this is altered to the milk that is a natural creation from nuts it would be much better; particularly as almonds and filberts, not so much of those that carry too much grease or oils in same as the Brazilian nuts, but particularly almonds and filberts will be helpful and carry with same elements that are much preferable to so much milk.

12/31/34
F. 22 yrs.
ELIMINATIONS: INCOORDINATION 480-13

Q. Please outline diet to be followed at present.

A. Tend to those foods more of the alkaline reaction, in a general diet; bewaring of too great quantities of sweets at any time. Quantities of nuts—any of these may be taken. Not nuts in great quantities, but especially almonds, filberts or the like.

Q. How are my teeth, and should any be extracted?

A. Only local attention, as we find, is particularly needed at this time; especially if there is included plenty of calcium either in the treatments of same or in the diets—which is included specifically, of course, in the almond and filbert.

7/4/40
F. 30 yrs.
ELIMINATIONS: INCOORDINATION 2072-2

Fruits and nuts in their season should be taken, especially almonds and filberts.

2/8/36
F. 47 yrs.
CANCER: TENDENCIES 1000-11

Q. Are there any foods that should be eliminated, and if so, suggest diet?

A. Rather use the fruit and vegetable diet. The fats should be more from nuts than meats; for these, as we find, would be most helpful—and especially cashew nuts, almonds, filberts, and the like.

12/11/37
M. 30 yrs.
ARTHRITIS 849-23

Keep to those things that will aid in the eliminations. Build up the body with more of iron, as may be had from nuts and the like. Let these form a part of the daily diet.

11/21/34
ASSIMILATIONS: INCOORDINATION M. Adult
ACIDITY & ALKALINITY 741-1

As to the matter of the diet, keep rather to the *alkaline*-reacting foods; and where acids of any building foods are used let them be specifically in nuts. Naturally, the normal vegetable reaction would be kept in at least one meal during the day.

Q. Will outline a specific diet for the body?

A. As indicated. Those foods that have a tendency towards an alkaline reaction, but let the proteins be taken rather in the form of nuts, for the fats and oils, you see; these are much more preferable.

1)—Almonds

12/21/43
F. 20 yrs.
TUMORS 3180-3

Especially almonds are good and if an almond is taken each day, and kept up, you'll never have accumulations of tumors or such conditions through the body. An almond a day is much more in accord with keeping the doctor away, especially certain types of doctors, than apples. For the apple was the fall, not almond—for the almond blossomed when everything else died. Remember this is life!

8/31/41
ARTHRITIS: PREVENTIVE F. 51 yrs.
BODY: GENERAL 1158-31

And, just as indicated in other suggestions—those who would eat two to three almonds each day need never fear cancer.

12/28/43
F. 56 yrs.
CANCER 3515-1

Eat an almond each day—one almond—the body will have no more trouble or recurrence of this nature through the system.

3/16/36
ANEMIA F. 38 yrs.
DEBILITATION: GENERAL 954-2

In the afternoon (middle of the afternoon) eat half an ounce of almonds; just almonds, you see.

3/21/39
F. 49 yrs.
RELAXATION 1158-21

Q. Almonds?

A. These may be taken as a part of the diet preferably between meals, about three or four times a week; about ten at a time.

1/22/37
F. 39 yrs.
ACNE 1293-2

Q. Can you give the entity a recipe for a skin lotion?

A. The better skin lotion is the powder as we have indicated or a lotion with an almond base.

4/19/41
F. 51 yrs.
ASSIMILATIONS 1158-30

Q. Shall I resume peanut oil rubs?

A. There is nothing better. They supply energy to the body. And just as a person who eats two or three almonds each day need never fear cancer, those who take a peanut oil rub each week need never fear arthritis.

11/23/41
F. 16 yrs.
CANCER: PREVENTIVE 1206-13

Q. What can I do to improve skin condition of face and back, and of scalp and hair?

A. And know, if ye would take each day, through thy experience, two almonds, ye will never have skin blemishes, ye will never be tempted even in body towards cancer nor towards those things that make blemishes in the body-forces themselves.

10/29/36
M. Adult
ANEMIA 1131-2

Q. In what minerals is the body deficient?

A. As indicated from the type of foods suggested; iron, calcium and phosphorus—these are the ones deficient.

Q. Please give the foods that would supply these.

A. The almond carries more phosphorus *and* iron in a combination easily assimilated than any other nut.

2)—Coconut

2/6/31
F. 22 yrs.
EPILEPSY 543-7

Q. How often could coconut be eaten?

A. Not at *all!* No nuts, or bananas, or apples.

2)—Nut Butters

2/19/29
M. 48 yrs.
ELIMINATIONS 91-2

Not too much of grease of any nature, though butter—preferably those of the nut variety may be used.

1)—Peanut Butter

10/23/39
M. 20 yrs.
ASSIMILATIONS: POOR **984-3**

Peanuts are very good and peanut butter is especially very good for the body.

12/2/43
F. 39 yrs.
COLD: CONGESTION **1747-6**

Do refrain from eating too many peanuts with candy. Peanut butter will be found to be better, for this has those combinations that would be better for the body, but do not take it too often—for this only adds elements that are supplied in KalDak especially that active principle for working with the liver in its activity of secretion and of supplying elements for better assimilation.

3—Nut Oils

12/17/31
F. Adult
ACIDITY & ALKALINITY: PSORIASIS **5557-1**

In the matter of the diet, be mindful that these are both blood and nerve building, keeping an even balance in the alkaline- and acid-producing forces for the system. *Particularly,* should there be much of—at one period, at least, of the day—the *oils* of *nuts.* These are good for this body, *rathe*r than meats.

7/29/29
M. 50 yrs.
ULCERS **5641-2**

Morning—Much of the oils of nuts may be taken as will be well assimilated—not overtaxing same, see?

7/22/31
F. 28 yrs.
ASSIMILATIONS: ELIMINATIONS: INCOORDINATION **2261-1**

Those foods as would be taken would be the oils of nuts, or nuts and oils.

1)—Peanut Oil

10/27/41
F. 31 yrs.
ELIMINATIONS **1688-8**

Q. Is peanut oil taken internally good for my body?

A. Not good if taken by itself. If this is taken in combination with olive oil, or alternated, it would be very well.

7/17/44
M. 51 yrs.
ANEMIA **5334-1**

Also take internally once a day about a teaspoonful of peanut oil. Let this be taken in very small sips, assimilated. Do this just before retiring at night.

XII

Seafood—Fish, Shellfish & Snails

1)—Seafood: General

3/22/38
F. 29 yrs.
ACIDITY & ALKALINITY: MINERALS: CALCIUM: TEETH **1523-3**

Q. Suggest diet beneficial to preserving teeth.

A. Seafoods—all of these are particularly given to preserving the teeth; or anything that carries quantities of calcium or aids to the thyroids in its production would be beneficial—also it is not overbalanced, see?

Q. Is calcium taken in pills advisable?

A. That taken from vegetable matter is much more easily assimilated; or from fish AND seafoods.

3/30/44
F. 32 yrs.
SPINE: SUBLUXATIONS **4031-1**

Use only kelp salt or deep sea salt or the health salt, rather than plain calcium chloride that is mined internally in portions of the country.

Have plenty of seafoods. These should be the only characters of meats. Do not change wholly to the vegetable diet, for this would be too weakening for the body conditions.

9/29/36
F. 33 yrs.
PREGNANCY **540-7**

Those of the bi-valves of the seafoods are the preferable for the body. These as we find will make for developments and produce assimilations better for the body.

8/11/36
ANEMIA **F. Adult**
CIRCULATION: INCOORDINATION **1247-1**

Throughout the whole period we would be mindful that the diet is ever that which is easily assimilated. Do not attempt to have too much at the beginning, but all seafoods should be a portion of the diet; not every meal nor every day but just as it will assimilate or agree with the body. Sometimes it may be able to take more than others, but all characters of seafoods.

11/24/37
ANEMIA: TENDENCIES **F. 9 yrs.**
APPETITE: BODY-BUILDING **1179-3**

We would keep the activities as related to body-building forces. There may be taken at times those properties carried in the very seafoods themselves, if used often during such periods; especially swordfish. These, of course, are not to be all the diet, but these often included in the diet will be effective for this particular body.

Q. Should she also take A B D G capsules?

A. This depends upon whether or not the diets are indicated are a part of the regular diet. If those properties are supplied through that particular class or character of seafood mentioned, then the other vitamins are *NOT* near so necessary.

Q. How can her appetite be improved?

A. Too oft we find there is anxiety about appetites for growing individuals especially as may be about this body—as the body is rather "fussy," as it would be called, about what it eats.

As we find, where there is being supplied the necessary vitamins by properties given in the system, this then cuts off the desire for the supply to the body, see?

Hence as has been indicated, we would use certain characters of foods—especially in seafoods of the natures indicated—to supply the elements in such manners that they are assimilated and thus make for the increasing of the appetite, or the desire for the supply of elements that would make for body-building.

Too oft we find that where properties are supplied in the concentrated vitamin contents they take the place of foods; hence the appetites apparently are NOT active, when the real reaction is in the CANNED or pill activity and not from BODY reactions, see?

11/3/43
M. 54 yrs.
GLANDS: ADRENALS: THYROID: GLAUCOMA **3276-2**

Q. Should I eat meat of any kind, like fowl or fish?

A. Seafoods and shellfish will be advantageous to the body. Let's consider why. Of course, there are variations as to systems of different individuals. Here we are speaking of this individual body: There has been and is a lacking in the supply of energies or those elements that aid in the activity of the thyroid glands. Seafoods will supply elements tending towards a helpful influence, and also will aid in stimulating the draining of poisons from the alimentary canal, or kidneys and bladder. Activities in kidneys and bladder are directly associated with the eyes, or the nerves that are active from the third cervical to the adrenals and the glands controlled by or through kidney circulation.

Hence these (seafoods) would be beneficial.

3/15/44
F. 26 yrs.
PARALYSIS **3694-1**

Add to the body all of the seafoods that may be easily assimilated; deep sea fish . . .

ANEMIA: TENDENCIES **10/2/43**
ASSIMILATIONS: ELIMINATIONS: INCOORDINATION **F. 37 yrs.**
KIDNEYS **1695-2**

Do take D and G, but these more in the foods than supplementing in the combinations. These will bring better forces to the body; that is, in the food values take seafoods.

1/20/33
F. 18 yrs.
GLANDS: INCOORDINATION **951-2**

Be mindful that the diet is kept in a manner that does not work crosswise with the elements that are being created in the system. As much of seafoods as convenient will work *with* the balancing of the forces in system, for they create a character of element in the minutia, and supply to the blood and nerve forces of the system, to the active forces in the principles of the blood supply and the functioning organs, an assimilated character of force that works with the activities of the body. Those foods that carry sufficient elements of gold and phosphorus are found partially from seafood.

7/10/30
BLOOD-BUILDING **M. 65 yrs.**
ASSIMILATIONS **4806-1**

We would be mindful of the diet, that there are those of the full rebuilding—especially of those that build for the blood supply.

In the noon meal, those preferably of the vegetables that are raw, in part—and there may be added some seafoods, with oils as dressings for same.

12/30/42
M. 21 yrs.
BODY-BUILDING: LOCOMOTION: IMPAIRED **2873-1**

The food values should be those fully well balanced with calcium, iron, and especially the vitamins B-1 and the B-Complex. Those are much preferable for the body.

At least three times each week, then, supply these from the foods rather than the reinforced vitamins (though these reinforcements may be desirable if there is the inability of the body to assimilate foods that carry excesses or the full quantity of such vital forces).

To be sure, these are not all the foods that are to be taken:

Evenings—At least three times a week have fish or seafoods of any character, and occasionally a little beef and lamb—but these seldom.

9/23/43
F. 49 yrs.
ANEMIA: MULTIPLE SCLEROSIS **3232-1**

Q. Do I have an anemic condition as told I have?

A. There is an anemic condition. Hence the supplies of seafoods are especially good for this body—particularly after there has been the reduction of that plethoric condition in the ascending colon.

2/8/43
M. 37 yrs.
CIRCULATION: INCOORDINATION **2772-4**

Q. Am I allergic to seafood; if so, which kinds?

A. As we find, not allergic to seafoods; it is rather allergic to combinations of foods that are taken with seafoods. These cause the tendencies for a quick superficial circulation. It is the excesses of an activity of the vital forces that come from seafood combinations.

Q. What combination has this effect with seafoods?

A. Any sort of sweets or any of those foods that are of an acid nature.

4/5/29
CIRCULATION: LYMPH: TOXEMIA **F. Adult**
ACIDITY & ALKALINITY **5558-1**

Beware of how the diet is used in the eliminants. Keep closer to those of the alkaline-forming diet. Little of meats other than that of the seafoods. These may be taken in moderation.

7/7/30
DIGESTION: INDIGESTION: PELVIC DISORDERS **F. 22 yrs.**
ACIDITY & ALKALINITY **5621-2**

Beware of meats, save those of certain of the seafoods, or of such natures, as will add for the iodines and the reactory forces of potashes in the system.

8/12/43
M. 33 yrs.
GENERAL **2981-2**

Q. What kind of a diet? Include meat? Mild alcohol?

A. A regular or well-balanced diet is well for this body. Keep plenty of foods that carry iodine, both as to vegetables and as to seafoods. These, the seafoods we would have at least twice each week. This is best for this body as well as for most bodies.

Q. Should the diet include meat?

A. Seafood is a form of meat, but keep away from any hog meat or any beef.

7/12/43
GENERAL **F. 75 yrs.**
MULTIPLE SCLEROSIS **3097-1**

Q. What caused the nerve and heart condition?

A. Overstrain without proper balance in the diet to supply the elements necessary. As should be indicated, the diet for one that labors in the field is one thing. The diet for one who labors at drawing or writing or painting is another. The diet for one who does nothing is something else (except think about having a good time)! But the diet for one who uses the brain forces in his activity should be something entirely different! Seafoods are better for this body, taken often; not these alone, but plenty of seafoods . . .

NERVOUS TENSION **6/17/41**
RHEUMATISM **F. 26 yrs.**
2517-1

As to the diet throughout the period—keep close to those foods that will supply the greater quantity of B-1 vitamin.

Evenings—Especially seafoods, as oft as practical just so they do not become obnoxious to the body. Vary them of all characters. Fish or shellfish, or any of all of these at various times, and prepared in varied manners; though never too much of these fried. Rather have them broiled, boiled, baked, stewed, scalloped or the like.

PARALYSIS **6/24/43**
M. 68 yrs.
3056-1

Do have oft for the body those properties that carry a great deal of iodine and calcium; or seafoods often.

These, of course, are not all that should be taken, but these should be a part of the diet from day to day; not every day, but sufficient that these carry their influences in the body.

DIABETES **3/27/44**
SPINE: DISK: SLIPPED **M. 38 yrs.**
4020-1

In the diet be mindful that plenty of seafoods are taken. These carry those elements that will supply chemicals needed in the body.

ARTHRITIS **7/19/43**
F. 33 yrs.
3134-1

Take seafoods, prepared in some manner at least three times each week. Do not take too much of juices, yet do not take too much of solid foods; though as indicated, seafoods may be prepared in stews, soups, or in whatever manner is most satisfactory to the body.

ANEMIA **7/28/43**
GENERAL: MULTIPLE SCLEROSIS **F. 56 yrs.**
3118-1

Keep to those things that heal within and without. Have seafoods often. These we would give as the main portion of the diet, or the things to be stressed.

APOPLEXY: AFTEREFFECTS **4/23/30**
BLOOD BUILDING **F. Adult**
5667-1

We would be mindful of the diet, that it consists principally of those of seafoods as the flesh.

ANEMIA **10/17/34**
M. Adult
698-1

Q. Should he be given any iron?

A. *Rather* would we change, now, to the silicon and the phosphorus—as we have indicated—*only* through the vegetable forces, and the seafoods.

Nothing more effective in the blood supply than gold, that we obtain from the seafoods.

3/16/44
F. 31 yrs.
ASSIMILATIONS: POOR **3696-1**

It will be necessary to supply more calcium either in foods or in supplementary ways.

In the supplying of elements for the body increase the amounts of seafoods in the diet.

5/6/43
F. 37 yrs.
OBESITY **2988-1**

Do not eat too much of any form of meats. Seafoods are the better, this at least two or three times each week; fowl, if other meats are taken.

7/6/43
F. 32 yrs.
INJURIES: MINERALS **3076-1**

In the matter of the diet for the body—keep plenty of seafoods of all characters about three times a week.

Seafoods carry a great deal of the iodines as well as calcium.

4/28/43
F. 36 yrs.
ELIMINATIONS: POOR **2977-1**

Keep seafoods as a good part of the diet.

Not too much of fats. Never hog meat.

4/29/42
F. 37 yrs.
GLAUCOMA **630-3**

The condition to aid, then, is the DIET—AND that which IS a stimuli to the glandular forces AND the forces of body where assimilations are carried on.

Do have quantities of fish in the diet and seafoods.

3/15/44
F. 26 yrs.
PARALYSIS **3694-1**

Add to the body all of the seafoods that may be easily assimilated; deep sea fish.

9/28/41
ANEMIA **M. 8 yrs.**
ASSIMILATIONS: POOR **2595-1**

Q. What causes and what should be done for lack of appetite?

A. Keep away from too much sweets, but take all that is possible of the meat and vegetable juices, and fruit juices. Of course, fish—or any seafood the body desires will be well for the body; for he will not overeat of it.

4/6/44
F. 62 yrs.
NERVE-BUILDING **4033-1**

Q. Please suggest foods to stress and foods to avoid in the diet.

A. In the diet there should be the stressing of those that are nerve building; such as fish, especially seafood—not fresh water fish.

6/6/44
M. 11 yrs.
BODY-BUILDING **2890-3**

As we find, there are many changes for the betterment with this body. As we find, there needs to be kept some of those suggestions occasionally, and we would add reinforcements in the amounts of calcium which would be taken into the system; as is indicated in some of the structural portions of the body, as teeth and as a condition in the general blood supply.

We would include some fish; seafoods, not fresh water fish.

12/15/43
F. 23 yrs.
PARKINSON'S DISEASE **3405-1**

Have a great deal of raw foods, fish, seafoods; not fresh water fish.

9/5/29
M. 55 yrs.
SPINE: SUBLUXATIONS **5459-5**

Q. Will the elimination of meat from my diet have a weakening effect temporarily?

A. No. Only so far as the mental forces allow same, for there is as much *vitality* in the outline of those things the body *should* eat as would be with the meats, and when conditions are of the nature as has been given, *meats* aggravate, while vegetables, or characters of meats that build—that is, such as fish, shellfish. These do not carry those vibrations that aid in accentuating such pressures as disturb this body—but rather give the tendency to give more strength and endurance to a physical body.

7/20/25
F. 20s
INJURIES: SPINE: LUMBAR **49-1**

The diet free from meats as much as possible, save fish or seafoods.

10/24/30
F. 59 yrs.
ANEMIA **501-1**

In the noon or lunch, plenty of the shellfish—or fish proper. These are good, whether in the dried or in the fresh. The fresh carry more of that vitamin as makes for stamina in the vital forces of reproduction of *every* form *of* life in the system. Remember, this is for good and bad influences or bacilli as may be in body! Hence, these should be carefully selected, and be *very* fresh, and not from polluted waters.

2/22/44
F. 26 yrs.
CIRCULATION: LYMPH: TUBERCULOSIS **3687-1**

Do eat quantities of seafoods, not fresh water fish, but seafoods, including salt water fish, oysters, clams, lobster and the like. Not large quantities but have these often.

10/21/32
ELEPHANTIASIS: TENDENCIES **F. 18 yrs.**
ARTHRITIS: GLANDS: INCOORDINATION **951-1**

Supply an overabundant amount of those foods that carry iron, iodine and phosphorus in the system. The meats should be preferably (when taken at all) of fish, or oysters, or seafoods.

2)—Fish: General

9/19/35
ASSIMILATIONS: POOR **F. 80 yrs.**
CANCER **975-1**

Evenings—When meats are taken let them be preferably small quantities of fish. These should never be fried. These would only be those that were prepared very thoroughly, and in most instances after preparation be *chilled* almost, as it were, that they may be the easier assimilated by the gastric forces that have had so much disturbance; but these will be aided by the properties we have indicated in the compound for the body.

7/26/32
ANEMIC **M. 25 yrs.**
ASSIMILATIONS: POOR **481-1**

We would be mindful of the diet, that those foods are taken that are easily assimilated. Do not take quantities of grease of any nature. When meats *are* taken, they should be those of fish. It should be either baked or broiled.

Evenings—Cooked vegetables, and the meats *when* these are taken. Do not eat meat more than three times each week, and don't gorge self when this is done!

12/29/41
M. 40 yrs.
ASSIMILATIONS: POOR **826-14**

Have fish but these prepared with the reinforced vitamins in the flour, the meal or the like.

1/20/24
F. Adult
BLOOD-BUILDING **4120-1**

The diet should be watched closely, taking those properties that will create stimulation to blood supply, especially nerve-building forces in blood. Meats only that of fish. Vegetable matter that grows above the ground.

5/11/42
F. 74 yrs.
BODY-BUILDING **2074-2**

Give foods that are very stimulating. Every form of better stimulant that is for building strength, as fish.

11/3/42
F. Adult
ANEMIA **2843-3**

In the matter of the diet, for the strength of the body use fish and fish soups—all of these take in varied quantities according to the appetite of the body.

8/25/39
F. 39 yrs.
TOXEMIA **1985-1**

The activities of red meats would become more disturbing to the body. Fish should be a portion of the diet as the meats, if there is any of these taken.

1078-1
M. 17 yrs.
GLANDS: INCOORDINATION: HYPOTHYROIDISM **10/14/35**

In the general diet have always those things for the meals that are in accord with body, blood and nerve building. But not great quantities of meats. No red meats. No fried meats nor fried foods of any kind. Let these when taken be roasted or broiled or prepared in such a manner. Fish should be the principal food taken in place of meat. Broiled or boiled fish.

8/14/36
M. Adult
BLOOD: HUMOR **862-2**

Refrain from most any meats, only those at times of the boiled or baked fish or the like.

4/23/42
F. 34 yrs.
CONCEPTION **457-8**

Q. Should meat be entirely eliminated?

A. No. Fish food is the character of meats to be taken.

3/15/40
M. 45 yrs.
BODY-BUILDING **2146-1**

This has much to do with the general building up of the body. Keep away from meats, of course; that is, rare meats. Fish is preferable when meats are to be used at all.

7/30/40
F. Adult
OBESITY **2315-1**

Each meal should be preceded by the grape juice—thirty minutes before eating.

Evenings—Take a little of one or the other of the raw vegetables as a salad; with baked, broiled fish but NOT any fried. All cooked vegetables should be cooked in their own juices (as in Patapar paper), rather than with meats or fats.

5/22/44
F. 56 yrs.
1895-2

ARTHRITIS: TENDENCIES

Do decrease any red meats. Fish, we would take but none of any heavy foods, none of these fried.

6/25/40
M. Adult
2288-1

ARTHRITIS

As to the diet, refrain from any foods carrying any elements as of silicon, lime or the like. Hence not much meats unless fish. No fried foods of ANY character.

8/28/28
F. 48 yrs.
569-16

CANCER

Beware of meats. This has caused the greater distress at the present time.

Q. What would be a correct diet for the body at this time?

A. Vegetable diet, or pre-digested foods. No meats though fish may be taken.

7/25/39
M. 24 yrs.
1967-1

CANCER

Do not eat meats of any great quantity. A little fish would be very well at times provided it is VERY fresh.

8/5/29
F. 43 yrs.
2713-1

NEURASTHENIA

Q. Would you specify the necessary diet?

A. It's been given! As outline for such, it was given in that it should carry more of the iodines. All manners of fish should be taken at least once each day. Leave the meats alone, save fish. In the evening meal more of the fish.

1/17/43
F. 6 yrs.
2883-1

CIRCULATION: IMPAIRED
BODY-BUILDING

In the diet—have plenty of calcium; the foods that carry plenty of calcium; especially fish in small quantities, to be sure, but not large quantities. These should be a part of the diet for the body.

3/16/43
F. 21 yrs.
2937-1

ASSIMILATIONS: POOR
BODY-BUILDING

Do give vitamin-rich foods; such as fish. Season with butter or the like, rather than with other forms of greases.

3/31/43
ASSIMILATIONS: ELIMINATIONS: INCOORDINATION **F. 18 yrs.**
BODY-BUILDING **2947-1**

Keep the diet body-building. Plenty of vitamins A and D; plenty of B-1 and the B-Complex or plenty of fish.

No hog meat of ANY character. Let there be plenty of fish.

This is not to be all the diet, of course, but these should form a great part of the diet—just so often as not to become obnoxious to the body; altering in the manner of preparation.

Q. What causes pain in arms, shoulders and back, and what can be done for relief?

A. The lack of sufficient energies being supplied to the nerve forces and the stimulation of the nerve plexus calling for more activity. AND at times a pressure in the assimilating system.

Thus the needs of keeping good eliminations.

Q. How can she best overcome constipation?

A. By the diet; and, as indicated, these are taken into consideration.

10/6/43
DEBILITATION: GENERAL **F. 31 yrs.**
BODY-BUILDING **3267-1**

In the diet, do keep body-building foods.

Not too much of fats, but foods that are easily assimilated; plenty of fish, both canned and fresh.

Doing these, we should bring the better conditions for this body.

5/12/30
NERVOUS SYSTEMS: INCOORDINATION **F. 24 yrs.**
NERVE-BUILDING **2654-2**

We would be mindful of the diet and of the digestive system, as related to the nerve energies and nerve-building for the system. Be sure that the foods supplied are abundant with phosphorus, with those of properties that carry those that are nerve *building* in their reaction. Plenty of the foods that grow mostly above ground. Fish, these are good for the body, supplying the iodine necessary to overcome too much of a tendency of potashes in the body.

4/7/23
NERVOUS SYSTEMS: INCOORDINATION **M. Adult**
NERVE-BUILDING **4730-1**

The diet—all those that lend energy to nerve-building forces and those that give to the blood force the eliminating properties—vegetables, those that are green. Meats, very little. When used, only fish or the sinew of any other force. Do that.

2/5/36
M. 28 yrs.
ARTHRITIS **849-13**

Be most careful that there are not shellfish. Not too great a quantity of meats, and when meats are taken let same be *broiled* fish. These, we find, with *quantities* of the green vegetables, would supply greater quantities of those elements to create this balance in *conjunction* with the indicated manipulative and electrical treatments and the baths.

4/18/35
ANEMIA **M. Adult**
ASSIMILATIONS: POOR **898-1**

Evening meal—In the meats have those especially, whenever possible, of fish.

Keep these consistently, persistently; we will gain weight, we will put off this dullness, this tendency for catching cold, this weakness throughout the whole system; and bring the body—in six to eight months—to its normal weight of about a hundred and fifty pounds.

7/1/26
F. 37 yrs.
BLOOD-BUILDING **5739-1**

The diet should be kept in accord with the rebuilding of a cleansed blood system. Not overamount of meats. Fish may be taken in small quantities.

8/27/40
F. 40 yrs.
ATHLETE'S FOOT: ECZEMA **2332-1**

If meats are taken, only take such as fish and these broiled, baked, stewed or the like.

4/15/38
ASTHENIA: TENDENCIES **M. 20 yrs.**
BODY-BUILDING **487-22**

In the diet, keep to those foods that are body-building. When there IS the taxation through the physical exercise, have plenty of meats—as fish, but let these be WELL DONE. Preferably not the fried foods.

4/25/40
CATARACTS **F. 3 yrs.**
EYES: INJURIES **2178-1**

Two or three days each week we should have small quantities of fish—not fried, but rather broiled or boiled or baked. Not such large quantities as to become abhorrent to the body; but fish assimilated with the food values is especially helpful in such conditions—aiding in the blood supply, for the general health and welfare of the body in the present; as the body tends towards deficiency in the blood-building forces as well as the nerve forces.

ALLERGIES: METALS: ECZEMA **12/29/43**
DERMATITIS **M. 32 yrs.**
ECZEMA **3422-1**

In the diet refrain from any meats other than fish for at least ten days. Do include in the diet during those periods a great deal of raw vegetables.

3/21/39
F. 49 yrs.
RELAXATION **1158-21**

Q. Fish, fowl or lamb?

A. Fish about twice a week, and this a piece about two by three, about a quarter or half inch thick, broiled, if so desired.

4/14/43
M. 5 yrs.
CHILDREN: ABNORMAL **2963-1**

As to the foods, plenty of the iodine-producing or iodine-giving goods—as fish.

1/6/42
M. 57 yrs.
GENERAL **462-14**

Noons—Fish at least twice each week, even with the surroundings* for there is needed the reaction in the system of this nature of food. These with plenty of vegetables should supply sufficient needs for the body.

2/5/42
F. 24 yrs.
INJURIES **2679-1**

In the diets, also, much may be accomplished. Necessarily, there must be plenty of those properties that aid in keeping a correct balance in the production of Iymph, leucocyte AND the red blood supply.

Then, have especially those foods that carry more of the calcium and the vitamins A, D, B-1 and other B Complexes.

Hence we would have plenty of fish; these alternated as parts of the diet.

9/28/41
ANEMIA **M. 8 yrs.**
ASSIMILATIONS: POOR **2595-1**

Evenings—If it is practical or possible, have the body eat fish two or three times a week. These are the foods to be stressed in the diet.

11/16/22
BLOOD: OXIDIZATION **F. Adult**
BLOOD-BUILDING **4810-1**

Q. Should this body eat any meats, Mr. Cayce?

A. Very little meats. When meats are eaten, preferably those of fish and those not in large quantity, but something of those that carry the sinew and vital forces—no hot meat.

4/27/42
F. 33 yrs.
ASSIMILATIONS: ELIMINATIONS: INCOORDINATION **2737-1**

Fish, should be the principal fresh foods. These should never be fried.

INCOORDINATION **5/19/35**
GLANDS: SALIVARY: DIGESTION: GENERAL **F. 27 yrs.**
DIET: PREGNANCY **808-3**

As indicated, keep a tendency for alkalinity in the diet. This does not necessitate that there should *never* be any of the acid-forming foods included in the diet; for an overalkalinity is much more harmful than a little tendency

---

*A few miles from Atlantic Ocean.

occasionally for acidity. The meats should be such as fish, or the like. A well balance between the starches and proteins is the more preferable, with sufficient of the carbohydrates. And especially keep a well balance (but not an excess) in the calciums necessary with the iodines, that produce the better body, especially through those periods of conception and gestation.

8/12/37
F. 36 yrs.
LACERATIONS: STOMACH **1422-1**

No food that makes for a quantity of alcohol in its activity in the system.

Meats—never rare meats. Rather use those that are broiled or roasted; preferably only fish.

7/26/40
F. 12 yrs.
EPILEPSY **2153-2**

Evenings—A little fish (not fried), with mashed potatoes, sweet potatoes, squash or the like.

3/30/38
F. 36 yrs.
TUBERCULOSIS **1560-1**

Have fish once or twice or three times a week; preferably this also baked or broiled. Do not have it altogether as seafood nor altogether as fresh fish; but have quite a variation in same. And those that are the larger, the better. And when this is eaten, especially the larger bone in the back of the fish—baked—should be EATEN for the calcium that is in same. Do not take calcium separate.

11/23/37
M. 13 yrs.
MENU: PSORIASIS **1484-1**

Evenings—Fish, these would be taken in moderation, with any of the vegetables that are grown UNDER the ground, with one or two of the green variety or nature that grow above the ground.

7/28/34
F. 54 yrs.
RHEUMATISM **133-4**

Between the periods of the grape and grapefruit diet, in the beginning use a liquid diet consisting of the citrus fruit juices of mornings and the vegetable juices at other meals; gradually—that is, in eight to ten days—beginning to add to the semi-solid foods as in this manner.

Evenings—(these foods only added gradually, after the eight- to ten-day period)—A little chicken or mutton broth, but very little of the meat itself. A little later the body may begin with broiled fish, and well-cooked vegetables—but not with too much grease in same. Even these vegetables and the fish would be better cooked in the Patapar paper or a steam cooker.

2/11/37
CIRCULATION: POOR **F. 40 yrs.**
ACIDITY & ALKALINITY **1337-1**

Do not have any fried foods, especially as of steak or things of that nature—but broiled, boiled or the like; and especially fish should be used if meats at all are taken.

12/9/36
ARTHRITIS: TENDENCIES **F. 63 yrs.**
BODY-BUILDING **1302-1**

In the matter of the diets: Here we need body-building foods but those that tend to be more alkaline-producing than acid. For the natural inclinations of disturbed conditions in a body are to produce acidity through the bloodstream. Hence we need to revivify same by the use of much of those that produce more of the enzymes, more of the hormones for the blood supply; yet not overburdening the body with those unless the balance in the vitamin forces is carried.

Hence as we will find, not heavy foods or fried foods ever, nor combinations where there are quantities of starches or quantities of starches with sweets taken at the same time. But fish, preferably as the meats.

10/17/34
F. 40 yrs.
HYPOCHONDRIA **1000-2**

In the matter of diets—those of the phosphorus nature, and of those that carry these properties as are necessary—the creation with the chlorine foods carry the gold in its combination—follow these closely.

Q. What foods contain gold, silicon and phosphorus?

A. These are contained more in the fish.

8/13/30
M. 42 yrs.
DEBILITATION: GENERAL **2335-1**

Fish may be taken in moderation, as may also any of those properties that will furnish both iodine and phosphorus for the system. Keep the activities as near normal as possible.

7/31/39
F. 71 yrs.
HYPERTENSION: TOXEMIA **1973-1**

Fish would be very well to supply more calcium; as well as those bony portions of same that are cooked to such an extent that these may be masticated also—that is, the heavy bones, not the small ones. Hence these boiled or broiled or roasted would be preferable for the body, and of the larger varieties. Fish carry a great quantity of those properties for body and blood building.

5/14/34
ANEMIA **F. Adult**
INTESTINES: COLON: PLETHORA **549-1**

The meats should only include lamb, fowl or fish. Do not take shellfish, but the fresh water fish would be preferable to the salt fish, see? Mackerel, and the like, don't take; but the fresh water fish will be much better for the body. Some little condiments may be taken at this meal, if so desired.

10/29/43
ASTHMA **F. 36 yrs.**
ASTHMA: ELIMINATIONS **3331-1**

Fish—preferably for this body, *not* salt water fish but fresh fish.

9/15/43
F. Adult
ANEMIA **2843-4**

Q. As I can seldom get fish, and sometimes not enough vegetables, should I take any sort of vitamins? If so, what?

A. It will be very much better if there is still the attempt to obtain salt water fish.

Q. Are all organs functioning fairly well? and how may they be kept so?

A. As indicated there is a form of anemia. Hence the suggestion to have fish that supply the vitamins missing in the system. Add these that may be gathered at this particular period, and these will contribute to the helpful forces that may come with the keeping consistent with applications suggested.

10/16/41
F. 30 yrs.
ANEMIA **2293-2**

In the diet—keep close to those foods that carry plenty of A, D and B-1 vitamins. Do use plenty of fish and fowl in the diet; preferably salt water fish for the body, rather than fresh fish.

6/9/44
M. 12 yrs.
ASTHMA **5192-1**

Q. What causes the deep ridges in thumbnail and what treatments should be followed?

A. These are the activities of the glandular force, and the addition of those foods which carry large quantities of calcium will make for bettered conditions in this direction. Eat bones of fish, as in canned fish.

9/2/29
CHILDREN: ABNORMAL **M. 7 yrs.**
NERVOUS SYSTEMS: INCOORDINATION **758-2**

Fish, and *all* of the ones that carry iodine would he well, but in moderation. These, and those elements as are for the changes in vibration, will bring the near normal and the proper corrections for this body.

4/12/35
F. Adult
TUMORS: LYMPH **889-1**

Q. Will seafoods be all right for the body, and which one of these should be avoided?

A. Shellfish should be avoided. Seafoods or fish would be very good; especially deep sea fish.

12/8/39
M. 32 yrs.
PINWORMS **1597-2**

As to the diet, following the three-day apple diet, let there be more of the supplying forces as will create iron, silicon and the like for the system.

Not too much of meats, though fish may be taken.

1)—Gefilte Fish

5/12/28
M. 33 yrs.
LIVER: KIDNEYS: INCOORDINATION **900-383**

Q. Is the albumin on the decrease or increase in the urine?

A. On the decrease. Little fish occasionally, but none ever fried. Gefilte is well, provided not spiced too highly.

2)—Salmon

6/6/44
M. 11 yrs.
BODY-BUILDING **2890-3**

As we find, there are many changes for the betterment with this body. As we find, there needs to be kept some of those suggestions occasionally, and we would add reinforcements in the amounts of calcium which would be taken into the system; as is indicated in some of the structural portions of the body, as teeth and as a condition in the general blood supply.

We would include some fish. When eating canned salmon eat the bony portion; don't take it out, as it will aid with the oil in same, to supply elements necessary for the body-building forces.

3)—Sardines

5/7/30
M. 22 yrs.
EPILEPSY **1001-1**

In the evenings—there may be small quantities of fish, or shellfish, or of those that are of the appetizing nature. Sardines in oil, *never* in mustard, may be used sparingly.

3)—Fish Oils: General

SPEECH: VOICE **5/12/30**
NERVOUS SYSTEMS: INCOORDINATION **F. 24 yrs.**
NERVE-BUILDING **2654-2**

The use of those properties as will be found in that of the *fish* oils, or of those that are mono-hydrated—*these* should be in the soft tissue of the *antrum* and of the *upper* portion of throat. These will *reduce* the pressure and relieve the strain. Do not *use* the throat or the bronchia or the larynx too severely, until there is *bettered* conditions in this direction. Do not *strain* the voice in the use of same, *especially* until the conditions in the digestive and the assimilating system are corrected—especially the *sympathetics* in the upper cardiac centers, or the *sympathetic* cardiac centers.

1)—Cod-Liver Oil

8/11/31
ELIMINATIONS: POOR **F. 42 yrs.**
BLOOD-BUILDING **484-1**

In the matter of the diet, keep those things that are *blood*-building . . . Cod-liver oil should be taken with most of the foods.

5/17/28
ENVIRONMENT: ALTITUDE: TUBERCULOSIS **M. 55 yrs.**
COLITIS **4874-3**

Well that as much of cod-liver oil as is easily assimilated be taken. Be governed as to the quantity, as to how same is assimilated—for this is detrimental when not being assimilated by the system, for it acts as an irritant to the gastric and to the juices of the intestines and digestion when not assimilated.

1/8/30
F. 29 yrs.
BLOOD-BUILDING: VITAMINS: DEFICIENT **5615-1**

Plenty of the vitamins as may be had in cod-liver oils.

5/14/34
ANEMIA **F. Adult**
INTESTINES: COLON: PLETHORA **549-1**

We find that it would be well also for the body to take at times small quantities of cod-liver oil and the Russian White Oil at times. These should preferably be taken of evening, just before retiring. Not large quantities, but small quantities taken should create the vitamins necessary to produce in the alimentary canal activities, in the organs of digestion and throughout the whole system, the proper relations of the bacilli as necessary for carrying on the activity of eliminations and actions through the whole of the alimentary canal.

12/2/37
F. 5 yrs.
COLD: COMMON **1490-1**

In the matter of the diets, keep these well-balanced in the body, blood and nerve-building. Here especially would we find that the cod-liver oil would be a beneficial condition in keeping away cold. This preferably as we find for this body would be taken in the White's Cod-Liver Oil tablets. This would be easy for the body to take and not hard to take.

9/11/31
M. 42 yrs.
CANCER **2097-1**

Beware of *any* element that carries too much alcohol in same. The foods would be those that are *nourishing,* as those of the oils, those of cod liver, cod-liver oils. Do this for at least twenty-one days, then we may alter or change as to meet the needs of the condition.

10/24/30
F. 59 yrs.
ANEMIA **501-1**

We would use—as those that carry the cod-liver oil, or cod-liver oil in an albumized state. This is as of *sunlight* taken into the gastric forces, of especially the duodenum.

10/26/36
F. Adult
DEBILITATION: GENERAL **1278-6**

The keeping of enzymes as in body-building forces, as from codfish or codfish oil, or the cod-liver oil and the like, these will make for the building up of resistance. But follow those suggestions as indicated. The properties in the cod-liver oil or halibut oil or those things that give co-resistances in the vitamins that such carry into the body.

4/24/26
COLD: CONGESTION **F. 7 yrs.**
MALARIA: AFTEREFFECTS **4281-12**

Q. Should she have any cod-liver oil now?

A. This is always good to build the system, yet do not *over*stimulate the system with drugs, or *any* nostrums that give an unbalanced condition for the system. Rather be controlled by the diet and by the activities of the system, see?

2/8/30
DEBILITATION: GENERAL: FLU: AFTEREFFECTS **F. 71 yrs.**
BLOOD-BUILDING **5604-1**

We would be first mindful or careful of the diet, that it consists of those foods that, while easily digested, are blood- and nerve-building in their nature. At least once each day take those of cod-liver oil.

2)—Halibut Oil

11/24/37
ANEMIA: TENDENCIES **F. 9 yrs.**
APPETITE: BODY-BUILDING **1179-3**

We would keep the activities as related to body-building forces, as may be had with those oils that produce the better vitamin reactions in the system; the halibut rather than the cod liver for this body.

Q. In what form should she take the halibut oil? What dosage and how often?

A. This as we find comes ready prepared in pellets, or the like; and these would be taken after the milk—one pellet mornings and evenings.

Q. Should she also take A B D G capsules?

A. This depends upon whether or not the halibut oils are a part of the regular diet. If those properties are supplied through that, then the other vitamins are NOT near so necessary.

4)—Shellfish: General

2/16/35
M. 45 yrs.
ACIDITY **829-1**

When meats are taken, preferably use shellfish or the scaly variety; none of the deeper sea variety. The lamb or veal are preferable to the heavier meats.

11/6/35
ANEMIA: TENDENCIES **F. 26 yrs.**
ACIDITY **1048-4**

The vitamins necessary in the system, and especially vitamin E—whose activity in the system is for reproduction of the activity through every *gland* of the body itself, or those forces that are from silicon, iron, gold, or the activities from phosphorus—as of shellfish. Especially clams, oysters, more than any of the others—unless it is lobster. These are well to be taken two to three times each week; but these should be boiled. These will make for those conditions that would be better.

ASSIMILATIONS: ELIMINATIONS: INCOORDINATION **2/18/28**
ASTHENIA **F. Adult**
TUMORS: TENDENCIES **4789-1**

Little fish, or any carrying iodine (as any of the shellfish) may be used in moderation. Do not mix same, however, with milk. The action of these would be detrimental to the system.

Do this as given and we will bring much better conditions for this body, preventing any accumulations in the form of tumor—as indicated in plethora condition existent in portions of the system—yet not well defined to that state where these may not be eliminated, were the proper precautions taken as given.

4/29/37
ASSIMILATIONS: ELIMINATIONS: INCOORDINATION **M. 45 yrs.**
BLOOD: HUMOR **877-16**

In the diet—of these things beware. Others may be taken very well. Do not eat shellfish of any kind.

2/27/37
COMBINATIONS: ASSIMILATIONS: ELIMINATIONS: **F Adult**
INCOORDINATION **1342-1**

The shellfish are very good but do not combine these with any of those fruits or vegetables that produce an acid reaction.

12/31/37
DEBILITATION: GENERAL **M. 41 yrs.**
ACIDITY & ALKALINITY **1476-1**

Noons—The shellfish may be taken at this time, in their various forms.

12/12/38
F. 51 yrs.
MEATLESS: NOT RECOMMENDED **1703-2**

Q. Why were meat and fish and milk prescribed in the reading, as I use no meat, now, and dislike shellfish?

A. It wouldn't be bad if you would use it! And the influences of same, in the CHARACTER or NATURE that is PURIFIED, for this body WOULD be better, as we have found and given, to build the proper activity for the system.

11/6/35
GLANDS: THYROID: HYPOTHYROIDISM **F. 63 yrs.**
MINERALS **1049-1**

In the matter of the diet, this would be rather important. Occasionally use a great deal of those things that carry quantities of iodine, for this the body requires. But for this body it will be most soluble from shellfish.

10/5/36
CIRCULATION: POOR **F. 42 yrs.**
UREMIA **1016-1**

Q. Any other advice as to diet?

A. As indicated from the slowed circulation, and the tendencies at times for the acidity, those things that pertain more to the alkaline-reacting diet would be the better. Rather would we give those things that the body should be warned against, and then most everything else may be taken . . . if it is taken in moderation, and *when* there is the *desire!* As there is the desire for food, whether it is the regular meal time or at others, it would be best for *this* body to eat! If it desires to eat this or that, eat it! but do not mix it with other foods! Beware of shellfish, though oysters may be taken . . . but not crabs nor shrimp nor any of those natures that make for a *humor* that works with the activity of a disturbed condition in the hepatic circulation.

10/14/35
M. 17 yrs.
GLANDS: INCOORDINATION: HYPOTHYROIDISM **1078-1**

In the general diet have always those things for the meals that are in accord with body, blood and nerve-building. But not too great quantities of meats. No red meats. No fried meats, nor fried foods of any kind. Let these when taken be roasted or broiled, or prepared in such a manner. Do not take too much of shellfish. To be sure, the shellfish carry iodine—but it is not so well for this body taken in that manner. However, *lobster* broiled or boiled may be included. Also broiled or boiled fish may be included but no shrimp, oysters, clams nor things of that nature.

5/7/30
M. 22 yrs.
EPILEPSY **1001-1**

In the evenings—There may be small quantities of fish, or shellfish, or of those that are of the appetizing nature. Or those of the lobster chilled.

1/22/37
F. 39 yrs.
ACNE **1293-2**

The diets as we find are very good that have been maintained by the body from time to time, but beware of some combinations—especially of shellfish of *any* nature with alcoholic influences for the system near the same time.

During days or periods when the electrical forces or the diathermy treatments are given, do not take alcohol into the system in any form!

8/5/29
F. 43 yrs.
NEURASTHENIA **2713-1**

Q. Would you specify the necessary diet?

A. It's been given! As an outline for such, it was given in that it should carry more of the iodines. All manners of shellfish should be taken at least once each day. Leave the meats alone, save shellfish.

In the evening meal more of the shellfish.

5/12/30
NERVOUS SYSTEMS: INCOORDINATION **F. 24 yrs.**
NERVE-BUILDING **2654-2**

We would be mindful of the diet and of the digestive system, as related to the nerve energies and nerve-building for the system. Be sure that the foods supplied are abundant with phosphorus, with those of properties that carry those that are nerve-*building* in their reaction. Plenty of the foods that grow mostly above ground. Shellfish—these are good for the body, supplying the iodine necessary to overcome too much of a tendency of potashes in the body.

8/28/41
M. 56 yrs.
ASSIMILATIONS: POOR **619-10**

We would keep those foods that carry full quantities (though not excessive) of calcium and iodine. These will be the more helpful if they are assimilated from foods than by the administration in other manners. For, the affectation or the helpful influence passes then through the entire activity of the assimilating and distributing of energies, BY that assimilation through the body.

Q. Are my teeth causing any ailments?

A. No; these—as indicated in the throat and mouth—are more from the disturbances of the glandular forces, or the thyroid activity in relationship to the metabolism. Thus the needs for supplying those foods that carry quantities of iodine and calcium. Salt water fish, or all of seafoods. All of these are the measures and means by which such elements are carried, and in which much of these influences as helpful forces will be found.

4/2/35
F. Adult
ACIDITY: ANEMIA: TENDENCIES **875-1**

Be very mindful that the diet is more of the alkaline-reacting in its nature than acid, and that there are not such combinations as starches with hydrochlorics or proteins with the alkaline foods that make for such reactions in the duodenum and those portions where the digestive forces regurgitate or produce gas, this filling up, this fullness in the stomach itself.

Q. Will you outline a specific diet for the body?

A. As we find, those activities of the body are such that to make a specific diet must become rote, which would become disturbing to the better conditions of the body. Then, we would give rather the things of which the body should be warned in regard to its diet, but combinations in other directions may be made. No fried foods of any kind. Beware of too great a quantity of shellfish of any kind; the baked are the more preferable.

1)—Clams

10/17/34
M. Adult
ANEMIA **698-1**

Q. Should he be given any iron?

A. *Rather* would we change, now, to the silicon and the phosphorus—as we have indicated—*only* through the vegetable forces, and the seafoods.

Q. You wouldn't give him anything for anemia?

A There is nothing better for anemia than phosphorus, with these conditions! *Nothing* more effective in the blood supply than gold, that we obtain from the seafoods; such as clams—but not crabs, not such natures as these.

11/27/34
M. 32 yrs.
KATABOLISM: METABOLISM: INCOORDINATION **749-1**

Q. Will you outline a diet for the body?

A. Beware rather of shellfish of certain natures, that produce the tendency towards irritation. Clams are good; fish of certain characters is very good . . . Keep a well-balanced diet that will make for the better assimilations; strengthening, of course, more in those things that carry phosphorus and iron—that are found much in foods just indicated.

2)—Lobster

10/17/34
M. Adult
ANEMIA **698-1**

Q. Should he be given any iron?

A. *Rather* would we change, now, to the silicon and the phosphorus—as we have indicated—*only* through the vegetable forces, and the seafoods.

Q. You wouldn't give him anything for anemia?

A. There is nothing better for anemia than phosphorus, with these conditions! *Nothing* more effective in the blood supply than gold, that we obtain from the seafoods, but not crabs, not such natures as these. Certain elements as we would find in the *lobster* would be well, but not the Maine lobster; preferably those of southern waters.

11/25/35
ANEMIA **F. Adult**
BODY-BUILDING **1065-1**

In the diet keep those that are blood- and nerve- and body-building. Once or twice a week have shellfish, especially as lobster.

3)—Oysters

4/18/32
DEBILITATION: GENERAL **F. Adult**
BLOOD-BUILDING **4164-1**

Evenings—A well-*balanced* diet, occasionally using the diet that is more blood-building in its nature. Plenty of oysters that carry the greater part of iron, and as little of copper or manganese as possible.

4/5/35
GLANDS: HYPOTHYROIDISM **F. 49 yrs.**
ACIDITY & ALKALINITY **800-1**

Be mindful through the whole period that the diets are more in the form of an alkaline-reacting; or a fruit and vegetable diet, with little of shellfish, especially, though oysters for a portion may be taken if they are roasted.

10/20/43
GLAUCOMA: HYPERTENSION **M. 46 yrs.**
VITAMINS: ONE-A-DAY: GLAUCOMA **3305-1**

We may apply food values that may aid in staying the condition; that is, extra quantities of B-1 and (niacin) and those foods in excess—such as oysters, and foods that are rich in those added principles that are active in the body forces pertaining to the optic centers or nerve centers.

Keep those foods that will carry such properties as indicated, adding in supplementary form the A, D and B.

10/17/34
M. Adult
ANEMIA **698-1**

Q. Should he be given any iron?

A. *Rather* would we change, now, to the silicon and the phosphorus—as we have indicated—*only* through the vegetable forces, and the seafoods.

Q. You wouldn't give him anything for anemia?

A. There is nothing better for anemia than phosphorus, with these conditions! *Nothing* more effective in the blood supply than gold, that we obtain from the seafoods; such as oysters, but not crabs, not such natures as these.

10/17/34
F. 40 yrs.
HYPOCHONDRIA **1000-2**

In the matter of the diets those of the phosphorus nature, and of those that carry these properties as are necessary—the creation with the chlorine foods carry the gold in its combination—follow these closely.

Q. What foods contain gold, silicon and phosphorus?

A. These are contained more in those of the varieties that are given as same. Oysters.

11/27/34
M. 32 yrs.
KATABOLISM: METABOLISM: INCOORDINATION **749-1**

Q. Will you outline a diet for the body?

A. Beware rather of shellfish of certain natures, that produce the tendency towards irritation. Oysters are good. Fish or certain characters is very good. No fried foods of any kind. Keep a well-balanced diet that will make for the better assimilations; strengthening, of course, more in those things that carry phosphorus and iron—that are found much in the foods just indicated.

11/19/42
CHOLECYSTITIS **F. 31 yrs.**
COMBINATIONS **2853-1**

Q. What effect has alcohol when you eat raw oysters?

A. It produces a chemical reaction that is bad for MOST stomachs. Oysters should never be taken with whiskey.

5)—Snails—Conch

1)—Conch Soup

1/30/31
ASSIMILATIONS: ELIMINATIONS: ASTHENIA **M. 35 yrs.**
ASTHENIA: SURGERY: AFTEREFFECTS **4791-1**

Q. Any advice regarding diet?

A. Necessary that those conditions from which the body has suffered, as respecting the digestion, the organs themselves, be taken into consideration. Keep those foods nearer of an alkaline reaction, and that are of easy assimilation—though blood- and nerve-building, adding plenty of those foods that carry the phosphorus. This is an indication or a condition wherein the conch would be excellent for a portion of the diet. Conch soup or conch broth.

4/15/44
ACIDITY **M. 32 yrs.**
INTESTINES: PYLOROSPASM **5010-1**

In the matter of the diet, keep great quantities of seafoods. Especially conch soup would be well for this particular body. These may be obtained, even though rare, in the southern and eastern coast of Florida.

11/27/34
M. 32 yrs.
KATABOLISM: METABOLISM: INCOORDINATION **749-1**

Q. Will you outline a diet for the body?

A. Beware rather of shellfish of certain natures, that produce the tendency towards irritation. Keep a well-balanced diet that will make for the better assimilations; strengthening, of course, more in those things that carry phosphorus and iron—that are found much in those foods just indicated as well to use—or in greater quantity may be found in conch soup taken occasionally; this would be *very* good, especially.

10/17/34
M. Adult
ANEMIA **698-1**

Q. Should he be given any iron?

A. *Rather* would we change, now, to the silicon and the phosphorus—as we have indicated—only through the vegetable forces, and the seafoods.

Q. You wouldn't give him anything for anemia?

A. There is nothing better for anemia than phosphorus, with these conditions! Conch soup would be the *more* effective. *Nothing* more effective in the blood supply than gold, that we obtain from the seafoods. But the conch would be excellent. This is best obtained from Miami or Bimini.

11/25/35
ANEMIA **F. Adult**
BODY-BUILDING **1065-1**

In the diet: keep those that are blood- and nerve- and body-building. Once or twice a week have shellfish, or those that are of the conch nature—as conch soups . . . But the broth of the conch is the most excellent for any body; for it carries the greater quantity of phosphorus than any food that may be assimilated by man—the conch! (This would be well to consider in some other directions.)

XIII

Sugars and Sweets

1)—Honey & Honeycomb

9/30/41
M. 11 yrs.
BODY-BUILDING: ELIMINATIONS **1188-10**

Q. What foods should be included in weekly diet and in what amounts?

A. As we have indicated again and again those that are body building and at the same time keep in the foods the correct balance of the vitamins for body (rather than in chemical additions) building. These are the better foods, and sufficient quantities to satisfy the appetite of the body. A growing body requires plenty of vitamins A and B and D and C, that the structural portions may also have sufficient from the assimilated foods, rather than being supplied from concentrated forms of same.

Do that rather in the body-building diet. Not too much of sugars, yet sufficient. Let the sweets be taken in such forms as of honey. This is body building, also supplies energies that are well for a growing, developing body.

4/5/41
M. 20 yrs.
ASSIMILATIONS: ELIMINATIONS: INCOORDINATION **2157-2**

Q. How much sweets should be taken by the body?

A. Not too great a quantity. If taking sweets, use honey.

ADHESIONS: LESIONS **10/26/40**
CANCER **M. 40 yrs**
BODY-BUILDING **2276-3**

Use honey as the sweetening for most things, whether this be with the cereals or upon cakes or in whatever pastry is prepared—make same partially with honey.

9/8/24
M. Child
LIVER: KIDNEYS: COLD: COMMON **4682-1**

Digestive tract very good. Should be warned with present conditions, and until the body is adjusted properly not too much sweets for the body, save honey, which is very good for the whole system.

4/9/44
F. 53 yrs.
ASSIMILATIONS: ELIMINATIONS: INCOORDINATION **4038-2**

Q. Any advice regarding diet?

A. Not too much meats of any kind nor sweets. Seldom take any sweets other than honey or such natural sweets—these are preferable for the body.

4/11/35
ARTHRITIS: TENDENCIES **F. Adult**
BLOOD: HUMOR **888-1**

In the matter of diet, be more mindful that there are less of the acid-producing foods; more of carbohydrates—that is, sweets—but sweets such as honey.

3/29/40
F. 14 yrs.
ASSIMILATIONS: ELIMINATIONS: INCOORDINATION **1206-11**

Q. Does body eat too much sugar and candy, or not enough?

A. This is very well balanced at present; and, as indicated, do not let the body become AWARE of an attitude as to too much sugar or the like, see? either by suggestion or by activity; though precautions generally are necessary, as for those in the environs of the body. When sweets are taken, we find that honey is preferable to cane sugar.

3/21/39
F. 49 yrs.
RELAXATION **1158-21**

Q. Honey?

A. About once a day, or four or five times a week. Small quantity, of course, either with the preparation of the foods or with buckwheat cakes or corn cakes.

10/11/38
CYSTITIS: TENDENCIES **F. 35 yrs.**
ACIDITY & ALKALINITY **540-11**

As to the diets—these are very well if kept in a balance of at least eighty percent alkaline-producing to twenty percent of the acid-producing. This would then indicate not great quantities of sugars or of sweets, though honey may be taken as the sweets.

11/9/38
ANEMIA: TENDENCIES **M. 7 yrs.**
BODY-BUILDING **773-16**

Q. Please outline diet for each of the three meals daily.

A Keep these rather generally well-balanced.

Eat that which the bodily forces call for that supply the necessary building; though do not, of course, overbalance same with too much sweets. Keep the natural sweets—as with honey when that character is desired.

11/1/40
M. 33 yrs.
ARTHRITIS **849-54**

Q. What caused the severe pain in the left knee and what should be done when this happens?

A. This is the breaking up of those crystallizations. It comes partially from cold, and from too much sweets.

Q. What should be done to relieve this when it occurs?

A. Leave off sweets, and increase eliminations!

Q. Any suggestions regarding diet, other than leaving off sweets?

A. As indicated, NOT TOO MUCH SWEETS! More fruits, more vegetables. All KINDS of fruits SHOULD be taken.

Q. What sweets may be taken, or are best for the body?

A. Honey, or those made with honey. Not cane sugars, NOT cakes, NOT pies! These should be taken very, VERY seldom!

11/23/37
M. 13 yrs.
PSORIASIS **1484-1**

Q. What sweets?

A. Only honey as sweets, or those that are prepared with same.

1/5/44
DEBILITATION: GENERAL **M. 27 yrs.**
ANEMIA **3535-1**

All the sugar the body will assimilate, but it will have to be in very small quantities. It is better taken in cereals or fruits—that is, the natural sweets in these, rather than adding sugar. Occasionally, if palatable to the body, eat rice cakes or buckwheat cakes, but do use only honey and butter, rather than other types of sweets. This is the manner to take the sugar, rather than large quantities of sweetening.

11/4/40
M. 56 yrs.
ARTHRITIS **2392-1**

Little of sweets, save honey in the honeycomb.

Q. Will this treatment if carefully carried out give permanent cure?

A. This will depend upon the body's returning to those things that would bring back the reaction. Keeping off of too much sweets, and these eliminated as indicated should be, we find that it should be a permanent cure.

3/15/37
BLOOD: HUMOR **F. 56 yrs.**
TOXEMIA **569-25**

Eat honey in the honeycomb as a sweet, and be sure there is the comb in most of that eaten; for this, with other conditions, will assist in better purifying through the alimentary canal, for it acts as an aid to better conditions, and will not disturb the pancreas and the kidneys—the activity of all of these being disturbed in the present; but works better with corn bread or whole wheat bread, that are better breads than the white bread.

2/18/26
M. 54 yrs.
DIABETES **953-21**

As regarding the honey and honeycomb, as is seen, a portion of this is of that same cellular nature. Small quantities may be taken with impunity, yet the greater portion of same *should* be *comb* made from clover and buckwheat, rather than from flower or herb, see? That is, see that the honeycomb as used is from the apiary that has this annex to same for the care of the bee making same.

7/26/40
F. 12 yrs.
EPILEPSY **2153-2**

Refrain from any large quantities of sweets. Most of the sweets, if any form is taken, should be in the fruits or honey with the honeycomb, but not in great quantities.

8/11/36
M. 68 yrs.
ACIDITY **1245-1**

Not too much of sugars, but honey as sweets is very good and will be found to agree with the body—especially honey *in* the honeycomb, with corn bread.

2/12/38
F. 61 yrs.
ARTHRITIS **1512-2**

Q. Is it best for me to have any sweets?

A. Any sweets would be only honey WITH the honeycomb.

3/7/35
F. 43 yrs.
COLITIS: TENDENCIES **846-1**

Honey in the honeycomb, and only with the comb, should be the greater part of that taken as sweets.

Q. Until I get better, when I have a headache what can I do to relieve it?

A. As we would find, if these are begun we will have very few returns of the headache—which comes from this heaviness upon the colon and the lacteal duct and the strain on the system.

11/22/34
DEBILITATION: GENERAL **F. 12 yrs.**
TUMORS: WILMS'S **632-8**

Q. What type of sweets or what sweets can the child take to satisfy her appetite?

A. What sweets can the *body* take; it's not a child! Honey! Preferably honey with the comb, or in the honeycomb.

3/26/25
ASTHMA F. Adult
ELIMINATIONS 85-1

First, as for the diet, let those be little of sweets, save as would be found in honey and honeycomb of the better nature. That is, as that produced by sweet clover, buckwheat, or such natures.

9/10/23
M. Adult
ELIMINATIONS: INCOORDINATION 4232-1

Let the diet be not of meats, or of sweets, except of the honeycomb, with very little honey in it. That's the only sweets the body should eat.

5/9/29
F. 64 yrs.
ACIDITY: ASSIMILATIONS: BLOOD-BUILDING 1377-3

Q. Will natural sweets, such as honey be detrimental?

A. Those of honey in the honeycomb are better.

4/12/35
F. Adult
TUMORS: LYMPH 889-1

Q. How much sweets can the body take?

A. If these are of honey, eat what the body requires. There will be periods when the body's appetite will desire these, but supply same not from cane sugar but from honey—and especially in the honeycomb.

8/31/40
F. 12 yrs.
EPILEPSY 2153-4

Q. Would Jerusalem Artichoke Flour take the place of the sweets she craves?

A. It might take the place, but would be too violent a reaction upon the pancrean system, and to the kidneys themselves.

The sweets should be rather in the nature of honey and the honeycomb. Once a day, early of morning, take a teaspoonful of honey (teaspoonful, not a tablespoonful), and there will not be the desire so much for other sweets.

INCOORDINATION 5/19/35
GLANDS: SALIVARY: DIGESTION: GENERAL F. 27 yrs.
PREGNANCY 808-3

Q. What type of sweets may be eaten by the body?

A. Honey, especially in the honeycomb. Not too great a quantity of any of these, of course, but the forces in sweets to make for the proper activity through the action of the gastric flows *are* as necessary as body-building; for these become body-building in making for the proper fermentation (if it may be called so) in the digestive activities. Hence two or three times a week the honey upon the bread for the food values would furnish that necessary in the whole system.

6/3/17
M. Adult
ACIDITY & ALKALINITY: ANEMIA 4834-1

Nothing that is actively acid should be taken. Take yogurt or simply honeycomb which has had the honey taken from it.

5/1/35
M. 1-1/2 yrs.
WORMS: PINWORMS: AFTEREFFECTS 786-2

Q. Any honey?

A. Honey in the honeycomb will be very good, but not large quantities.

1)—Honey, Egg, Lemon

1/22/36
F. 28 yrs.
COLITIS: TENDENCIES: COUGH 808-4

To quiet the mucous membranes and to relieve that tendency for irritation, or the cough, we would prepare a combination in these proportions (though a double quantity may be prepared at the time if desired, for it may be kept—and a dose taken two to three times a day):

Beat the white of an egg until it is very fluffy. Then, *as* it has been fluffed, beat into same a teaspoonful of honey and the juice of a whole lemon. The dosage would be one to two to three teaspoonsful at a time.

This will work well with the digestive system, if the fruit juices and vegetable juices are used—and a little bit later beef juice, and then the semiliquid foods; as the broth of chicken, or the broiled chicken or the like may be then taken.

Q. What is the difference in taking into the system the white of an egg raw, and cooked?

A. That depends upon the system, and upon the manner and with what combinations it is taken.

For, as we have indicated for this body, it is not well that the white of the egg be taken, for it tends to make for an acid reaction. But when it is beaten very thoroughly first, and then the honey and the lemon added, the reactions are entirely different; for the properties in same not only react upon the body through the mucous membranes of the digestive forces but through the whole of the Iymph circulation, also adding to the system a *necessary* force that *is* needed in the system for the assistance of coagulation of the Iymph flow in the creation of the blood cells themselves. It is as the *natural* reaction of the yolk of an egg. It isn't that there should be all acid in any system, nor all alkaline; but it is the *reaction* of these *upo*n the system that aids in *creating* the elements in the body, see?*

---

*11/9/65—Report from 808-4 on using the white of egg-honey-lemon to cut phlegm: "For 3 hours I had been trying to get up phlegm—couldn't talk for it. *Immediately* upon taking the 3 teaspoonfuls of the above-mentioned combination the phlegm broke and I spit it up. Several hours later I had another spell with the phlegm and it worked again, though it took 2-3 minutes this time. Next morning all was clear—no more trouble with it."

2/15/36
F. 37 yrs.
FLU: AFTEREFFECTS **845-3**

For any flu or cold, *this* would be well as an expectorant and as an eliminant, and to cause the clearing of hoarseness—made in this way and manner:

Take an egg that has *not* been in the refrigerator or cold storage. Take the white of same. Beat it. Then, to this white of egg, add:

Juice of one lemon, dropped very slowly into same.

About a teaspoonful of honey, dropped slowly into same also.

About *three* drops—one at a time—of glycerine.

Beat thoroughly together. Of course, it would be worked in together when the glycerine is added.

Take a teaspoonful every two or three hours.

We will find this will clear a cold, relieve stress through the throat and the nasal passages, bronchi and larynx, and be most helpful for this body.

2)—Honey & Milk

2/19/38
ASSIMILATIONS: ELIMINATIONS: INCOORDINATION **M. 60 yrs.**
HYPERTENSION **1539-1**

Honey and milk should be taken as a nightcap, as it were. Stir or dissolve a full teaspoonful of strained honey into a glass or tumbler of heated milk. Taking this about twenty to thirty minutes before retiring will be found to be most helpful, most beneficial.

9/16/42
M. 45 yrs.
ARTHRITIS: NEURITIS **2816-1**

Be mindful that not too much coffee or tea is taken. Take at least a glassful of milk each day, preferably at the evening meal. Even if this is warm (not hot but warm), so as to dissolve half a teaspoonful of honey in same, it would be all the better.

12/9/39
F. 52 yrs.
INSOMNIA **2057-1**

Also when the osteopathic treatments are begun, but not until then (for the system should be cleansed thoroughly first, by the taking of the two rounds of the properties indicated), we would begin taking each evening before retiring about a cupful of heated milk (raw milk, preferably), in which there would be stirred a level teaspoonful of pure honey. Do not boil the milk, but just let it come to the heating point, and then stir in the honey.

11/29/39
ELIMINATIONS: INCOORDINATION **F. 40 yrs.**
INSOMNIA **2050-1**

Q. What will help the body sleep better?

A. Eliminating the poisons and the tensions, or "buzz" as it were upon the nerve system, as indicated, will naturally make for easier sleep.

In the beginning of these, if there is the tendency for sleeplessness, or insomnia, stir a teaspoonful of pure honey in a glass of *hot* milk and drink same.

2)—Pastries: General

5/14/34
ANEMIA **F. Adult**
INTESTINES: COLON: PLETHORA **549-1**

Be mindful that not too much sweets are taken, but sufficient that there may be created a balance with the green vegetables for a sufficient fermentation in the proper proportion and nature. Hence tarts or fruit pies, or rolls, or the like; but not just cake alone, for this is not so well.

2/7/42
ANEMIA **F. 28 yrs**
ACIDITY **2680-1**

Q. Do I have ulcers of the stomach?

A. No. This is the thyroids causing a disturbance in the combination of the chyle and the acids in same. Or, the gastric flows being super-acid, these areas become raw or upset. Thus the needs that little fats be in the diet; that is, not entirely obliterated, but little butter, little sweets—such as pastries and the like. These symptoms will gradually disappear as the glandular forces are brought to normalcy.

2/22/34
ASTHENIA **F. 65 yrs.**
ACIDITY & ALKALINITY **509-2**

Do not take large quantities of candies or pastries or tarts that are used with meats.

1/10/41
M. 60 yrs.
ELIMINATIONS: INCOORDINATION **1963-2**

Refrain from any great quantity of butter or butterfats. None of pastries, or pies; though foods that are of the diabetic sugar-proof nature may be at times taken.

7/26/43
M. 2 yrs.
ELIMINATIONS: INCOORDINATION **3109-1**

Keep away from candies and pastries.

1/17/41
CANCER: TENDENCIES **F. 44 yrs.**
ELIMINATIONS: POOR **459-11**

Have the better elimination by some changes in the diet.

DO be consistent with the diets—keeping away from pastries, cakes and the like.

7/31/31
ANEMIA **F. Adult**
ASSIMILATIONS: ELIMINATIONS **4472-1**

Beware that not too much pastry or of confection are taken, though there will be periods when there will be the unusual desire for such.

3)—Sugar: General

2/2/39
M. 47 yrs.
DERMATITIS **877-28**

Q. What about starches and sweets?

A. As has been indicated, these are not to be entirely tabu, but as would be from a normal mental balance of consideration, take about eighty percent alkaline-producing foods to twenty percent acid-producing. Sugars are in the MAIN, combined with starches, acid-producing. Starches also produce energy, as does sugar. It is the combinations of these that become rather the hindrances than the INDIVIDUAL properties themselves, see?

8/27/41
M. 51 yrs.
BLEPHARITIS **2577-1**

As to those warnings concerning the pancreas condition—be mindful that in the diet there are not sugars taken.

1/2/44
M. 2 yrs.
EPILEPSY: SUGAR: NOT RECOMMENDED **3437-1**

For these lesions have been of such a length of period that corrections will necessarily have to be made, and these may cause reflexes such as to produce (the corrections) one or two violent reactions—though not as severe as some, provided sweets are kept from the body.

7/17/33
F. 44 yrs.
GLANDS: INCOORDINATION **757-4**

Sugars may be used in *small* quantities, but should never be excessive; nor sweets of *any* nature excessive for the body, else fermentation that will effect that which is being eliminated in the activity of those forces in the blood that need to be eradicated from the system.

5/4/31
F. 47 yrs.
BLOOD: OXIDIZATION: ELIMINATIONS **5502-2**

Q. What should body be careful of in her diet?

A. Too much of those forces as make for what is sometimes termed grape sugars in the system. Those forces or combinations that create too much sugar.

1/30/28
F. Adult
ELIMINATIONS: POOR: TOXEMIA **81-2**

No sugar as too much carbon must not be created when proper eliminations are to be established.

3/1/41
F. Adult
ARTHRITIS: NEURITIS: TENDENCIES **838-3**

We would not include too much of pastries or sugars. If sugars are desired, use rather beet sugar or saccharin as the sweetening—these are preferable to cane sugar.

10/24/30
F. 59 yrs.
ANEMIA **501-1**

In the evening, those of the sweetened foods should be preferably of saccharin or beet sugars; *not* cane.

11/4/35
F. 4 yrs.
GLANDS: INCOORDINATION **795-4**

As to the diets for this body: These should be somewhat out of the ordinary, as we have indicated; though not in such an extreme manner as to make for confining the body to activities that become as hardships. Beware of *excessive* acid-producing foods; though it must be considered that the body in its developing stage requires sufficient of those energies from sugars that are proper for the system. Hence the sweets should be of such natures that they do not form a character of acid that becomes detrimental to those very tendencies that are being overcome by the supplying of acid in the body through the metal forces.

Hence sweets or sugars from the sugar cane should be tabu. Use rather those that are of a vegetable or fruit nature, or the sweets that are contained in such.

Hence the Health Foods that are combined with beet sugar, or with saccharin, may be used in the candies or the pastries; that may be a part of the diet.

1)—Beet Sugar

10/29/36
M. Adult
ANEMIA **1131-2**

Q. Suggest best sugars for body.

A. Beet sugars are the better for *all,* or the cane sugars that are not clarified.

3/29/40
F. 14 yrs.
ASSIMILATIONS: ELIMINATIONS: INCOORDINATION **1206-11**

Q. Does body eat too much sugar and candy, or not enough?

A. This is very well balanced at present; and, as indicated, do not let the body become AWARE of an attitude as to too much sugar or the like, see? either by suggestion or by activity; though precautions generally are necessary, as for those in the environs of the body. When sweets are taken, we find that candies made with beet sugar are preferable to cane sugar.

INCOORDINATION **5/19/35**
GLANDS: SALIVARY: DIGESTION: GENERAL **F. 27 yrs**
PREGNANCY **808-3**

Q. What type of sweets may be eaten by the body?

A. Preserves made with *beet* rather than cane sugar. Not too great a quantity of any of these, of course, but the forces in sweets to make for the proper activity through the action of the gastric flows *are* as necessary as body-building; for these become body-building in making for the proper fermentation (if it may be called so) in the digestive activities.

2)—Brown Sugar

12/13/40
M. 33 yrs.
ARTHRITIS: ELIMINATIONS **849-55**

Q. Any suggestions for improving the diet?

A. Be warned as to too much sweets, as indicated. Of course, honey may be used; or the pastries made with BROWN sugar and not with the white or cane would be preferable, if there is the insistence upon having same.

3)—Maple Sugar

3/29/40
F. 14 yrs.
ASSIMILATIONS: ELIMINATIONS: INCOORDINATION **1206-11**

Q. Does body eat too much sugar and candy, or not enough?

A. This is very well balanced at present; and, as indicated, do not let the body become AWARE of an attitude as to too much sugar or the like, see? either by suggestion or by activity; though precautions generally are necessary, as for those in the environs of the body. When sweets are taken, we find that maple sugar is preferable to cane sugar.

5/9/29
F. 64 yrs.
ACIDITY: ASSIMILATIONS: BLOOD-BUILDING **1377-3**

Q. Will natural sweets, such as maple sugar be detrimental?

A. May be taken in moderation early in the day.

4)—Sugar Substitute: Saccharine

1/10/41
M. 60 yrs.
ELIMINATIONS: INCOORDINATION **1963-2**

The use of beet sugar is preferable to cane; or still more preferable is saccharin as sweetening.

4/17/31
DEBILITATION: GENERAL **M. 19 yrs.**
CHOREA **1225-1**

Evenings—Much of the sweets may be taken provided (that, at this period) these are not of the cane sugar variety. Those that are of the saccharine—these may be taken. Not too much of pastries that carry the cane sugars, but those that make for lime, silicon, magnesia—these will be well.

4/12/35
F. Adult
TUMORS: LYMPH **889-1**

Q. How much sweets can the body take?

A. If these are of saccharine as their base, eat what the body requires. There will be periods when the body's appetite will desire these, but supply same not from cane sugar.

4)—Sweets: General

4/29/37
ASSIMILATIONS: ELIMINATIONS: INCOORDINATION **M. 45 yrs.**
BLOOD: HUMOR **877-16**

Not too much sweets but sufficient for the supply of the energies used by activity. Depend on how physically active the body has been as to how much of sweets of any nature are taken.

2/2/37
OBESITY: TENDENCIES **F. 57 yrs.**
ACIDITY & ALKALINITY **1125-2**

Do not combine *any* of starches with any quantities of sweets. Do not take food values that cause great quantity of alcoholic reaction. This does not refer to alcohol, but sweets *and* certain starches produce a character of fermentation that is alcoholic that makes for excess of fatty portions for the body.

6/29/26
M. Adult
ASTHMA **90-1**

First, do not take sweets to *any* excess in the body. Not things with too much sugar, for this tends to irritate this condition. Do not overload the kidneys, for sugars will, you see.

10/17/35
ANEMIA **F. 49 yrs.**
ACIDITY & ALKALINITY **1023-1**

Do not take large quantities of sweets at the same period that starches are taken; or do not have these combined in the digestive area during the same period. However, starches should be used in moderation—as well as sweets. But have more of the natural sweets, as from fruits—or the salts from vegetables supplying the carbohydrates.

These will be found to bring near normal conditions for this body.

3/20/35
M. Adult
ASTHMA **861-1**

In the matter of the diet, be rather particular, rather insistent. Beware of sweets, for these—too—act upon the mucous membranes that are affected by the pressures from the congestion in the dorsal area, as congestion in reflexly the bronchi and the trachea area.

ASSIMILATIONS: ELIMINATIONS: INCOORDINATION **5/30/36**
CIRCULATION: IMPAIRED **M. 47 yrs.**
ACIDITY & ALKALINITY **1151-2**

Not quantities of sweets *with* white bread. The meats and sweets should be preferably taken at the same meal. It isn't so much *what* the body eats as it is the *combinations* that are taken at times. Beware then of those things.

7/30/36
M. 30 yrs.
ATTITUDES & EMOTIONS: WORRY: GENERAL **416-9**

Q. What foods should I avoid?

A. Rather is it the combination of foods that makes for disturbance with most physical bodies, as it would with this.

In the activities of the body in its present surroundings, those tending toward the greater alkaline reaction are preferable.

If sweets and meats are taken at the same meal, these are preferable to starches. Of course, small quantities of breads with sweets are all right, but do not have large quantities of same. These are merely warnings.

8/29/35
F. 45 yrs.
COLITIS **404-4**

When sweets are taken, eat all sweets; or don't eat so much of other things with them! Sweets are made more harmful (for they do furnish elements necessary) when they are taken with starches. Proteins are made more harmful when they are taken oftentimes with sweets.

8/11/31
ELIMINATIONS: POOR **F. 42 yrs.**
BLOOD-BUILDING **484-1**

Not sweets. Let the *system* create that as for the body.

8/24/35
F. Adult
ACIDITY & ALKALINITY: ANEMIA **978-1**

Be very mindful of the diet. Eat those foods that are alkaline in their reaction. Not too much sweets; for sweets occasionally tend to bring on those spasmodic conditions, *if* the system is the least bit acid, though these are not as bad if the system is alkaline.

12/17/36
M. 56 yrs.
KIDNEYS **1308-1**

And then be most mindful of the diet. These as we find to beware of, and those other things that agree with the body most any of these may be taken—but these leave off:

Not too much sweets or any that carry or produce alcoholic reaction (as combinations of white bread or certain sweets for the system). No strong drink—not with sweets.

7/11/36
F. 30 yrs.
EDEMA
ACIDITY & ALKALINITY **1201-1**

Keep the acid-producing or the necessity of the flow of the gastric juices, or of acid, which is for certain foods—combined properly. And do not mix starches with sweets.

1)—Blancmange

5/8/44
M. 4 yrs.
ASTHENIA **2299-13**

Blancmange or such may be given, that the body will take, and will give strength to the body.

8/28/35
F. 60 yrs.
NEPHRITIS **882-2**

Evenings—The sweets taken should be rather blancmange or such natures where the sugars carried in same may assimilate with the upper gastric flow, or the lacteals—from the assimilations through the flow of the gastric juices from the salivary glands and the upper portion of the stomach, rather than from the lower or the hydrochlorics. These will be found especially in those properties indicated, if the eliminations throughout the body are carried on as we have outlined.

10/6/42
M. Adult
STREPTOCOCCUS **2826-1**

Most of the food taken should be blancmange or such. And beef juice a little bit later, if the body responds.

2)—Candy

8/25/39
F. 39 yrs.
TOXEMIA **1985-1**

Refrain from those foods that produce alcohol. We do not mean so much the combinations of the alcohol, but those things that produce an alcohol reaction in the system; such as candies.

10/13/37
F. 45 yrs.
ARTHRITIS: TENDENCIES **1315-7**

Do not combine too much starches, nor too much of any of those things that will create too great a quantity of alcoholic reaction—such as candies with ANY of the starches; these produce that reaction with the system of the CHARACTER of fermentation that produces an alcoholic reaction which is disturbing to the system . . .

8/30/40
F. 33 yrs.
ANEMIA **2336-1**

Q. What causes craving for candy?
A. The thyroid disturbances.
Q. Is candy harmful?
A. Only those that are not of the cane sugar nature are not harmful. Those of other natures are not harmful, if taken in moderation.

10/30/37
M. 48 yrs.
DIABETES: TENDENCIES **470-19**

Neither would there be the elimination entirely of candies . . . Those that are of the nature in which the greater portion of the sweet is supplied from the natural fruits are preferable, as would be candied fruits or the like—these are well.

ANEMIA
COLITIS **7/16/43**
ELIMINATIONS: INCOORDINATION **F. 54 yrs.**
3098-1

Hard candies may be taken occasionally, but not too much of chocolate for this body.

3)—Charlotte Russe

1/24/35
M. Child
COLD: CONGESTION **738-2**

With the cold and congestion in the present, almost an entire liquid diet would be the better. Also charlotte russe (not in such great quantities), these are well for the body, making for the sweets sufficient and keeping the strength and vitality without the use of cane sugar, and ridding the system of the cold.

4)—Chocolate

10/29/43
ASSIMILATIONS: ELIMINATIONS: INCOORDINATION **F. 13 yrs.**
HEADACHE: MIGRAINE **3326-1**

Keep away from excesses of sweets, especially chocolate.

4/17/31
DEBILITATION: GENERAL **M. 19 yrs.**
CHOREA **1225-1**

Evenings—Much of the sweets may be taken, provided (that is, at this period) these are not of the cane sugar variety, but chocolates—or those of the cocoa bean, these may be taken.

9/2/39
DERMATITIS **M. 2 yrs.**
BABY CARE **1990-1**

Q. Is there a candy or sweet that would not be harmful in the diet?

A. The chocolate or the fudge that is prepared at some institutions as preparations for such conditions would be very well. But that as would be prepared with honey and peanuts would not be harmful.

5/19/35
F. 27 yrs.
PREGNANCY **808-3**

Q. Would health chocolate be harmful?

A. These carry with same (the health chocolates) that which does not work for the best with the assimilations through the lacteal area, making for a hard activity of the gastric flow—especially in the duodenum.

1/31/44
F. 29 yrs.
FLU: AFTEREFFECTS **3622-1**

In the diet keep away from too much starches, especially chocolate, or foods prepared with chocolate—especially, considering the way chocolate is made in the present, and carbonated waters.

2/15/44
M. 60 yrs.
ASTHMA **3661-1**

In the diet beware of too much sugar. Beware of any chocolate or of any sweets of that nature or of too much starches.

4/27/42
F. 33 yrs.
ASSIMILATIONS: ELIMINATIONS: INCOORDINATION **2737-1**

Not too much sugars, to be sure, but at certain periods, say once or twice a month, eat some good chocolate. This adds energies and carbohydrates in a manner that is well.

1/13/41
F. 27 yrs.
DEBILITATION: GENERAL **2426-1**

Q. Is bitter chocolate or bittersweet chocolate hard for me to digest?

A. Any of the chocolates are hard to digest at the present. These may be taken in moderation as conditions progress, but should never be taken in any large quantity.

5/25/44
HAY FEVER **F. 55 yrs.**
COMBINATIONS **5148-1**

Q. Any particular diet recommended?

A. Keep away from sweets and from too much starches. It's combinations, rather than the diet. No chocolate . . .

5)—Fruit Sherbet

9/6/33
ASSIMILATIONS: POOR **F. 3 yrs**
MALARIA: TENDENCIES **402-1**

Evenings—Properties that are easily assimilated. Ice creams or sherbets are very good; preferably the fruit sherbets would be well for the body.

6)—Ices & Ice Cream

12/31/34
F. 22 yrs.
ELIMINATIONS: INCOORDINATION **480-13**

Q. Please outline diet to be followed at present.

A. Tend to those foods more of the alkaline reaction, in a general diet; bewaring of too great quantities of sweets at any time, either as at breakfast in syrups and cakes or at other periods. Not too great a quantity of sweets at any period, as desserts; though ice cream, ices or the like may be taken in moderation. Divide in a normal manner the small quantity of sweets taken.

6/17/44
ARTHRITIS **F. 63 yrs.**
ELIMINATIONS: POOR **3395-4**

Ices, ice cream; these may be taken.

7)—Ices: General

7/30/40
F. Adult
OBESITY **2315-1**

Evenings—Not very much ice cream should be taken; but ICES—as fruit ices or sherbet—may be taken.

5/18/43
F. 66 yrs.
ASSIMILATIONS: ELIMINATIONS: INCOORDINATION **3008-1**

Beware of too much sweets. Ices are very well.

8/15/25
COLITIS **F. 6 yrs.**
MALARIA: TENDENCIES **4281-6**

As much ice as the body may desire. Ices, fruit ices, very good for the system, especially pineapple and orange ices, see?

i)—Pineapple Ice

11/28/33
M. Adult
ANEMIA **461-1**

Noons—Fruit ices are *very* good for the body at any time; especially pineapple.

8)—Ice Cream

5/8/44
M. 4 yrs.
ASTHENIA **2299-13**

Ice cream or such may be given, that the body will take, and will give strength to the body.

9)—Junket

4/12/27
ASSIMILATIONS: ELIMINATIONS **F. 22 yrs.**
ASTHENIA **5714-2**

Keep as much of the stimulant for the body as may be possibly given, see? using the junket and those properties as have been given, *occasionally,* to change and alter the action of these conditions through that portion of the system, where *assimilation* must take place, would we build strength and resistance for this body, see?

1/22/36
F. 38 yrs.
TUBERCULOSIS **1045-5**

For the assimilations, we find that the varied forms of junket would be helpful.

8/28/35
F. 60 yrs.
NEPHRITIS **882-2**

Evenings—The sweets taken should be rather junket, or such natures where the sugars carried in same may assimilate with the upper gastric flow, or the lacteals—from the assimilations through the flow of the gastric juices from the salivary glands and the upper portion of the stomach, rather than from the lower or the hydrochlorics. These will be found especially in those properties indicated, if the eliminations throughout the body are carried on as we have outlined.

9/22/36
M. 75 yrs.
CANCER **1263-1**

In the matter of the diet, keep more to the liquids and semi-liquids. Junket . . . properties of this nature would be better for the body for the first week or ten days.

8/15/25
COLITIS **F. 6 yrs.**
MALARIA: TENDENCIES **4281-6**

In the other forces, junket (not too much sugars with same, see? Beet sugar used in preference to cane sugar).

4/15/35
F. 56 yrs.
ASTHENIA **895-1**

In the matter of the diet, be very mindful that in the beginning this consists much of pre-digested foods. Junket, and things of such nature would be the first characters of food.

5/4/39
M. 31 yrs.
LIVER: KIDNEYS: INCOORDINATION **1885-1**

Junket, even those principles as from gelatin and the like are to be desired—if they agree with the body or if the appetite will take portions of same.

9/29/24
ULCERS: STOMACH **M. 45 yrs.**
ELIMINATIONS **4709-5**

Take no foods save those that carry the incentive for the proper producing condition in the system. Namely these . . . Junket may be used. This we find will also assist the conditions in the liver's action in the body.

5)—Syrups: General

9/30/41
M. 11 yrs.
BODY-BUILDING: ELIMINATIONS **1188-10**

Q. What foods should be included in weekly diet and in what amounts?

A. As we have indicated again and again, those that are body building and at the same time keep in the foods the correct balance of the vitamins for body (rather than in chemical additions) building. These are the better foods, and sufficient quantities to satisfy the appetite of the body. A growing body requires plenty of vitamins A and B and D and C, that the structural portions may also have sufficient from the assimilated foods, rather than being supplied from concentrated forms of same.

Do that rather in the body-building diet. Not too much sugars, yet sufficient. Let the sweets be taken in such forms as corn or Karo syrup. These are body building, also supply energies that are well for a growing, developing body.

3/28/44
M. 41 yrs.
ACIDITY & ALKALINITY **4008-1**

Q. What healthful sweets should I use?

A. . . . Karo syrup or corn syrup.

1)—Karo Syrup

4/5/41
M. 20 yrs.
ASSIMILATIONS: ELIMINATIONS: INCOORDINATION **2157-2**

For at least a week or ten days be especially precautious regarding the diet; easily assimilated foods.

Q. How much sweets should be taken by the body?

A. Not too great a quantity. If taking sweets, use Karo.

6/29/42
F. 25 yrs.
ANEMIA **2376-2**

Mornings—A little syrup may be taken—preferably Karo rather than other combinations, for this carries some carbohydrates that are well for the body.

2)—Maple Syrup

1/5/44
DEBILITATION: GENERAL **M. 27 yrs.**
ANEMIA **3535-1**

All the sugar the body will assimilate, but it will have to be in very small quantities. It is better taken in cereals or fruits, that is, the natural sweets in these, rather than adding sugar. Occasionally, if palatable to the body, eat rice cakes or buckwheat cakes, but do use only maple syrup and butter, rather than other types of sweets. This is the manner to take the sugar, rather than large quantities of sweetening.

XIV

Vegetables

1)—Vegetables: General

MUSCULAR DYSTROPHY **3/12/36**
INTESTINES: GAS **M. 43 yrs.**
1127-1

In the diet keep to those things that cause less and less of the gas to form in the digestive system, through a very depleted or very ineffective activity of a peristaltic movement. Hence use green or fresh vegetables, vegetable juices prepared in their own salts—these would be better for the body. Hence do not cook the vegetables together that are given the body, but separate—in Patapar paper; or serve each one separate, and it will be found to be more helpful, more beneficial to the body.

If the body responds, we may be able to give further suggestions.

3/8/35
F. 37 yrs.
ARTHRITIS **631-6**

Evenings—Rather the vegetables that are prepared in their own salts, or *own* fluids; *not* as cooked other than in a steamer or in Patapar paper. And use the juices of same as a portion of the diet, for the vitamins and the necessary salts that will create the fluids in the system are found in these.

1/19/35
CONSTIPATION: TENDENCIES **F. Adult**
ASSIMILATIONS: ELIMINATIONS: INCOORDINATION **796-2**

Evenings—Whole-cooked vegetables, but preferably cooked in their own juices—or cook them in Patapar paper, so that all of their juices are retained in same. Thus we will find that much that has disagreed will become helpful in the building up of the body. By using these in this way and manner, do not disturb self that poisons will come from the cooking pots or pans—but in the *cleansings* for the intestinal tract these will be eliminated.

Remember, the body rebuilds and replenishes itself continually. What portion would be the more active in its changes than those that *are* the channels for these very changes—the *digestive* forces of the body; the lungs, the liver, the heart, the digestive system, the pancreas, the spleen? All of these change the more often, so that when it is ordinarily termed that the body has changed each atom in seven years, these organs have changed almost *seven* times during those seven years!

Hence these should not disturb the body, provided the proper balances are being kept in the system.

4/26/35
F. 53 yrs.
GLANDS: INCOORDINATION: COOKING UTENSILS: GENERAL 906-1

No fried foods of any kind. Baked, broiled or boiled, or preferably the vegetables cooked in their *own* juices—as in Patapar paper or *steamed* in a manner as to retain their own salts, their own vitamins, and not combining them together. All seasoning should be done with butter and salt or paprika (or whatever may be used as the seasoning) *after* the foods have been cooked! The cooking of condiments, even salt, *destroys* much of the vitamins of foods.

3/20/35
M. Adult
ASTHMA: COOKING UTENSILS 861-1

The vegetables that are taken should be preferably cooked in their *own* juices, as in Patapar paper. This will make a vast difference in the building of resistance.

6/16/44
F. 54 yrs.
DERMATITIS: ACIDITY 1158-38

Q. Should certain vegetables always be cooked in Patapar paper?

A. There are certain vegetables that, with the processes in Patapar paper, the mineral salts which are most active with the human body are preserved.

Q. Have I arthritis in right finger joint?

A. As indicated, there is neuritic rather than arthritic tendency. Thus the need for better eliminations to be established. That is why the altering in the mineral salts and vegetable laxatives is suggested.

5/1/38
F. Adult
ARTHRITIS 932-1

Evenings—The vegetables that are well cooked, and *only* in their *own* juices; preferably in Patapar paper—each cooked separate, *then* they may be combined as they are eaten if so desired, seasoned while hot with salt, pepper and butter.

Adhere to this.

6/6/38
COLD: CONGESTION **F. 41 yrs.**
TEMPERATURE: FEVER **459-9**

Have plenty of vegetables cooked in their OWN salts, preferably; rather than with meats or fats—and not in open water but in their own juices (as in Patapar paper).

11/23/37
M. 13 yrs.
PSORIASIS **1484-1**

Noons—Vegetables that are preferably of the leafy variety; or those that are of the bulbous nature, but these should be thoroughly cooked and ONLY in their OWN juices (as in Patapar paper).

4/2/27
F. 37 yrs.
TOXEMIA **121-1**

In the diet, then, there should be kept that that will give to the digestion and the assimilation, with the blood corrected and with the nerves acting in the correct vibration, that that will be assimilated and will produce *elimination* in its proper way and manner. Vegetables—especially those that grow above ground. Not those that grow below. Leaves of every nature. Pod vegetables that grow above the ground only, and as much green and as much raw as the body will assimilate. Taking *all* with PLENTY of water!

11/25/33
F. 26 yrs.
TEETH: GENERAL **457-3**

Q. Any specific suggestions regarding diet in relation to teeth?

A. See that there is the proper amount of iron and silicon, that comes from vegetables—not from minerals; they are minerals, but vegetable minerals for the body.

6/6/34
F. Adult
ANEMIA **574-1**

Q. In what minerals am I deficient?

A. Silicon and iron. These are best supplied through the vegetable forces, for these are more easily assimilated.

4/27/35
ASSIMILATIONS: ELIMINATIONS: INCOORDINATION **F. 39 yrs.**
NEURITIS **908-1**

Evenings—Vegetables that are cooked only in their *own* juices, each one separate—in their *own* juices. The salt that these are to be seasoned with should preferably be of the kelp nature.

12/10/37
ADHESIONS: CHILDBIRTH: AFTEREFFECTS **F. 37 yrs.**
ANEMIA: TENDENCIES **1498-1**

Noons—Preferably either green vegetables raw or soups or broths from vegetables, or meat stock; but not mixed. That is, do not have grease with the vegetables in the noon meal whether cooked or raw; though salad dressing may be taken but not with vinegar.

4/29/38
F. 77 yrs.
TOXEMIA **1586-1**

Do not cook vegetables with meats to season them; only use a little butter, with pepper or salt or such. And preferably use the sea salt entirely, or iodized salt—this is preferable.

9/15/35
F. 44 yrs.
TUMORS **683-3**

Let the general diet at other periods be body-building. Not meats, only fowl or fish along this line would be taken at all. Principally vegetables. And, as we find, these would eliminate and make for a building of a near normal body.

Q. Is this growth in my breast cancerous?

A. No. Tumorous.

Q. It can be eliminated without an operation?

A. It can be eliminated *without* an operation. As indicated, the activities of the glands through all portions of the system have made for segregations of those conditions that have acted as a throw off from a catarrhal condition which has existed—and settled in the mammary glands.

Then, the application of those things indicated will create activities in the blood supply, *with* the keeping of the eliminations, that the condition may be absorbed and thrown off from the system.

3/15/29
M. 40 yrs.
ACIDITY & ALKALINITY **5567-1**

Let the diet be those of the vegetables that create the more salts and the more alkaline forces in the system.

12/1/30
COLD: COMMON: SUSCEPTIBILITY: WORMS **M. Child**
WORMS **203-1**

Beware of sweets for some time. Preferably would be as this:

Evenings—A *vegetable* diet well balanced between those that grow above and below the ground.

8/15/38
M. 54 yrs.
KIDNEYS: STONES **843-7**

Q. Will a substance known as "Mineral Food" be of value for my condition?

A. Not necessarily. The food values from fresh vegetables that are prepared are better than all the combinations of those that are allowed to set or rest. While it is necessary for the vitamin activities through the system, these may be obtained by a better balance being kept in the vital forces as may be obtained from fresh vegetables than from concentrated forces such as those.

8/29/40
M. 27 yrs.
PSORIASIS: TENDENCIES **641-5**

Q. Please outline proper diet that can be followed, considering my being on the road traveling so much.

A. This has to be considered from the mind, and not from the diet; because it has been outlined as to WHAT things! Then, don't eat those that are not consistent with that! Have plenty of vegetables. To be sure, the trouble here is in their being prepared properly; but the correct vegetables are obtainable in most of the places where the eating is done—unless it's a hot dog stand or at a drug store or the like. But go to an eating place—being consistent—and you'll get something to eat!

2/18/35
ASSIMILATIONS: POOR **M. 29 yrs.**
GLANDS: INCOORDINATION **831-1**

Noons—Not *strained* vegetable juices, but rather the juices of vegetables *and* the vegetables cooked together; which would include preferably only the leafy vegetables. These may be combined or altered at times with only green *raw* vegetables.

11/7/38
M. 33 yrs.
ELIMINATIONS: POOR **1467-4**

Precautions should be taken that there is sufficient of the laxative foods, or plenty of such as fresh vegetables well-cooked, as a part of the diet; so as to make for plenty of iron as well as the activities for resistances through the system.

11/24/24
ANEMIA **F. Adult**
BLOOD-BUILDING **2221-1**

Take care that the system is supplied with those properties of iron and the food values that dilate the system in its course through the system. Vegetables. These carry the necessary properties.

12/6/43
COLD: CONGESTION: PELVIC DISORDERS **F. 15 yrs.**
BODY-BUILDING **2084-15**

Q. Any changes in her diet other than the vitamins?

A. No great changes in diet, except don't get too much fats for the body. Don't have too much starches. Vegetables and such foods are better for the body.

3/26/38
F. 47 yrs.
MEATLESS **1554-6**

Q. Is my vegetarian diet good for me, and should I stick to it?

A. Rather as has been indicated, this from the material angle is not an absolute necessity—but in all good conscience keep that as thy SOUL (we didn't say HEART)—thy SOUL—desires.

Vegetables are nature's way, the natural, the correct, the cleansing. Keep it, then; but these are as to the needs of the self depending upon the manner of expending energies. So long as there is the expending of self in mental, yes. When it becomes active in great physical exertion—as it will, in thy experience—then there will be the needs for some changes to be made.

5/20/27
M. 57 yrs.
MEATLESS: ELIMINATIONS: POOR **3727-1**

First, be careful of the diet. While the body has come to realize there are certain conditions and elements that the body absorbs or digests better than others, *do not* partake of meats! Rather the vegetable, and at least one raw vegetable each day. Broths or soups of meats may be taken occasionally, but not too much!

1/8/31
F. 24 yrs.
ACIDITY & ALKALINITY **4172-1**

In the matter of the diet—be mindful that the foods taken are those of the non-acid producing in the system. Beware, then, of meats to any great extent—and especially of those vegetables of the tuberous nature. Then, the leaves or those of the pod nature will be found the better for the body, as will be those of the citrus fruits or those that grow from the vine. Beware, though, of those that carry too much of the seed itself.

10/20/32
BRONCHITIS: ELIMINATIONS: POOR **F. Adult**
ELIMINATIONS **4293-1**

Be mindful of the diet, that there are less of the acid-producing foods than have been taken. This means to beware of too much starches, too much of the greater and heavier proteins, or proteins that carry a great amount of dross that is to be eliminated. The following would be an idea as to the character of diet:

Evenings—Well-cooked vegetables that grow *above* the ground; none that grow below the ground—none! Those that are of the activity as to make for tuberous forces and heavy starches (as all of these are) make for heaviness that is hard to eliminate.

3/23/35
ANEMIA: TENDENCIES **F. 47 yrs.**
BLOOD-BUILDING **865-1**

Q. Would you recommend any specific diet?

A. As given, we would keep an alkaline-reacting diet. The fresh vegetables, raw vegetables, are preferable to meats for the body needs the balancing throughout the system. The centralizing system must be kept ironized as related to the eliminations of the body.

6/26/39
F. 21 yrs.
ENVIRONMENT: HAY FEVER **1771-3**

Beware of sweets in the diet. Have vegetables preferably as the main portion of the diet. Not too much of these things that are of the starchy nature.

9/4/37
DEBILITATION: GENERAL **F. 60 yrs.**
ASSIMILATIONS: POOR **1409-5**

Q. What diet will be most beneficial?

A. That which will be assimilated, which necessitates that they be tried from time to time. Those that are of the vegetable nature and that are body-building without too much grease. No fried foods, and not too much grease. These become hard for the assimilating in the system.

4/2/36
BRAIN: CLOTS: TENDENCIES **F. 60 yrs.**
MALNUTRITION **1137-1**

Have a well-balanced cooked vegetable diet for the evening meal, using three vegetables grown above the ground to one grown below with lamb, fowl or fish.

2/18/23
M. 3 yrs.
CANCER **3751-6**

Let the diet be not of meats or too much sweets, but of vegetables—no tomatoes or any other fruits of the acid state. But vegetable matter of all character. Let it be changed entirely so that the body receives influence of all. Cooked well, but not with fats. Season well, but not with black pepper, but with salt and cayenne.

11/11/38
F. 13 yrs.
GLANDS: INCOORDINATION **1206-9**

Vegetables that are of the leafy nature are the more preferable to any dried foods or beans. The green vegetables are well, so long as they are not treated with any chemical for preserving of same or for the color of same.

2/16/43
F. 50 yrs.
COMBINATIONS: TOXEMIA **2881-2**

Noons—At least some portions of raw vegetables, and a soup or broth of such natures as not to carry too much fats, but the salts of cooked vegetables—though they may be seasoned with mutton, beef, fowl or the like, or they may include just the vegetables with rice, barley or the like.

Evenings—At least three meals during the week should include vegetables. Be mindful of combinations more than other things to produce disordered conditions; that is, do not take too much of the vegetables that grow under the ground in proportion to those that grow above the ground, however these may be prepared. Have two above to one below—in that ratio.

4/26/27
M. 41 yrs.
PLETHORA **39-1**

Q. What foods can be eaten and what foods should be avoided?

A. The body may under these conditions take those foods as have been found good for the body. As *we* would find here, there is necessary the change, as is seen, from time to time to meet the needs. Vegetables—especially those that grow above the ground. Tomatoes (potatoes may be taken in moderation), celery, lettuce, beans, lentils, and greens of every nature, see?

5/12/28
M. 33 yrs.
LIVER: KIDNEYS: INCOORDINATION 900-383

Q. Is the albumin on the decrease or increase in the urine?

A. On the decrease. Eat more of the vegetables as of lentils, beans, spinach, collards, kale or such.

2/17/31
F. 22 yrs.
OBESITY 2096-1

Of evenings, we would take fish, *cooked* vegetables; no potatoes of *any* character; no tuberous roots of any character, but any of the green vegetables *cooked,* or of the *dried* vegetables that grow above the ground—*cooked.* Little or no butters.

1/7/34
F. 21 yrs.
GLANDS: INCOORDINATION 480-3

Lunch—Rather green vegetables entirely. Among the vegetables may be included spinach, lettuce, celery, carrots, peas (half cooked, or as canned)—or beans that have been cooked may be added, or beets. Mayonnaise or oil dressings may be used.

7/17/43
F. 69 yrs.
ARTHRITIS 3138-1

Leafy vegetables rather than the bulbous variety; carrots, radishes, onions, celery, lettuce, should be a part of one meal each day.

10/29/43
ASTHMA F. 36 yrs.
ASTHMA: ELIMINATIONS 3331-1

Do include leafy vegetables such as red cabbage, spinach, all forms of leafy greens—as mustard, lamb's tongue, as dock.

8/31/41
ARTHRITIS: PREVENTIVE F. 51 yrs.
BODY: GENERAL 1158-31

Q. What is best source of nicotinic acid?

A. Of course, the greater source is from smoke. But in vegetables—carrots, squash, pumpkin, and especially in what is called the oyster plant (salsify).

12/10/37
ADHESIONS: CHILDBIRTH: AFTEREFFECTS F. 37 yrs.
ANEMIA: TENDENCIES 1498-1

Noons—Preferably either green vegetables raw or soups or broths from vegetables, or meat stock; but not mixed. That is, do not have grease with the vegetables in the noon meal . . . whether cooked or raw; though salad dressing may be taken but not with vinegar.

5/7/30
M. 22 yrs.
EPILEPSY **1001-1**

In the evenings—These should be of the vegetable, with little of the meats. These well cooked first, with small quantity of some liquid or soup—but never use for the body those of the *canned,* unless they are those that are free of the benzoate character of a preservative. Do not use those!

8/27/32
F. 72 yrs.
CIRRHOSIS OF LIVER **2092-1**

Noons—Green vegetables. These will be well. The green vegetables would include lettuce, celery, tomatoes, spinach and water cress, or the like. These would be well seasoned with olive oil or tapioca or paprika, that there may be the proper toning of the digestive system for those cleansings that would take place to make for resuscitation in the system.

2/16/35
M. 45 yrs.
ACIDITY **829-1**

Evenings—If that is when the dinner is taken—principally this meal should consist of three leafy vegetables to one vegetable that grows under the ground, or two of the pod vegetables to one that grows under the ground. They would be combined such as spinach, lettuce, celery, raw white cabbage, red cooked cabbage, beans, lentils—these preferably of the green variety, but when they are dried (beans, etc.) only use two of these to one of any that grow under the ground; carrots, salsify and these natures, with the potatoes, but not so much of the pulp of the potato—rather eat the jackets of same. These would be preferable.

5/3/32
F. 49 yrs.
TOXEMIA **5647-1**

In the evening, then, there would rather be more of the vegetable with a little of the meats, *but do not eat heavy meals!* Rather eat four times a day than three times a day, see? Eat a small quantity.

1)—Canned Vegetables

1/27/40
F. 11 yrs.
KIDNEYS: INFECTIONS **2084-1**

Do not eat quantities EVER of meats. Fish, fowl—these occasionally, but preferably have the diet depend a great deal upon vegetables of all characters. Of course, all green vegetables early of spring, but not so much of dried vegetables—rather the fresher variety. However, those that are canned without benzoate of soda as a preservative may be taken through such seasons or periods when these are not obtainable fresh. As to the brand of vegetables canned that carries the least benzoate of soda—those that carry same are marked. As we find, though, Libby's is an excellent brand.

12/29/41
M. 40 yrs.
ASSIMILATIONS: POOR **826-14**

The vegetables should not be those that have been frozen but those that are preserved either in their own syrup or in the regular cane syrup and NOT those prepared with benzoate or any preservative—for the benzoate becomes hard upon the system.

2)—Frozen Vegetables

1/6/42
M. 57 yrs.
GENERAL **462-14**

Q. Considering the frozen foods, especially vegetables that are on the market today—has the freezing in any way killed certain vitamins and how do they compare with the fresh?

A. This would necessitate making a special list. For some are affected more than others. Much of the vitamin content of these is taken, unless there is the reinforcement in same when these are either prepared for food or when frozen.

3)—Green Vegetables

11/13/23
BLOOD: OXIDATION **F. Adult**
ASTHMA **4810-2**

Much of the condition in the bronchials and lungs is produced by the diet the body takes. Hence we have through the pneumogastric, with the cardiac expression to the lungs in the circulation, as is carried through the arterial forces from the lungs, becomes overcharged by the pressure produced down the canal itself in the end of the stomach proper, see? The cardiac end. This produces much of the distress to the body. No sweets should be taken for this reason, no meats of the nature of pork or of hog flesh, see? Rather that of the green vegetables carrying more acids that will become the form of alcohol in the digestive forces to carry out in the system that of vital forces necessary in the blood to meet the conditions in the system.

4/30/31
F. Adult
ELIMINATIONS: POOR **4178-1**

Noons—Preferably green vegetables combined in a salad, which may be followed with broths of any character just so they do not have too many condiments in same.

4/13/35
F. 36 yrs.
BLOOD-BUILDING **890-1**

In the matter of the diet, well that this be that which would supply a sufficient quantity of those vitamins necessary for increased blood and nerve energies for the system; and should naturally be of the alkaline type. That is, green vegetables.

7/1/26
F. 37 yrs.

BLOOD-BUILDING **5739-1**

The diet should be kept in accord with the rebuilding of a cleansed blood system. Not overamount of meats. Fowl or fish may be taken in small quantities. As much green vegetable food as can be well taken by the body. Never take too much acid with any of them. Little or no vinegar, then, with any of the foods.

2/18/25
F. 33 yrs.

ANEMIA **2457-1**

Then, the diet should be the principal care and attention of the body, for the condition depends upon that food value given the body and that which will be assimilated in the system. Hence giving the greater resistive force. The body should be more regular with the food taken, and taking the green vegetable as much as possible.

7/25/39
M. 24 yrs.

CANCER **1967-1**

Do not eat meats of any great quantity. Mostly use the leafy vegetables as the diet.

5/4/44
F. 31 yrs.

ARTHRITIS **5034-1**

Leave off any stimulants such as seasonings of any kind, except cayenne pepper. Use this in the preparation of leafy vegetables.

12/17/38
M. 45 yrs.

TUBERCULOSIS **1564-3**

Use all those influences which carry a great deal of the sunshine vitamins, as much as the body assimilates. But whenever there is any food taken that becomes a reactionary influence, ease off in the use of such foods.

Beware of any fried foods. Leafy vegetables—those that carry a great deal of the vital forces as are active by the sunshine are well.

Do not use ANY vegetables, however, that have been colored by the use of ANY coloring matter for their preservation or for their color.

10/11/37

DIABETES: TENDENCIES **M. 67 yrs.**
ACIDITY **1454-1**

Hence we would have the stimulating foods such as leafy vegetables—these in their combinations.

4)—Root & Tuberous Vegetables

4/26/27
M. 41 yrs.
PLETHORA **39-1**

Q. What foods can be eaten and what foods should be avoided?

A. The body may under these conditions take those foods as have been found good for the body. As *we* would find here, there is necessary the change, as is seen, from time to time to meet the needs. Vegetables—especially those that grow above the ground. Those of the tuberous nature avoid, unless these conditions are corrected, for tuberous vegetables, with a plethora condition, not good, though they may be taken in moderation. But make these corrections—then eat anything!

11/5/42
ASSIMILATIONS: ELIMINATIONS **M. 36 yrs.**
LIVER: KIDNEYS: INCOORDINATION **416-17**

Do have those properties such as rutabaga, turnips, artichoke in the diet some time during each week. These are combinations that will tend to purify such conditions.

11/29/37
M. 42 yrs.
GENERAL: RHEUMATISM **1334-2**

Hence we will find for this particular body that ALL the vegetable forces almost that may be considered which grow UNDER the ground would be the more beneficial; those of all the tuberous natures, but prepared in such ways and manners that the very activities or vibratory forces from same in the assimilations become as portions of the body. Hence prepare these preferably in their OWN juices, their own salts being retained that they may become a portion of the bodily forces themselves (as when prepared in Patapar paper).

Hence the assimilation of the activities from all forms of such vegetables would become portions of the diet for the body whether it be the artichoke or the turnip or the radish (which would be taken raw, and not all of these cooked necessarily), or the potato, or the oyster plant, or those that carry more of such influences.

Not that the leafy vegetables are to be left out entirely; but these would preferably be taken raw.

2/19/38
ASTHENIA: ANEMIA **M. 60 yrs.**
ASSIMILATIONS: ELIMINATIONS: INCOORDINATION **1539-1**

Hence those things that grow UNDER THE GROUND should supersede or be more abundant in the diet than those that grow as leafy or pod vegetables. This is because of the vibratory influence needed, that comes from the tuberous vegetables and their influence as from the earth itself.

11/1/30
F. 21 yrs.
EPILEPSY **543-4**

Potatoes, turnips, beets, and such should be taken from the diet.

3/31/43
ASSIMILATIONS: ELIMINATIONS: INCOORDINATION F. 18 yrs.
BODY-BUILDING 2947-1

Beets and beet tops should be included in the diet; radishes and the yellow yams should be included.

6/11/43
M. 36 yrs.
ASSIMILATIONS: POOR 3047-1

The foods that are of the nature of leafy vegetables, both raw and cooked, are preferable to those of the tuberous nature; though carrots—both raw and cooked—are well. Potatoes should be very sparse, not more than once or twice a week.

5)—Yellow Vegetables

7/10/42
CHILD TRAINING M. 9 yrs.
INJURIES: BIRTH: AFTEREFFECTS 2780-1

Q. Are there any suggestions as to diet?

A. Get him to eat whatever you can, but keep plenty of vitamin B; that is, not in concentrated form as in tablet or capsule, but in the foods—that is, plenty of every sort of yellow vegetable.

7/18/41
F. 77 yrs.
DEBILITATION: GENERAL 2538-1

Give all the foods that are rich in the vitamin B-1, with iron, with all the forms of nerve-building energies and blood-coagulative properties. These as we find will be found principally in vegetables that are yellow in color. All such should be taken in extra quantity.

8/31/41
ARTHRITIS: PREVENTIVE F. 51 yrs.
BODY: GENERAL 1158-31

Q. What foods are best source of vitamin B?

A. And B-1. All of those that are of the yellow variety, in vegetables. Also in many of those are the acids that go with same.

Q. How often should these foods be used weekly?

A. Have rather regular days or periods in which these foods are taken, or take some portion of them every day. This is a vitamin that is not stored as is A, D, C or G, but needs to be supplied each day.

7/18/41
F. 77 yrs.
DEBILITATION: GENERAL 2538-1

Give vitamin B-1 in pellet or capsule form, under the direction of physician—NOT by injection.

Give all the foods that are rich in the vitamin B-1, with iron, with all the forms of nerve-building energies and blood-coagulative properties. These are we find will be found principally in fruits and vegetables that are yellow in color. All such should be taken in extra quantity.

7/6/41
F. 46 yrs.
ADHESIONS: LESIONS **2529-1**

In the matter of the diet throughout the periods—we would constantly add more and more of vitamin B-1, in every form in which it may be taken; in the types of vegetables that may be prepared for the body. Be sure that there is sufficient each day for the adding of the vital energies. These vitamins are not stored in the body as are A, D, and G, but it is necessary to add these daily. All of those vegetables, then, that are yellow in color should be taken; yellow squash, yellow corn, all of these and such as these; beets—but all of the vegetables cooked in their OWN juices, and the body eating the juices with same.

2)—Raw Vegetables: General

3/23/35
ANEMIA: TENDENCIES **F. 47 yrs.**
BLOOD-BUILDING **865-1**

Q. Would you recommend any specific diet?

A. As given, we would keep an alkaline-reacting diet. The fresh vegetables, raw vegetables, are preferable to meats for the body needs the balancing throughout the system. The centralizing system being kept ironized as related to the eliminations of the body.

11/8/35
ANEMIA **F. Adult**
ASSIMILATIONS: ELIMINATIONS: INCOORDINATION **1051-1**

Throughout the period be very mindful of the diets, that these are kept *tending* toward the alkaline-reaction; but of sufficient body and blood building—that may be found through the food values that carry not only the vitamin E but those also of A and B. Or those forces that make for creating of the effluvium that is *productive* in its activity with the glands of the system (the E). Or those activities in the A that would make for an aid in the *draining,* as it were, or the eliminations as related to the activity of all *structural* portions of the body

Hence one meal each day we would have raw vegetables.

6/14/44
GLANDS: INCOORDINATION **F. 15 yrs.**
VITAMINS **1179-11**

Q. Should the body continue taking Vitamin Plus?

A. The Vitamin Plus is well in or through the seasons when the body is indoors much, but when the body is able to be in the open, as in the present and then exercise is taken, that is preferable. Then take the vitamins in the general diet for the body. Keep these well balanced with plenty of raw vegetables.

5/2/44
M. 33 yrs.
PARKINSON'S DISEASE **3491-2**

Q. Please suggest foods to stress and foods to avoid in the diet.

A. Do stress B-1 and E. Do leave off too much starches. Have plenty of raw vegetables.

11/7/38
M. 33 yrs.

ELIMINATIONS: POOR **1467-4**

Precautions should be taken that there is sufficient of the laxative foods, or plenty of such as raw vegetables, as a part of the diet; so as to make for plenty of iron as well as the activities for resistances through the system.

6/12/39
F. 40 yrs.

ANEMIA **1387-2**

In the matter of the diets—these have been very well balanced—but occasionally, especially in the early fall, include plenty of raw vegetables. Let one meal each day consist principally of raw fresh vegetables—not that this should consist entirely of such, but the principal portion of same. These will tend to aid in purifying as well as creating, through the activity of the assimilating forces, the vital energies to resist the tendency or inclination for inflammatory forces through the system—especially if the subluxations are removed in the osteopathic manner as we have indicated.

2/22/44
F. 46 yrs.

ACIDITY **1713-23**

Q. Are raw vegetables harmful to me?

A. Certain vegetables are all right. Prepare them oft with gelatin or various types of salad dressings that are not acid-producing, and we will find these will be well. Grate, slice and prepare them in varied manners.

12/31/34
F. 49 yrs.

MENOPAUSE **601-6**

We would be mindful that there is a lack of accumulations of acids, and not too much of fats taken in the system—or starches. This will prevent those tendencies for the system to take on weight at this time.

Let it be rather as one meal, at least, each day consisting entirely of raw vegetables, see?

4/16/42
M. 43 yrs.

COMBINATIONS: ELIMINATIONS: INCOORDINATION **2732-1**

Have plenty of vegetables, and especially one meal each day should include some raw or uncooked vegetables. But here, too, combinations must be kept in line. Do not take onions and radishes at the same meal with celery and lettuce, though either of these may be taken at different times, see?

4/24/34
M. 43 yrs.

ACIDITY: ALKALINITY: ANEMIA **642-1**

At least one meal each day should consist of only fresh green vegetables; not cooked, but all raw. This is for creating a balance. At first it will tend to appear to create gas, but keep on using.

11/13/37
F. 57 yrs.
ELIMINATIONS 1472-2

Have a portion of one meal each day to consist of raw vegetables; not the whole meal but a portion of same, combining in such a salad as many of the fresh raw vegetables as may be had that are PURIFYING to the bloodstream yet that will agree with the system. Some of these will be found to at times disagree; then leave these off until there has been a better readjustment through the activities of these influences upon the body-forces.

8/27/35
F. 61 yrs.
ARTHRITIS 983-1

Keep to those things that are body and blood building. But let *one* meal each day, whether noon or evening, be only of fresh green, raw vegetables; any or all of these combined. An oil or salad dressing may be used, just as preferable to the body. Keep rather an alkaline diet, adhering to the one raw vegetable meal each day.

2/11/37
CIRCULATION: POOR F. 40 yrs.
ACIDITY & ALKALINITY 1337-1

One meal each day should have at least a green, raw vegetable. Raw vegetables may be combined and used as a whole meal, or a quantity of one raw vegetable used at a meal; but the raw vegetables at least once during a day combined with some meal, whether noon or at the evening meal.

10/23/36
BLOOD: HUMOR F. 35 yrs.
OBESITY 1276-1

No fried foods at all. There should be at least one meal a day of only raw fresh vegetables, whether in the middle of the day or whether in the evening; preferably in the noonday time would this meal be taken.

12/12/38
F. 51 yrs.
INTESTINES: GAS 1703-2

Q. Since I get gas, seemingly, from cooked foods, would I do well to eat more and more raw and less cooked?

A. As we find, it is the matter of the BALANCE in same, rather than the cooked foods. For NATURAL sources should indicate to the body that raw foods, unless there is a great deal of physical exertion, are inclined to make gas more than cooked foods—if the cooked foods are properly balanced.

6/16/34
M. 44 yrs.
INJURIES: ACCIDENTS: AFTEREFFECTS 478-3

Keep those things that are the more easily assimilated by the body; that is, not merely the liquid diet or of such nature but that which carries with same the iron, the silicon, the blood- and nerve-building influences. And let at least one meal each day, whether the noon or the evening meal, be entirely of green fresh *raw* vegetables; such as any that are cleansing for the blood supply and act with the gastric juices of the stomach to make for better assimilation through the activity of the pancreas, as well as the lacteal ducts and those ducts that make for an activity in the kidney and the areas throughout the hepatic circulation.

5/4/41
BURSITIS: TENDENCIES **M. 52 yrs**
KATABOLISM: METABOLISM: INCOORDINATION **1151-28**

If there is the desire for the greater vitamin energies, those mostly needed for the body, as we find, or that are the more deficient, are the E and B-2; which may be obtained most through the raw vegetables.

7/6/38
F. 48 yrs.
MENOPAUSE **1158-18**

Q. It is difficult for me to arrange one daily meal of salad only; therefore, might I supplement my diet by tablets recommended by Dr.———?

A. These may be taken if there is a lack of those activities from the raw salad; but they do not, WILL not, supply the energies as well or as efficaciously for the BODY as if there were the efforts made to have at least one meal each day altogether of raw vegetables, or two meals carrying a raw salad as a portion of same—each day.

3/4/35
F. Adult
KATABOLISM: METABOLISM **844-1**

Noons—Preferably (if this is taken as the lunch) *only* raw vegetables; such as lettuce, tomatoes, celery, peppers, beet tops, beets, spinach, onions, radish, carrots—any of these, that may be grated well. But one meal each day, at least, should be of *only* RAW vegetables, and this doesn't mean raw apples, either!

5/23/43
F. 42 yrs.
ARTHRITIS **3014-1**

Do use raw vegetables where they are not too much roughage. Take often such as celery; lettuce, tomatoes and such; also carrots and beets and beet tops.

7/18/42
ASSIMILATIONS: ELIMINATIONS: INCOORDINATION **F. 2-1/2 yrs.**
ELIMINATIONS: POOR **1521-6**

Rest, and do not overload the body: especially not upon raw vegetables, but rather using the easily assimilated or pre-digested foods—until there is a thorough stirring of the liver, and then allowing time for a coordination between lungs liver, heart and kidneys, through the stimulations given.

11/30/42
F. 3 yrs.
PINWORMS **2015-10**

Q. How did the trouble of pinworms originate, or what caused it?

A. Milk! You see, in every individual there is within intestinal tract that matter which produces a form of intestinal worm. This is in everyone. But with a particular diet where the milk has any bacillus, it will gradually cause these to increase, and they oftentimes develop or multiply rapidly; and then they may disappear, IF there is taken raw, green food.

A. Would you change the kind of milk she drinks?

A. It isn't so much the change in the kind of milk that is needed. Either add the raw, green foods as indicated, or give those properties as would eliminate the sources of same. But it is better, if it is practical, to induce the body to eat lettuce and celery and carrots—even a small amount. One leaf of lettuce will destroy a thousand worms.

5/21/42
CONCEPTION **F. 34 yrs.**
COOKING UTENSILS: PATAPAR PAPER **457-9**

Q. Do raw foods carry more of the calcium; such as lettuce, cabbage, carrots and cauliflower? Does cooking destroy the calcium in foods?

A. To be sure. At times, but if the cooking is done in Patapar paper, so that all the juices are saved with same, then these are just as well—and, as indicated—at times more preferable, for they are more easily assimilated, and especially so during pregnancy.

4/29/38
F. 77 yrs.
TOXEMIA **1586-1**

In the matter of the diets, these as we find would become rather specific.

Noons—ONLY raw vegetables. These may be combined in many varied ways. Celery, lettuce, tomatoes, radish, peppers, cabbage, spinach, mustard, leeks, onions. Any or all of these may be combined. These may be taken with an oil or salad dressing, but not that which has very much of any vinegar or acetic acid in same.

7/30/40
F. Adult
OBESITY **2315-1**

Each meal should be preceded by the grape juice—thirty minutes before eating.

Noons—Either cooked vegetable juices as in soups or the like, or an altogether raw salad consisting of such as celery, lettuce, tomatoes, carrots and the like. All of these when taken raw should be grated, or a little of one or the other may be taken with the raw juices from one or the other of these vegetables indicated—the juice extracted by use of a juicer, see?

12/9/39
ASSIMILATIONS: ELIMINATIONS: INCOORDINATION **F. 52 yrs.**
CIRCULATION: IMPAIRED **2057-1**

Eat plenty of well-cooked vegetables. And let one meal each day consist principally of raw, fresh vegetables. Many of these may be combined and used with or without dressing, to suit the taste of the body; as lettuce, spinach, celery, tomatoes and the like. Let such a raw salad form the basis of at least one meal each day.

Do these, and we will find we will bring better conditions for the body.

Because meats or other foods were not mentioned does not mean that these should not be taken at all, but do not make a meal upon same; take these rather sparingly. Let the greater portion of the diet consist of those things indicated.

1/26/35
F. 59 yrs.
INJURIES **3823-2**

Noons—Whole green vegetables are more preferable to heavier foods, especially at noontime; and these should be taken raw, in the form of a salad such as celery, lettuce, onions, leeks, tomatoes, peppers, radish, carrots and the like—raw cabbage, especially the sprouts or the like. An oil or salad dressing may be used that will make it more palatable for the body; and this should be with calcium—rather sodium chloride, that is iodized and more preferable for the calciumizing or working with the conditions necessary for recuperative forces of the body. During those periods when there is little of the activity, so that there are not the normal eliminations, well that the vegetables that are the more laxative in form be used.

6/29/42
F. 25 yrs.
ANEMIA **2376-2**

Do have one meal each day consisting principally of raw vegetables; not all of the meal, but the greater portion, while the other part should he preferably soups, stews or the like. Include all of the vegetables that may be eaten raw—tomatoes, carrots, lettuce, celery, mustard, onions, radishes—all of such use; peppers and the like. Not necessarily all at once, to be sure, but some of these, or their combinations. Each day have one meal when these form the principal part. The rest may be the vegetable soups or the condensed soups, or tomato or cream of tomato, or any of those kinds.

6/7/44
M. 34 yrs.
ARTHRITIS: RHEUMATOID **5169-1**

A great deal of raw vegetables as cabbage, lettuce, celery, carrots, all forms of water cress. Leafy vegetables are preferable to the pod or tuberous variety.

1/11/37
ELIMINATIONS: POOR **M. 61 yrs.**
ACIDITY & ALKALINITY: GENERAL **1217-2**

For this body, eat more vegetables grown above the ground than those below the ground. Each day, though, have at least two or three raw vegetables; whether celery, lettuce, tomatoes, carrots, turnips, or any of these. These may be grated together and combined with a salad dressing that is of an olive oil base.

12/29/43
ALLERGIES: METALS: ECZEMA **M. 32 yrs.**
DERMATITIS **3422-1**

In the diet refrain from any meats other than fish or fowl, for at least ten days. Do include in the diet during those periods a great deal of raw vegetables, especially water cress, celery, lettuce, carrots, onions and the like.

6/24/38
ARTHRITIS: TENDENCIES **F. 68 yrs.**
TOXEMIA **1622-1**

Noons—or one meal each day—should consist only of raw vegetables. This may be done at the noon meal or the evening meal, as suits the convenience or the better taste of the body itself. These vegetables may be combined. It is preferable that they be grated or ground together and—though cleansed—the peels should be with each of the vegetables used; whether carrots, onions, lettuce, celery, thyme, or whatever character of vegetables used. Use the tops of radishes, when these are combined, as well as the radish itself. With such a salad there may be used salad dressing, preferably, rather than oil; though oil may be taken occasionally if desired by the body.

5/1/36
ANEMIA: TENDENCIES **F. 46 yrs.**
CIRCULATION: INCOORDINATION **1158-1**

Q. Should I take Dermetic's Vegetable Tablets?

A. Not necessary with one meal of raw fresh vegetables. For, although compounds are well, these in their natural state are better. Lettuce, celery, onions, tomatoes, peppers, carrots, spinach, mustard—any of these are much preferable *green,* fresh, than prepared in a preservative of any kind.

2/21/34
M. 20 yrs.
EPILEPSY **521-1**

Noons—Preferably fresh vegetables, as carrots, lettuce, celery, leeks, onions and the like.

At this meal there may also be had oils, as olive oil or the dressings that make such a meal more palatable.

3/16/44
ASSIMILATIONS: POOR **F. 31 yrs.**
MINERALS: CALCIUM **3696-1**

It will be necessary to supply more calcium either in foods or in supplementary ways.

In the supplying of elements for the body increase the amounts of raw foods or vegetables. These should include every character of raw vegetables that may be prepared, either with gelatin or in salads at times.

4/26/35
F. 53 yrs.
GLANDS: INCOORDINATION **906-1**

Be mindful that there is at least *one* meal each day taken of *raw* green vegetables; this doesn't mean green in color only but those that are raw and fresh, not stale vegetables. These may include such as lettuce, celery, tomatoes, carrots (these all raw), pepper, onions, radish; which may be mixed or may be taken any one or two or three of these. A dressing or mayonnaise may be used; but these should be well ground or mixed together or shredded; and may be taken at the noon meal or in the morning or in the evening.

6/12/34
CANCER: TENDENCIES **F. 42 yrs.**
TUMORS **583-8**

As to the diet, there should not be too great quantities of meats at any time; rather the vegetable, fruit, citrus fruit and nut diet—these would be the better for the body. Have at least one meal each day wholly of green vegetables; that is, *fresh*—not green in color necessarily, but green, fresh, *raw* vegetables; combining such as lettuce, celery, carrots, cabbage (both the green and red), tomatoes, peppers, and the like. These may be taken with mayonnaise.

6/14/35
M. Adult
GLANDS: INCOORDINATION **935-1**

Noons—Principally (very seldom altering from these) raw vegetables made into a salad. Use such vegetables as cabbage (the white, of course, cut very fine), carrots, lettuce, spinach, celery, onions, tomatoes, radish; any or all of these. It is more preferable that they all be grated, but when grated do not allow the juices in the grating to be discarded; these should be used upon the salad itself. Preferably use the *oil* dressings; as olive oil with paprika, or such combinations.

5/5/44
F. 40 yrs.
TUBERCULOSIS **5053-1**

Vegetables are very well, especially those that may be eaten raw. Prepare the raw vegetables with gelatin often. This may be used with salad dressing, if this is desirable, or with salad oils.

12/15/27
M. 30 yrs.
ASTHENIA **4605-1**

As for the diet, let that be principally of that as almost pre-digested foods—though as much of raw vegetables as may be well taken, carrying plenty of iron and of salts; such as carrots, celery, lettuce.

3—Vegetables—Various

1)—Artichokes

3/17/38
CANCER **F. 52 yrs.**
GENERAL **601-29**

Q. What other artichokes are there besides Jerusalem and Green California?

A. The Jerusalem, the Green California and the Tubular. Only the Jerusalem variety AND the bulb or the Green are to be eaten by THIS body, but NOT very often.

6/12/39
F. 40 yrs.
ANEMIA **1387-2**

Occasionally, especially in the early fall, include all characters of artichoke.

7/23/40
F. 37 yrs.
ACIDITY **2310-1**

Also use artichoke, both the bulbous (or the Jerusalem) and the leaf-eating character. This taken at least once or twice a week will clarify the glandular forces of the system, equalizing that pressure, and aiding the activity of the pancreas, the spleen, with the general circulation.

4/28/43
CIRCULATION: INCOORDINATION **F. 36 yrs.**
ELIMINATIONS: POOR **2977-1**

DO take artichokes in ALL their forms, for this will aid in keeping a better balance in those tendencies for disturbances of circulation between the pancreas and the liver, as well as the kidneys. These should to taken raw at times, and cooked at times, when the Jerusalem artichoke is taken. Vary these. When the French or the bulb character of artichoke is used, have plenty of butter with same. But these are good for the body.

6/1/39
F. 52 yrs.
GLANDS **1904-1**

Especially we would have in the diet all forms of artichoke—the American, the bulbular, as well as occasionally the Jerualem artichoke. Not so often either of these, but about once or twice a week.

4/1/43
POLIOMYELITIS **F. 11 yrs.**
KIDNEYS: BODY-BUILDING **2948-1**

Do have at least once a week, some form of the vegetable known as artichoke, that is an active principle in producing the energies for eliminating through the kidneys. Whether this is the Jerusalem artichoke or the French or the bud these should be taken at least once each week. Alternate these for the body.

12/9/36
ARTHRITIS: TENDENCIES **F. 63 yrs.**
BODY-BUILDING **1302-1**

In the matter of the diets: Here we need body-building foods but those that tend to be more alkaline-producing than acid. For the natural inclinations of disturbed conditions in a body are to produce acidity through the bloodstream. Hence we need to revivify same by the use of much of those that produce more of the enzymes, more of the hormones for the blood supply; yet not overburdening the body with those unless the balance in the vitamin forces is carried.

Hence as we will find, not heavy foods or fried foods ever, nor combinations where there are quantities of starches or quantities of starches with sweets taken at the same time. But fish, fowl or lamb preferably as the meats.

The leafy vegetables preferably to the tuberous, though certain tuberous ones are necessary—as the artichoke, both as to the bulb and the root, for the very effect of the phosphorus for the system

2/27/42
F. 52 yrs.
COLD: CONGESTION **404-10**

Q. What vegetables are especially good for my body, considering the condition of kidneys?

A. Artichoke—these cooked.

i)—Jerusalem Artichokes

7/27/39
DEBILITATION: GENERAL **F. 27 yrs.**
DIABETES: TENDENCIES **480-52**

Keep a general upbuilding in the diet, by the body-building influences. Occasionally have the artichoke, to keep down those inclinations for the lack of the proper activity in the pancreas.

These as we find should bring much better results and experiences for the body.

12/17/40
F. 45 yrs.
PRURITIS **1100-30**

Q. Is the Bragg dehydrated artichoke all right for [470] to use, instead of the fresh artichoke?

A. Not as efficacious or efficient in its activity in the system as the fresh. For, dehydration—especially of artichoke—is to lose not only the vital forces of its activity upon the system, but to produce an effect in the functioning of the system such that it requires a continued usage of same, or it becomes something upon which the body is dependent, rather than attuning the functioning of the organs—as the liver, pancreas and spleen—to the needs, or to the ability to produce—through the activity of the glands through these—that necessary for keeping a balance in the body.

Use the fresh, rather than the dehydrated.

12/2/37
F. 5 yrs.
DIABETES **1490-1**

The oyster plant, the Jerusalem artichoke occasionally—once a week sufficient for this; this adds adrenalin and is that which will keep down accumulations and prepare the activity of the glands—especially the spleen, the liver, the pancreas—and work well with the balancing of the sugar content for the system.

3/4/40
F. 53 yrs.
GLANDS: ADRENALS: BODY-BUILDING **2025-3**

Q. What can I do to get rid of gas in my stomach, which often keeps me from eating, and occasionally causes vomiting?

A. The artichoke will aid in this especially.

4/8/40
F. 58 yrs.
ANEMIA **2164-1**

At least once a week (but not more than that) we would add the Jerusalem artichoke in the diet. This preferably for this body would be taken raw; one not larger than a guinea egg or the like, and taken WITH the regular meal.

4/23/43
M. 4 yrs.
ACIDITY: KIDNEYS: INCOORDINATION **2542-3**

Q. What can be done to help control the kidneys?

A. We would give the body occasionally, say once a week, the Jerusalem artichoke.

2/18/39
CHILD TRAINING **F. 10 yrs.**
ASSIMILATIONS **1179-5**

And at LONG intervals, say once every ten days, give the body a small raw artichoke (Jerusalem artichoke). This will tend to make for a better coordination in the activities of the pancreas as related to the kidneys and pelvic organs; that produce an irritation upon the nervous system.

We will BEST see the indications of the EFFECT of this—particularly—in the eradicating of the tendencies for the little dark circles that come occasionally under the eyes.

6/24/43
M. 68 yrs.
PARALYSIS **3056-1**

These, of course, are not all that should be taken, but these should be a part of the diet from day to day; not every day, but sufficient that these carry their influences in the body.

Occasionally the Jerusalem artichoke, cooked only in its OWN juices, or in Patapar paper, should be eaten. The effect of the insulin in this is needed in the system, in the activity created in the pancreas and its effect upon the liver and the kidneys as the poisons are eliminated by the activity of the glandular forces producing those influences to be eliminated.

4/2/39
F. 38 yrs.
CHOLECYSTITIS **1857-1**

Once a week have artichoke, the Jerusalem type, as this will aid in cleansing, easing the activity of the kidneys with the disturbance that has been with the circulation, and with the liver disturbance. This will also purify the activity through the bladder, aiding in the relief of those tensions when the acidity causes disturbance through portions of the system.

3/21/39
M. 9 yrs.
DIABETES: TENDENCIES **415-7**

Q. What is cause and cure for overactivity of kidneys and bladder?

A. Too much sugar. The inclinations as indicated from the character of foods. This would indicate that it would be well, at least twice a week, that there be the artichoke—either raw or cooked as would be a potato, but preferably cooked in Patapar paper.

Also this arises from some of those disturbances in the cerebrospinal system that should be corrected by the adjustments.

Q. What is the cause of the body having an aversion to all foods except starches?

A. Because it has been unbalanced in such a way and manner as to cause the activities to become such that there is the desire or inclination in this direction. And these very things then tend to make for greater distresses. And unless there are corrections, it may bring on a greater disturbance in the diabetic tendency.

12/20/37
M. 46 yrs.
ELIMINATIONS: INCOORDINATION **1502-1**

We would add to the diet the Jerusalem artichoke. This should be taken at least for one meal each week, or at one meal each week. Preferably take same cooked as potatoes; not cooked too much but sufficiently that they may retain all of the active principles. Hence we would cook them in their OWN juices, or in Patapar paper. This is to add that stimulation necessary for the activity of the pancreas and the flow of these through the activity to the reduction of those tendencies for the inflammatory conditions to the kidneys and the bladder, and the activity of the lower hepatic circulation.

Beware of too much of fats of any nature.

10/12/38
M. 61 yrs.
LIVER: KIDNEYS **1708-1**

If these additions indicated here DO NOT make for a distributing of the energies to the system in such a way as to eliminate the necessity for an operative method, they would at least segregate and build up the system so that the operative forces would not be as severe as if they were undertaken in the present condition of the blood supply and the general system itself.

Then, as we find:

We would keep very well towards the diet which has been indicated. However, one specific change we would make; that there be added at least once a week the Jerusalem artichoke. This would be most beneficial, from the very activity of the properties in this as related to sugar, and as related to the activities of the pancreas and kidneys. This may be taken either raw or cooked, one way at one time and the other the next. When cooked, however, it would be boiled in its OWN juices—that is, in Patapar paper; and would not be boiled so *much* that it becomes hard or stringy, but just so it may be taken and well assimilated if it is eaten right. Use one about the size of an egg or a little larger.

12/27/41
F. 19 yrs.
PREGNANCY **711-4**

Do also supply the insulin needed for supplying activities for the glandular force as related to the activity between the liver and the kidneys. Besides in the other foods, this should be supplied by the use of a Jerusalem artichoke once each week, with the meal—say Wednesdays; one about the size of a hen egg. Cook this in Patapar paper. Put it in with the water cold, and after it has begun to boil, let it boil at least twenty-five minutes. When taken from the hull, prepare the artichoke with the juices in same, seasoning with a little butter, salt and pepper if desired, to make it palatable.

DIABETES: TENDENCIES **1/10/41**
MALARIA: TENDENCIES **F. 60 yrs.**
ELIMINATIONS: INCOORDINATION **1963-2**

Q. Is the body diabetic?

A. A tendency.

We find that these conditions exist: There is too much sugar in the activities of the kidneys. There is a torpidity in the activity of the liver. There is a slowing of the circulation to the head and to the heart AND the general chest.

This, to be sure, with the slowing activity, tends to leave a toxic condition; not that may be termed of a malarial-producing nature, but would eventually cause a strep formation in the blood, with the conditions which exist in the blood flow itself, and the excess tendency of activity of kidneys.

Q. What can he do to protect himself against it?

A. As indicated, the diet—and exercise of specific characters that tend to tone up and to create a balance.

And twice each week take the Jerusalem artichoke, about the size of a hen egg; first raw—say on Tuesdays—and the next time cooked, say on Thursdays, but cooked in its own juices (as in Patapar paper). Only eat one each time, you see. When cooked, season it to make it palatable, but do not eat the skin—save the juices and mash with the pulp when it is to be eaten. Eat it with the meal, of course; whether it is taken raw or cooked. Do not take it between meals, but at the regular meal.

DO NOT take injections of insulin. If more insulin is necessary than is obtained from eating the amount of artichoke indicated, then increase the number of days during the week of taking the artichoke, see?

9/19/39
F. 59 yrs.
DIABETES **2007-1**

Have more of the raw and leafy vegetables than others.

At least four meals each week should include the Jerusalem artichoke in the diet. One time this should be taken cooked, the next time raw. When cooked, prepare as you would a boiled potato; not boiled too much, but sufficient that it crumbles—and keep the juices of same in same. Hence, cook in Patapar paper. This may be given with a little salt, no pepper, and not too much butter. Butter should not be taken in any quantity, though a little for seasoning vegetables is better than the fats or oils, see?

COLITIS **7/16/43**
ANEMIA **F. 54 yrs.**
ELIMINATIONS: INCOORDINATION **3098-1**

Occasionally—about once a week when it is in season, or when obtainable—we would take the Jerusalem artichoke, cooked in its own juices—as in Patapar paper, and these juices mixed in same when prepared to eat. This will work with the pancreas, also the adrenals and the digestive forces for this body, as related to sugar and the activity of same in the blood supply. This is not good for the body prepared otherwise than as indicated—cooked in its own juices.

9/7/43
DEBILITATION: GENERAL **M. 40 yrs.**
CIRCULATION: LYMPH **3199-1**

In the matter of the diet—do add as soon as practical the Jerusalem artichoke twice each week: this cooked, however, in its own juices—as in Patapar paper. This will aid in bringing a better heart activity as well as the spleen's reaction to the digestive forces as stimulated from time to time.

If these are done, we should find much better conditions for this body.

10/9/43
CIRCULATION: POOR **F. 50 yrs.**
DIABETES **3274-1**

Q. Are the kidneys involved?

A. Naturally the kidneys are involved. With a disturbance of the circulation between heart and liver, it causes a reflex condition in the kidneys. Just keep away from sugar. Do use the Jerusalem artichoke at least once a week in the diet, but only cooked in its own juices—or mix the juices in which it is cooked with the bulk of the artichoke; that is, cook it in Patapar paper.

Q. Do I still have diabetes? What remedy?

A. A tendency towards same, as indicated from the amount of insulin to be given in the artichoke diet.

3/27/44
F. 66 yrs.
DIABETES **4023-1**

Instead of using so much insulin; this can be gradually diminished and eventually eliminated entirely if there is used in the diet one Jerusalem artichoke every other day. This should be cooked only in Patapar paper, preserving the juices and mixing with the bulk of the artichoke, seasoning this to suit the taste. The taking of the insulin is habit forming. The artichoke is not habit forming, not sedative-producing in the body as to cause accumulations of poisons as do sedatives; though it will be necessary to take a sedative when there are the attacks, but take a hypnotic rather than a narcotic—only under the direction, however, of a physician.

1/17/44
M. 57 yrs.
TOXEMIA **3063-3**

For it is the juice that contains the properties most needed to act upon the pancreas and spleen activity of the body. Season with a little butter, a little salt and pepper if desired but not too much. This will change a great deal the ability for activity, if the other treatments suggested are kept up.

3/15/44
F. 26 yrs.
PARALYSIS **3694-1**

Add all of the foods that carry silicon and the salts that may revibrate with the applications of the gold to the nerve centers for assimilation; as foods of the tuberous nature of every character—the ground artichoke (tuberous artichoke) . These should be parts of the foods for the body. Have at least five vegetables grown below the ground to one grown above the ground, or in that proportion.

12/2/40
F. 60 yrs.
538-66

DEBILITATION: GENERAL
APPETITE: DIGESTION: INDIGESTION: NERVOUS

Q. Any special foods at mealtime advised?

A. All of those that carry a great deal of iron and silicon, and things of that nature; that is—all of those that grow under the ground through the winter. Artichoke occasionally should be among them—Jerusalem artichoke, though cooked rather than raw.

2/25/41
F. 51 yrs.
454-8

DIABETES: TENDENCIES

The Jerusalem artichoke that has been indicated is for the pancrean activity with the kidneys; for, from the amount of insulin in same, this will be inclined to make for a change in this activity through the body, thus reducing the pressures in all of the blood supply and the general nerve system—that is, the pressures from poisons, see? Prepare the artichoke in Patapar paper. Do not attempt to eat the shell, of course, but cook the whole artichoke in the Patapar paper, then mash the inside of it as you would a potato and add a little seasoning—or a little butter—just to make it palatable.

11/12/41
F. 13 yrs.
2084-10

GENERAL

Q. What should the dose of artichoke now be, how often and on what days?

A. Once a week take an artichoke, this—for this body—on Thursdays; one not larger than a hen egg; preferably cooked in its OWN jacket and the juices from same mixed with it when prepared to be eaten.

Q. A previous reading recommended that artichokes be stored in earth. Should earth be moist or dry and should it be cool or warm, as indoors?

A. Just so it is stored in earth. Do not keep it too moist, but keep sufficiently dry that the artichoke is preserved. See, the vibration of this particular type of artichoke is insulin. Earth's forces keep it in its normal state. It may be buried indoors, but it would have to be kept near to normal temperature; else we would take much of the properties from the vegetable.

4/5/44
F. 39 yrs.
3386-2

DIABETES: TENDENCY

Q. Craving for sweets?

A. This is natural with the indigestion and the lack of proper activity of the pancreas. Eat a Jerusalem artichoke once each week, about the size of a hen egg. Cook this in Patapar paper, preserving all the juices to mix with the bulk of the artichoke. Season to taste. This will also aid in the disorder in the circulation between liver and kidneys, pancreas and kidneys, and will relieve those tensions from the desire for sweets.

10/5/38
DEBILITATION: GENERAL **F. 40 yrs.**
GLANDS: INCOORDINATION **1657-2**

Once a week—we would say (considering the conditions and surroundings) Thursday evenings, preferably—we would have a Jerusalem artichoke at least the size of a duck egg or the like, eaten either raw or cooked—just so it is thoroughly done but not overcooked; not roasted, but boiled, see—as a potato. This will tend to make for a better activity of the glandular system as related to the hepatic and the pancrean circulation.

5/12/44
F. 16 yrs.
DERMATITIS **2084-16**

Do add to the body Jerusalem artichoke, about once a week. This should be cooked in Patapar paper. Reserve or preserve all of the juices which cook from same and mix with the pulp as it is prepared. Once a week should be sufficient. Season with a little butter and a little salt and pepper.

Do use only the health salt or kelp salt or deep sea salt. All of these are of the same character.

5/20/38
F. 68 yrs.
TOXEMIA **1593-1**

At least a portion of the noon meal should consist of raw vegetables. Twice a week the Jerusalem artichoke would be taken; this to be cooked in its own juices—that is, when it is cooked put it in Patapar paper to boil, and this will preserve the juices of same and thus the insulin which is a component part of same will act upon the system when this is taken. Eat it as you would a boiled white potato.

6/1/39
F. 52 yrs.
GLANDS **1904-1**

Especially we would have in the diet all forms of artichoke as well as occasionally the Jerusalem artichoke. Not so often either of these, but about once or twice a week—this preferably boiled (the Jerusalem artichoke) as you would boil an Irish potato, but the WHOLE of this would be eaten, you see. When it is boiled, boil it in Patapar paper, and the juice which comes from same would be saved to be mashed with the pulp of the artichoke; and it should be mealy or crumbly just as the roasted or baked potato, see?

8/20/43
F. 54 yrs.
DIABETES: TENDENCIES **3166-1**

Do include in the diet, about once a week, the Jerusalem artichoke. Use one about the size of a hen egg, or a little larger, once each week for at least four or five weeks. Cook the artichoke in Patapar paper, so that the juices that are loosened in cooking may be preserved and mixed with the bulk of the artichoke when it is eaten, after it has been seasoned to the taste; this carries insulin in the correct quantity for this body, if not taken oftener than indicated.

4/20/40
F. 74 yrs.
ARTHRITIS **1224-3**

Three times a week the Jerusalem artichoke should be a portion of the diet; once raw, once cooked, and then once raw again. Only cook same, though, in its own juices—as in Patapar paper. Only ONE would be taken at the meal, you see—one meal of the day, three times a week; not a large one, but one about the size of a guinea egg. This also will aid in reducing the sugar, relieving the pressure on the bladder, and relieving the tendencies; for the insulin in the artichoke aids the general circulation.

5/4/39
M. 31 yrs.
KIDNEYS: INFECTIONS **1885-1**

The Jerusalem artichoke should be a portion of the diet each day. This would be taken preferably cooked, but it may be taken raw. The insulin from same—as it is easily assimilated for the activities not only of the pancreas and spleen and liver activity but—will aid in reducing the inclination for the inflammation and pus activity in the kidney itself. One artichoke the size of a duck egg or turkey egg, or thereabouts, should be taken each day—that is, the tuber of the Jerusalem artichoke.

11/23/40
F. 78 yrs.
DIABETES: TENDENCIES **2406-1**

Also include in the diet the Jerusalem artichoke. Do not give injections of insulin, but DO give the nervous shocks to the system by the use of these properties from which it is often extracted—that is, the Jerusalem artichoke. Give one of these (about the size of a guinea egg) EACH day for three successive days, leave off a week, then give for three successive days again, and continue it in this manner as a part of the diet, you see. This should be prepared by boiling it in Patapar paper, not overcooking nor undercooking it, but about as an Irish potato would be cooked. Let this be prepared and eaten with the meal, you see. And this shock—as from the activity to the pancreas and the general nervous system—WITH the other applications—will aid in better activity through the body.

Do these things, if we would bring the better conditions for this body.

5/18/43
F. 66 yrs.
ASSIMILATIONS: ELIMINATIONS: INCOORDINATION **3008-1**

Do have Jerusalem artichoke once each week, but cook this in its own juices; that is, in Patapar paper. One should be sufficient. For this supplies sufficient of insulin for the correcting of this disturbance between the pancreas and the liver activity, as with the cleansing of the system by the circulation through the kidney. This will also react upon both the thyroid and the adrenal activity in the circulation in this body.

12/5/39
ALCOHOLISM **M. 68 yrs.**
KIDNEYS: TOXEMIA **2055-1**

And after at least TEN of the osteopathic adjustments have been made in the manner indicated (not until then), we would use small quantities of Jerusalem artichoke in the diet occasionally, to aid in reducing the excesses of sedimentary forces that tend to work upon the supplying of greater quantity of sugar, also causing the dizziness and the tendency for sleepy conditions to arise from this toxic force. When begun, take only a Jerusalem artichoke about the size of a guinea egg, about once a week; and this would be better cooked in its own juices (for this body), or in Patapar paper.

1/27/40
F. 11 yrs.
KIDNEYS: INFECTION **2084-1**

Also once every ten days (and make it on the tenth day) eat one small Jerusalem artichoke; this to be cooked in its own juices (as in Patapar paper). This adds the adrenal reaction to the system in a manner that will keep the functioning of the kidneys without irritation, through the salts from same, and straining—as it were—the sugars from the activities in the system, keeping a balance with the activity of the glands—as the pancreas and spleen—in relation to its development and activity.

1/17/41
F. 44 yrs.
ELIMINATIONS: POOR **459-11**

At least once a week eat a Jerusalem artichoke about the size of a hen egg—not larger; and this preferably cooked (rather than taken raw), and cooked in its own juices (as in Patapar paper—letting the juices that come from it be mixed with the vegetable itself in its preparation, you see. This may be taken three to four times a week, but should be taken at least once each week—with the regular meal, you see, not eaten as a meal itself, but with other foods. Keep this consistently each week for three to four weeks, then leave off two weeks, and then take for another period, and so on. But when taking it, take it consistently once, twice, three or even four times a week, you see, for a three to four week period at a time.

7/31/39
F. 71 yrs.
HYPERTENSION **1973-1**

Have plenty of leafy vegetables; and occasionally the artichoke—especially the Jerusalem variety. These (the artichokes) would be cooked in their own salts, that is, cooked in Patapar paper; not too done nor too raw, though they may be eaten raw at times if so desired.

These done, we may bring better influences for this body.

11/20/37
CIRCULATION: INCOORDINATION **F. 30 yrs.**
ARTHRITIS **1482-1**

As has been indicated for the body, naturally the diet is an important factor in the effect produced upon the assimilating forces of the body itself. Keep away from great quantities of starches. Take those things where the activities for the system—as of the pancreas, the spleen, the liver activities—become as a greater portion of the activities to produce desired or effective activity in glandular reaction. Especially the Jerusalem artichoke should be a portion of the diet at least once or twice a week.

2)—Asparagus

3/18/32
F. 38 yrs.
ADHESIONS: BLOOD-BUILDING **5515-1**

Evenings—Cooked vegetables . . . those that are of the blood building in the vegetables as of asparagus. Not a great deal of any foods.

5/29/30
M. 28 yrs.
BLOOD-BUILDING **102-2**

Take those that are not just *fat* building, but *nerve* building, and those that carry some, as may be termed, *just fodder* in the system; as will be seen in those of lots of asparagus, and such—that are taken as *green* vegetables.

12/15/27
M. 30 yrs.
ASTHENIA **4605-1**

As for the diet, let that be principally of that as almost pre-digested foods—though as much of raw vegetables as may be well taken, carrying plenty of iron and of salts; such as asparagus, very little, but this has a diuretic that is good for the system. This, of course, cooked (the asparagus).

Do not take sedatives so much, though soda—plain bicarbonate of soda—may be taken in small quantities for same, *provided* the foods taken carry sufficient iron and salt and salts, or vegetables and fruit salts.

5/20/39
F. Adult
ANEMIA: ELIMINATIONS **1779-3**

These as we find we would take, now, rather in periods—not merely as a routine; for these will aid not only in building resistance through portions of the system where there is the greater need of the more perfect circulation but will enable the digestive system to assimilate more of the iron as well as silicon for the system. These are necessary elements.

Hence we will find that the fresh vegetables—especially such as asparagus and those of such natures will be especially good as a part of the diet, regularly.

And, most of all, keep that attitude of constructive thinking; making for that influence of no anxieties for self but more of the constructiveness in the experiences of others—as a helpful influence in every way and manner.

11/28/22
F. Adult
ANEMIA **4439-1**

Use whole wheat bread and vegetables that carry a high percentage of carbons such as asparagus.

4/1/31
APOPLEXY **M. 52 yrs.**
NERVE-BUILDING **3747-1**

The diets will be along those lines that made for nerve *building*. Plenty of the green foods—as asparagus. Not too much of the asparagus, but only those of the fresh or the green.

3)—Beans: General

8/19/35
ASSIMILATIONS: POOR **F. 80 yrs.**
CANCER **975-1**

Q. What diet should be followed, with specific recommendations for breakfast, dinner and supper?

A. Those foods, as we find, that are body building, but that carry very little of the tuberous growths; that is, no *dried* beans at any time. None of those things that make for the bulbous nature in the system; for each of these carries a chemical reaction that does not make for activity with the system. Hence we would give *this* as an outline, though, to be sure, there may be changes at times for these things would naturally become of such a rote as to be offensive to the body if they were continued in this manner alone.

Q. What foods should be avoided?

A. As indicated, those of the tuberous nature—or beans.

7/27/39
F. 27 yrs.
DEBILITATION: GENERAL **480-52**

Keep a general upbuilding in the diet, by the body-building influences. Plenty of all forms of the bulbular vegetables—beans and the like.

These as we find should bring much better results and experiences for the body.

10/4/35
M. 41 yrs.
DEBILITATION: GENERAL **1014-1**

Vegetables, especially beans, and such natures. These should be the principal foods for the evening meals. Not too much, but satisfy the appetite.

6/4/26
M. 54 yrs.
BLOOD-BUILDING **4769-2**

Let the diet be vegetable foods of that that grows *above* the ground. All that of the pod nature, see? Beans, and those of that nature. Not any of the tuberous nature.

9/15/31
DEBILITATION: GENERAL **F. 47 yrs.**
ACIDITY **1690-3**

Evening—Well-cooked vegetables, especially those of the *bean* variety, whether those of the snap, of the white, or the lima, or what nature—well cooked, with pig's feet, tripe, liver, oils of every nature are *well* to be taken.

7/23/43
ARTHRITIS **F. 59 yrs.**
ACIDITY **3110-1**

Some proteins should be taken, but these should be included in the vegetables—in the manner in which they are prepared. Use more of the leafy variety than those of the bulbular or seed nature. Take a great deal of beans. These especially should be often a part of the diet.

5/30/29
F. 31 yrs.
CONSTIPATION **1713-17**

Q. What should the body do to overcome constipation?

A. A great deal of vegetables, especially those that give iron, as beans.

3/25/30
ACIDITY & ALKALINITY **F. 45 yrs.**
DIGESTION: INDIGESTION **5625-1**

In the noon day those of the vegetables that care for the blood and nerve building, and that will produce not an overactivity but as a counter-*irritant* of activity in the kidneys, which will reduce the stimuli in the circulation in the hepatics. These we will find in those of the vegetable forces that grow especially in pods, as beans. These also may be added in a consistent manner with those of the non-acid or of the alkaline-*producing* conditions for the system.

3/17/38
F. 52 yrs.
CANCER **601-29**

In the matter of the diet—as has been indicated—whatever may be given is very well, provided such as the bulbous nature—as dried beans or the like—are not used as a portion of the diet.

A. Please itemize foods that allay inflammatory conditions?

A. As just indicated, most any of the foods desired may be taken except those of the bulbous natures as indicated.

3/21/39
M. 9 yrs.
DIABETES: TENDENCIES **415-7**

Evenings—Vegetables—preferably those that grow above the ground. Beans, these should be a part of the diet. No fried foods at any of the meals.

8/13/38
F. 45 yrs.
ARTHRITIS **1659-1**

As to diet, this should carry a great deal of the salts of vegetables AND fruits—rather than meats. Never any fried foods at any time. The vegetables would be cooked in their OWN juices—that is, in Patapar paper. The juices that come from same shall be well mixed with the vegetables themselves, so that the body gets the benefit of those; such as beans with their salts as come from same—after being well washed and cooked in the Patapar paper, but DO NOT put meat or anything of the kind in same. Season only with a little butter and sufficient salt or pepper to satisfy the appetite or to be palatable to the taste of the body.

6/3/41
DEBILITATION: GENERAL **M. 25 yrs.**
APPENDICITIS **1970-1**

(Do not begin this diet, of course, until after the period of the grape poultices and the grape diet.) Vegetables may then be taken, if cooked in their OWN salts, or their OWN juices—and eat the juices with same, cooking all in Patapar paper. Such as beans.

7/28/39
DEBILITATION: GENERAL M. 27 yrs.
ASSIMILATIONS: ELIMINATIONS: INCOORDINATION 1970-2

Use plenty of beans—but these cooked in their OWN juices (as in Patapar paper) and never those that have had any kind of preservatives on same.

9/1/39
M. 49 yrs.
PARKINSON'S DISEASE 1989-1

Be mindful of the diet—that there are plenty of vitamins. Have plenty of green vegetables as beans, these cooked in their own salts (as in Patapar paper) saving the salts or the water in which such are cooked as a part of the diet.

8/12/40
F. 33 yrs.
ANEMIA: DIGESTION: INDIGESTION 2320-1

Have beans well cooked, but in their own juices (as in Patapar paper). Not large quantities of these ever, but take a little at least three times each day—that is, each meal consisting of some.

11/18/30
F. 60 yrs.
ELIMINATIONS: POOR 505-1

In the matter of diet—these, as we find, will be more of the well balanced that carry more of the irons in their reaction—as will be found in those of all the vegetable forces, as of beans. Also it will be found that little of the meats should be taken.

10/21/32
ELEPHANTIASIS: TENDENCIES F. 18 yrs.
ARTHRITIS: GLANDS: INCOORDINATION 951-1

Supply an overabundant amount of those foods that carry iron, iodine and phosphorus in the system.

The evening meal may be of well-balanced vegetables that are of the leafy nature, and that carry more of those properties as given. Some characters of beans—provided they are well dried and grown in a soil that is different from that carrying iron, see? These will aid.

4/17/31
DEBILITATION: GENERAL M. 19 yrs.
CHOREA 1225-1

Evenings—When beans are used, eat those that carry as much rind as is possible.

ASSIMILATIONS: ELIMINATIONS: INCOORDINATION 11/9/40
CANCER: TENDENCIES F. 61 yrs.
ACIDITY & ALKALINITY 1697-2

Q. What foods may be taken that will digest properly?

A. Any of those that are easily assimilated, that is, three times as much alkaline-reacting as acid-producing foods. This means the alkaline-REACTING, and not acid-producing. For instance all the vegetables that are easily assimilated would be included; beans—provided they are not sprayed with preservatives—these either canned or fresh.

9/16/42
M. 45 yrs.
ARTHRITIS: NEURITIS **2816-1**

Eat plenty of corn bread, beans, but not cooked in or with meat. Rather cook the vegetables in plain water, with a little butter or seasoning put on after being cooked, see?

Be mindful of the diet for a LONG period—at least six months to a year to two years; and the body will improve and keep better through the period.

3/18/32
F. 38 yrs.
ADHESIONS: BLOOD-BUILDING **5515-1**

Evenings—Cooked vegetables . . . those that are of the blood building in the vegetables—as of beans.

10/20/34
ACIDITY: LESIONS **F. 48 yrs.**
ACIDITY **703-1**

Have at least three of the leafy vegetables to one below the ground, or with the leafy vegetables there may be one or two of the bulbous nature—as beans.

9/2/29
CHILDREN: ABNORMAL **M. 7 yrs.**
NERVOUS SYSTEMS: INCOORDINATION **758-2**

Those that are . . . stimuli for the nerve system; especially those of the elements in the vegetable forces that are of the pod nature as beans.

3/28/44
M. 41 yrs.
ACIDITY & ALKALINITY **4008-1**

Those foods that grow under the ground of certain characters, as beans supply certain sulphurs as well as other elements that are needed in the body for better chemical balance.

5/1/35
M. 1-1/2 yrs.
PINWORMS. AFTEREFFECTS **786-2**

Be very mindful that the diets are body and blood building.

All the vegetables may be taken that are *prepared* for the body; as beans, bean soup.

10/5/38
DEBILITATION: GENERAL **F. 40 yrs.**
OBESITY: TENDENCIES **1657-2**

Have more of the vegetables—the leafy variety would be preferable to those of the bulbular nature or such as beans (that is, the dried, see?).

3/30/38
F. 36 yrs.
TUBERCULOSIS **1560-1**

Then the foods for weight and that will aid in caring for the activities through the absorptions and through the digestive forces.

Beans in their season, these are well.

5/20/35
M. Adult
ACIDITY **926-1**

Do not combine quantities of starches with proteins; as beans (white beans), lima beans, or roughage—do not combine these with quantities of bread. When these are taken, do not eat bread.

5/30/24
M. Adult
ASTHMA **4740-2**

To give then the relief to this body, first we would not eat meats, save fish or fowl and that not of too large quantities. Beans, that character of foods may be eaten. Not much sweets but those that add nutriment to the system, without overtaxing the digestive organs in elimination.

ASSIMILATIONS **7/22/31**
DEBILITATION: GENERAL **F. 28 yrs.**
BLOOD-BUILDING **3842-1**

We would give a diet that is easily assimilated. Let the diet be that as is nerve and blood building. Of vegetables, beans, and the like.

1/26/35
F. 59 yrs.
INJURIES **3823-2**

Evenings—A well-balanced vegetable diet. Fresh beans, may be a part of the diet provided it is prepared in its *own* source—as cooked in Patapar paper, so that all the juices and vitamins may be retained in same.

12/2/37
F. 5 yrs.
COLD: COMMON **1490-1**

In the matter of the diets, keep these well balanced in the body, blood and nerve building. Especially vegetables of the bulbous nature as beans.

2/23/25
M. 20 yrs.
BODY-BUILDING **77-2**

Q. What special foods should be given the body that would give to the mind and body strength, endurance and activity?

A. Green vegetable forces of every character, especially those of the tuberous nature. Of course some portions of them cooked, the greater number eaten raw. Beans, those of that nature.

4/1/31
APOPLEXY **M. 52 yrs.**
NERVE-BUILDING **3747-1**

The diets will be along those lines that make for nerve *building*. Plenty of beans, and such may be taken.

i)—Green Beans

3/15/37
BLOOD: HUMOR **F. 56 yrs.**
TOXEMIA **569-25**

Q. What cooked vegetables may be taken?

A. Any of the leafy vegetables. The beans, green beans but not dried beans.

DEBILITATION: GENERAL **1/12/44**
GLAUCOMA **F. 58 yrs.**
EYES **3552-1**

And then in the general diet add a great deal of vegetables that have a direct bearing upon the optic forces through the general system; such as green beans. These have a direct bearing upon the application of that assimilated for the optic forces.

6/8/40
M. 55 yrs.
ANEMIA **2273-1**

Very green foods, take these freely with the meals whenever practical. Green beans are good, but these should be well cooked and not with grease. Butter and a little seasoning is preferable.

10/11/37
DIABETES: TENDENCIES **M. 67 yrs.**
ACIDITY **1454-1**

Hence we would have the stimulating foods such as green beans in their combinations.

2/19/29
M. 48 yrs.
ELIMINATIONS **91-2**

The diet should be, little of meats—preferably those of vegetables that carry plenty of iron, and *no* pod vegetables—though beans—*green* beans—may be eaten, and the meats should be left from the system.

2/27/42
F. 52 yrs.
COLD: CONGESTION **404-10**

Q. What vegetables are especially good for my body, considering the condition of kidneys?

A. Cooked beans (and these should be green beans, or canned green beans—though not preserved with any preservative such as benzoate of soda).

ii)—Lima or Butter Beans

3/28/44
M. 41 yrs.
ACIDITY & ALKALINITY **4008-1**

Q. What combinations of foods are good and what combinations are bad for my system? What foods should I avoid?

A. Avoid too much starch or too much proteins without consideration of the sufficient calories or carbohydrates; that is, do not overburden the system with acid-producing foods. As an illustration—these are not the only foods to take or to leave off, but:

Do not take quantities of such as beans, dried or the dry or fresh beans where they are shelled—as butter beans or lima beans with white bread. Do not take such in combinations with macaroni and cheese.

3/15/37
BLOOD: HUMOR **F. 56 yrs.**
TOXEMIA **569-25**

Canned butter beans in minute quantities may be taken; that is, once or twice a week and not large quantities then.

8/27/40
F. 40 yrs.
ATHLETE'S FOOT: ECZEMA **2332-1**

Have plenty of vegetables. Little of the beans that are dried—as butter beans.

7/25/26
F. 32 yrs.
KIDNEYS: PREGNANCY **540-6**

Keep a well balance between the diets for sufficient calcium and lime; as in butter beans. Things of that nature carry these in such quantities that they may be easily assimilated. So let the foods that are prepared occasionally have more and more of these.

iii)—Wax Beans

6/6/40
ASSIMILATIONS: POOR **F. 19 yrs.**
ANEMIA **2277-1**

Then the diet: Eat all of the vegetables that are especially YELLOW in color—even the yellow beans, the wax beans are preferable to the green variety.

4)—Beets & Beet Tops

ANEMIA: TENDENCIES **10/2/43**
ASSIMILATIONS: ELIMINATIONS: INCOORDINATION **F. 37 yrs.**
KIDNEYS **1695-2**

Then take at least once each day the vitamins B-1. Do not take A. Do take D and G, but these more in the foods than supplementing in the combinations. These will bring better forces to the body; that is, in the food value take plenty of beets.

8/10/43
CHILDBIRTH: AFTEREFFECTS **F. 44 yrs.**
ELIMINATIONS **3148-1**

Q. Should any particular foods be avoided or stressed in the diet?

A. Stress the raw foods as indicated, especially beets. Avoid macaroni, and white potatoes. That character of food should be avoided.

1/10/42
M. 12 yrs.
DIABETES: TENDENCIES **415-8**

Have plenty of those foods that carry some calcium; as beets and the like. The beets, as soon as possible, should be preferably the fresh—but those that are preserved or canned are good, provided these are not preserved in benzoate of soda. This would be indicated on the labels.

6/24/43
M. 68 yrs.
PARALYSIS **3056-1**

. . . Do have oft for the body those properties that carry a great deal of iodine and calcium; or seafoods often. Those that carry the elements indicated are especially in beets and beet tops. These are healing in their activity upon the lymph circulation. They are even capable of destroying certain characters of bacilli in the system.

12/2/40
DEBILITATION: GENERAL **F. 60 yrs.**
APPETITE: DIGESTION: INDIGESTION: NERVOUS **538-66**

Q. Any special foods at mealtime advised?

A. All of those that carry a great deal of iron and silicon, and things of that nature; that is, all of those that grow under the ground through the winter—as beets and the like, see? these are beneficial.

10/20/41
F. 64 yrs.
ARTHRITIS **1512-3**

Do not take too much of turnips nor of other root vegetables, such as potatoes of any kind, rutabagas or any of those natures. The oyster plant as a root vegetable, however, is not so bad. The only root vegetable that should be taken plentifully is beets.

7/31/43
M. 39 yrs.
CANCER **3121-1**

In the diet—do live mostly, for a while on beets; having these almost daily. The beets are for the purifying of the blood, as combined with the plaintain tea and ointment.

DEBILITATION: GENERAL **1/12/44**
GLAUCOMA **F. 58 yrs.**
EYES **3552-1**

And then in the general diet add a great deal of vegetables that have a direct bearing upon the optic forces through the general system; such as beets. These have a direct bearing upon the application of that assimilated for the optic forces.

5/30/24
M. Adult
ASTHMA **4740-2**

Beets, that character of foods may be eaten. Not much sweets but those that add nutriment to the system, without overtaxing the digestive organs in elimination.

5/30/29
F. 31 yrs.
CONSTIPATION **1713-17**

A great deal of vegetables, especially those that give iron, as beets.

6/23/43
ATTITUDES & EMOTIONS: FEAR **F. 38 yrs.**
BODY-BUILDING **3061-1**

And in the diet do add often beets and beet tops. These will aid in so purifying the bloodstream that there may be at least the hindering of the spreading of those activities in the structural body itself.

4/29/42
F. 37 yrs.
GLAUCOMA **630-3**

The condition to aid, then, is the DIET—AND that which IS a stimul[us] to the glandular forces AND the forces of body where assimilations are carried on.

Beets and beet tops also should be part of the diet.

3/22/44
M. 79 yrs.
APPETITE: CATARACTS **3288-2**

Do keep a great quantity of raw, fresh vegetables as part of the diet. Beets, beet juices—with the tops a little later will be excellent also for the body. Have the raw vegetables often with gelatin.

10/27/43
ANEMIA: TENDENCIES **F. 53 yrs.**
ELIMINATIONS: POOR **3316-1**

Do have plenty of beets. It would be well to prepare these with the gelatin, by juicing or scraping them. These should never be combined with any vinegar or acetic acid. To be sure, these would not be all the foods that should be taken, but have plenty of these vegetables. Use more of the leafy than the pod or bulbular nature. Vegetable juices, soups or broths will be well.

12/15/43
F. 23 yrs.
PARKINSON'S DISEASE **3405-1**

Have a great deal of raw foods, beets also, preferably not those that have been pickled but fresh beets. Include the tops with these when at all practical. Beets should be in the diet at least two or three times a week.

9/13/43
M. 41 yrs.
ARTHRITIS **3077-1**

Liquids and semi-liquids for the present—beef juices. These will be the better, with the regular vegetables that are beneficial. Do include in these a great deal of beet tops and beets.

10/6/43
DEBILITATION: GENERAL **F. 31 yrs.**
BODY-BUILDING **3267-1**

In the diet, do keep body-building foods; including plenty of beets—but not with vinegar. These should be a portion of the diet regularly.

Doing these, we should bring the better conditions for this body.

2/23/35
DERMATITIS **M. Adult**
BLOOD: HUMOR: MENU: PSORIASIS **840-1**

Noons—preferably raw fresh vegetables; none cooked at this meal. These would consist of beet tops, that make for purifying of the *humor* in the lymph blood as this is absorbed by the lacteal ducts as it is digested. We would not take any quantities of soups or broths at this period.

7/28/43
ANEMIA **F. 56 yrs.**
GENERAL: MULTIPLE SCLEROSIS **3118-1**

In the diet—keep to those things that heal within and without. Use plenty of beets, and especially beet tops. These, of course, are to be used in sufficient quantity to satisfy the appetite but not to make them become as something disliked. So prepare them in many different forms.

4/14/43
M. 5 yrs.
CHILDREN: ABNORMAL **2963-1**

Especially have beets, particularly those that are fresh and young. And do train the body to eat the beet tops as well as the young beets themselves. Cook them in their own juices. Use Patapar paper for cooking, and mix the juices with the vegetables when they are eaten.

10/7/43
M. 68 yrs.
NEPHRITIS: TENDENCIES **1112-9**

Eat plenty of beets. These will aid the body in the regular diet and will make for much better conditions.

5/20/39
F. Adult
ANEMIA: ELIMINATIONS **1779-3**

These as we find we would take now, rather in periods—not merely as a routine; for these will aid not only in building resistance through portions of the system where there is the greater need of the more perfect circulation but will enable the digestive system to assimilate more of the iron as well as silicon for the system. These are necessary elements.

Hence we will find that the fresh vegetables—especially such as beets and those of such natures—will be especially good as a part of the diet regularly.

1/12/40
F. 27 yrs.
NEURASTHENIA **2076-1**

Throughout this period the diet should consist more of the forces as in vitamin B-1. Plenty of beets. These especially should be taken daily, either in a raw salad or cooked, or the juices extracted in a juicer and taken in small quantities.

6/14/43
F. 47 yrs.
ARTHRITIS: TENDENCIES **585-11**

Add to the diet a great deal of beet tops, and we will find it will change a great deal of these disturbances.

2/21/34
M. 20 yrs.
EPILEPSY **521-1**

Evenings—Vegetables at this meal may include any of those that are well-cooked in their *own* sauce, or their *own* liquid, not adding waters nor seasoning until after they are cooked. And have three that grow *above* the ground to one that grows below the ground, but may include the tops and the roots of such; as beets, or the like, *when* such below the ground are prepared. Not at all times, but that the vitamin forces of these may carry the necessary elements for creating a balance in the system that has long been lacking in sufficient of the phosphorus, silicon, iron and iodine. Hence all the vegetables that carry these properties should be included in the meals from day to day; for they are more easily assimilated by the body or system from vegetable matter than from any other source or character. And do not use great amounts of high seasoning in any of the foods.

12/12/31
F. 46 yrs.
ULCERS: STOMACH **482-3**

In the evening meals, those of the well-cooked vegetables, but only those of the leafy nature—or that grow in pods; not the bulb nature. No beets, nothing of that nature. The *tops* of these may be taken, and may be eaten, but not the bulb nature.

5)—Black-Eyed Peas (Cowpea)

7/15/30
F. 55 yrs.
ACIDITY **760-16**

Peas—those of the lady peas, or black-eyed as called—are good, provided not too much grease is cooked with same.

2/27/42
F. 52 yrs.
COLD: CONGESTION **404-10**

Q. What vegetables are especially good for my body, considering the condition of kidneys?

A. Cooked black-eyed peas.

6)—Cabbage: General

9/12/37
BLOOD: COAGULATION: POOR **F. 62 yrs.**
ACIDITY & ALKALINITY **1411-2**

Q. What would be the most appropriate vegetables or foods to build up my blood supply so as to maintain the same pressure throughout?

A. As indicated, those that make for the keeping of a normal balance in the acids and alkalines of the system.

Study just a bit the vegetables and the general food values of ALL foods; as to how they react to the body.

As WE would then find, this would be a good GENERAL outline, though this to be sure would not include ALL, that may be eaten or all that would be eliminated; for we would find at times there are various conditions and various foods that produce, under the stress and strain of activity, a varied effect; that is: (this is not the food list as yet, but now here are the variations.)

When the body is under stress or strain by being tired, overactive, and then would eat heavy foods as cabbage boiled with meat—these would produce acidity; yet cabbage WITHOUT the meats would produce an alkaline reaction UNDER the same conditions!

5/30/29
F. 31 yrs.
CONSTIPATION **1713-17**

Little of meats. A great deal of vegetables, especially those that give iron, as cabbage.

3/21/39
M. 9 yrs.
DIABETES: TENDENCIES **415-7**

Evenings—Vegetables—preferably those that grow above the ground. Cabbage, these should be a part of the diet. No fried foods at any of the meals.

8/13/38
F. 45 yrs.

ARTHRITIS **1659-1**

As to diet, this should carry a great deal of the salts of vegetables AND fruits—rather than meats. Never any fried foods at any time. The vegetables would be cooked in their OWN juices—that is, in Patapar paper. The juices that come from same shall be well mixed with the vegetables themselves, so that the body gets the benefit of those; such as cabbage with their salts as come from same—after being well washed and cooked in the Patapar paper, but DO NOT put meat or anything of the kind in same. Season only with a little butter and sufficient salt or pepper to satisfy the appetite or to be palatable to the taste of the body.

9/1/39
M. 49 yrs.

PARKINSON'S DISEASE **1989-1**

Be mindful of the diet—that there are plenty of vitamins. Have plenty of green vegetables as cabbage—these cooked in their own salts (as in Patapar paper), saving the salts or the water in which such are cooked as a part of the diet.

9/16/42
M. 45 yrs.

ARTHRITIS: NEURITIS **2816-1**

Eat plenty of cabbage, all leafy vegetables, but not cooked in or with meat. Rather cook the vegetables in plain water, with a little butter or seasoning put on after being cooked, see?

Be mindful of the diet for a LONG period—at least six months to a year to two years; and the body will improve and keep better through the period.

1/10/42
M. 12 yrs.

DIABETES: TENDENCIES **415-8**

Have plenty of those foods that carry some calcium; as cabbage. The cabbage should be taken cooked and raw, but not cooked with grease.

9/26/28
F. 30 yrs.

ASTHENIA: NEURASTHENIA **1713-16**

Q. Should I eat cabbage and carrots?

A. Carrots. *Not* the raw cabbage. Cabbage as prepared *without* too much grease is well, for it carries a great deal of iron and silicon, as well as traces of active forces in the system that are good so long as they digest well with the body.

3/28/44
M. 41 yrs.

ACIDITY & ALKALINITY **4008-1**

Q. Is there any combination of foods that could be truthfully called Brain Foods, Nerve Foods, Muscle Foods?

A. Those that are body building; those that are nerve building and those that supply certain elements. Those foods that grow under the ground of certain characters, as cabbage supply certain sulphurs as well as other elements that are needed in the body for better chemical balance.

5/1/35
M. 1-1/2 yrs.
PINWORMS: AFTEREFFECTS 786-2

Be very mindful that the diets are body and blood building. A little cabbage at times—both raw and cooked.

3/30/38
F. 36 yrs.
TUBERCULOSIS 1560-1

Then the foods for weight and that will aid in caring for the activities through the absorptions and through the digestive forces.

Pot liquor and cabbage raw and cooked, but NOT WITH MEATS—cook them in their OWN juices, and with butter—these are well.

3/22/32
F. 42 yrs.
COLITIS 404-2

Q. Why cannot this body eat a cooked green vegetable, such as cabbage, etc.?

A. It may, well these be added in the system—so that they will act with the gastric juices.

9/27/37
F. Adult
DEBILITATION: GENERAL 1419-5

Noons—at this meal the leafy vegetables that are well cooked in their OWN salts, or cooked in Patapar paper and retaining the juices of same for the salts of same. Such vegetables may be included in this meal as red cabbage, the white cabbage, the celery cabbage or the like—not too much of these.

4/1/31
APOPLEXY M. 52 yrs.
NERVE-BUILDING 3747-1

The diets will be along those lines that make for nerve building. Plenty of cabbage and such may be taken.

i)—Cabbage—Raw

7/30/41
M. 26 yrs.
ANESTHESIA: AFTEREFFECTS 1710-6

Q. Please give further corrective diet.

A. As indicated, it is necessary in the present to add plenty of the elements found in raw cabbage, and occasionally salads. Not that the body is to live off these entirely, to be sure, but these are to be in the diet often—two to three times a week as a part of some meal during the day. The general diet should be for body-building. Be sure that most of the foods carry especially vitamin B.

Q. What should be done to relieve the discomfort in small of the back, apparently resulting from spinal injections?

A. This has been indicated, as to the use of the corrective gases that will relieve gas in stomach, as well as to the general character of foods that will work with same through the intestinal tract—if combined with the character of adjustments indicated.

8/19/35
ASSIMILATIONS: POOR **F. 80 yrs.**
CANCER **975-1**

Noons—Preferably only the juices of, or very finely grated raw vegetables; such as cabbage. These may be taken with or without the salad dressing. Or this may be altered at times to the juices only of the *cooked* vegetables; or there may be had two or more vegetables combined to make for balancing of the elements in the body that are necessary, carrying silicon and iron that are as resistive forces and aids in the blood supply to eradicate these disturbing forces in the system.

ASSIMILATIONS **7/22/31**
DEBILITATION: GENERAL **F. 28 yrs.**
BLOOD-BUILDING **3842-1**

We would give a diet that is easily assimilated. Let the diet be that as is nerve and blood building. If cabbage is taken let it be raw, rather than cooked.

6/14/35
F. Adult
GLANDS: INCOORDINATION **935-1**

Noons—Principally (very seldom altering from these) raw vegetables made into a salad. Use such vegetables as cabbage (the white, of course, cut very fine). It is more preferable that they be grated, but when grated do not allow the juices in the grating to be discarded; these should be used upon the salad itself. Preferably use the *oil* dressings; as olive oil with paprika, or such combinations.

8/5/29
F. 43 yrs.
MENU: NEURASTHENIA **2713-1**

Q. Would you specify the necessary diet?

A. It's been given! As an outline for such, it was given in that it should carry more of the iodines and vegetables that grow above the ground. Raw cabbage, but not cooked cabbage. At least each day have a vegetable that is raw. In the evening meal more of the raw vegetables again, see?

11/18/30
F. 60 yrs.
ELIMINATIONS: POOR **505-1**

In the matter of diet—these, as we find, will be more of the well balanced that carry more of the irons in their reaction—as will be found in those of all the vegetable forces, as of cabbage (not cooked). Also it will be found that little of the meats should be taken.

1/25/33
F. 44 yrs.
GLANDS: INCOORDINATION **757-3**

Noons—Preferably a whole *green* vegetable diet as well as a balance of the diets that produce the *cleansing* effects throughout the system, see? Raw cabbage. And there may be used with these a French dressing or mayonnaise, to make them more palatable.

12/18/30
M. 24 yrs.
BACILLOSIS: POLIOMYELITIS **135-1**

Noons—More of the vegetables that are *raw*. These may be made into salads with salad dressings, especially with as much of the olive oil as is palatable and that will be assimilated with the character of foods. This would include cabbage, and all of those that may be used as such.

3/21/39
F. 49 yrs.
RELAXATION **1158-21**

Q. Raw cabbage?
A. This about three or four times a week.

2/26/38
ANEMIA **F. 10 yrs.**
PINWORMS **1401-2**

To do this, then, we would—before beginning the other treatments—have one whole day, morning, noon and evening meal, with practically nothing save raw cabbage; this eaten slowly, chewed very, VERY well.

There may NOT APPEAR a quantity at ALL of the worms, for the same will be reacted upon by the day's use and activity of the cabbage upon the system.

7/30/41
M. 26 yrs.
ANESTHESIA: AFTEREFFECTS **1710-6**

Q. Please give further corrective diet.

A. As indicated, it is necessary in the present to add plenty of the elements found in raw cabbage, and occasionally salads. Not that the body is to live off these entirely, to be sure, but these are to be in the diet often—two to three times a week as a part of some meal during the day. Then general diet should be for body building. Be sure that most of the foods carry especially vitamin B. These are best found in vegetables of the yellow variety.

ii)—Cabbage—Red

10/4/35
ANEMIA **M. 41 yrs.**
DEBILITATION: GENERAL **1014-1**

Evenings—Vegetables, especially red cabbage. These should be the principal foods for the evening meals. Not too much, but satisfy the appetite.

11/12/35
M. 50 yrs.
ADHESIONS: LESIONS **1055-1**

In the diets, be mindful that we keep those things that add iron, silicon, and gold in the system. It may be necessary later to change some of these, but in the present let the diet consist greatly of vegetables that are of the leafy nature as red cabbage, and things of that nature, but *not* with grease in same. These should be cooked in their *own* juices. Preferably cook each in Patapar paper, or in a fireless or waterless cooker. These are preferable, but *not* in aluminum.

4/18/35
ANEMIA **M. Adult**
MENU: ASSIMILATIONS: POOR **898-1**

The evening meal should consist of the vegetables, especially such as red cabbage, all the leafy vegetables and all the bulbular natures save the white potatoes.

Keep these consistently, persistently; we will gain weight, we will put off this dullness, this tendency for catching cold, this weakness throughout the whole system; and bring the body—in six to eight months—to its normal weight of about a hundred and fifty pounds.

3/18/32
F. 38 yrs.
ADHESIONS: BLOOD-BUILDING **5515-1**

Evenings—Cooked vegetables . . . those that are of the blood building in the vegetables—as of cabbage, the red cabbage only. This taken in small quantities. Not a great deal of any foods.

10/17/34
F. 40 yrs.
HYPOCHONDRIA **1000-2**

Q. What foods contain gold, silicon and phosphorus?

A. These are contained more in those of the vegetable, of those varieties that are given as same. Cabbage, much of these depend upon where the vegetation is grown, as to the character of forces that are carried in same. Raw cabbage at times carry these properties—especially the red cabbage.

1/26/35
F. 59 yrs.
INJURIES **3823-2**

Evenings—A well-balanced vegetable diet. It would be especially well at the evening meal to have *red* cabbage, provided it is prepared in its *own* source—as cooked in Patapar paper, so that all the juices and vitamins may be retained in same.

5/1/38
F. Adult
ARTHRITIS **932-1**

Evenings—The vegetables that are well cooked, and *only* in their own juices; preferably in Patapar paper—each cooked separate, *then* they may be combined as they are eaten if so desired, seasoned while hot with salt, pepper and butter. Red cabbage, the small. If *any* meat is taken, let it be only the broiled or boiled lamb, fowl or fish.

Adhere to these.

iii)—Cole Slaw

1/10/41
APPENDICITIS: TENDENCIES **M. 33 yrs.**
ULCERS: DUODENAL **481-4**

Plenty of cabbage in slaw, thoroughly grated, and used with whatever character of dressing is desired.

4/7/37
F. 29 yrs.
COLD: CONGESTION: AFTEREFFECTS **808-6**

Q. Is my present diet correct?

A. As indicated it is very good, though there may be a little change to the fresh vegetables. Cole slaw may be taken in whatever way is most palatable for the body.

iv)—Sauerkraut

4/28/31
M. Adult
ULCERS: DUODENAL: TOXEMIA **719-1**

Beware of stimuli, especially of an alcoholic nature or content, but these as an example: No highly seasoned foods. No kraut, or such.

7)—Carrots: General

5/21/42
PREGNANCY **F. 34 yrs.**
VITAMINS **457-9**

Q. Do carrots carry vitamin B? Does it make any difference whether they are raw or cooked?

A. They do. If cooked, be sure they are cooked in their own juices to preserve the greater portion of same, but there's quite a variation as to that that is released for digestive forces by being cooked. There are periods when they are better assimilated cooked than raw, but the juices are the source of the vitamin—and that, of course, close to the skin.

3/28/44
M. 41 yrs.
ACIDITY & ALKALINITY **4008-1**

Q. Is there any combination of foods that could be truthfully called Brain Foods, Nerve Foods, Muscle Foods?

A. Those that are body-building; those that are nerve-building and those that supply certain elements. Vegetables that carry certain chemicals, as carrots are especially nerve-building and supply the vitamins called the B and B-Complex, or B combinations.

2/21/34
M. 20 yrs.
EPILEPSY **521-1**

Evenings—Vegetables at this meal include any of those that are well cooked in their *own* sauce, or their *own* liquid, not adding waters nor seasoning until after they are cooked. And have three that grow *above* the ground to one that grows below the ground, but may include the tops and the roots of such; as carrots, or the like, *when* such below the ground are prepared. Not at all times, but that the vitamin forces of these may carry the necessary elements for creating a balance in the system that has long been lacking in sufficient of the phosphorus, silicon, iron and iodine. Hence all the vegetables that carry these properties should be included in the meals from day to day; for they are more easily assimilated by the body or system from vegetable matter than from any other source or character. And do not use great amount of high seasoning in any of the foods.

7/31/43
M. 39 yrs.
CANCER **3121-1**

In the diet—do live mostly, for a while, on carrots, having these almost daily. The carrots are for the purifying of the blood, as combined with the plantain tea and ointment.

8/23/43
F. 42 yrs.
LOCOMOTION: IMPAIRED **3173-1**

We would also take into the system extra quantities of vitamins D, B and B-1. These may be had in carrots.

7/27/39
F. 27 yrs.
DEBILITATION: GENERAL **480-52**

Keep a general upbuilding in the diet, by the body-building influences. Plenty of raw as well as cooked carrots.

These as we find should bring much better results and experiences for the body.

12/2/37
F. 5 yrs.
COLD: COMMON **1490-1**

In the matter of the diets, keep these well balanced in the body, blood and nerve-building.

Especially vegetables of the bulbous nature as carrots.

1/20/33
F. 18 yrs.
GLANDS: INCOORDINATION **951-2**

Have green vegetables. Also those foods that carry sufficient elements of gold and phosphorus which are found partially from the characterization of vegetable forces—as in carrots.

4/28/42
F. 7 yrs.
EYES **2004-4**

Q. What further treatment should be applied for her eye condition?

A. A gentle massage given of evenings would be very well . . . And give the body PLENTY of carrots. Have some of these in the meal each day—both raw and cooked.

DEBILITATION: GENERAL **1/12/44**
GLAUCOMA **F. 58 yrs.**
EYES **3552-1**

And then in the general diet add a great deal of vegetables that have a direct bearing upon the optic forces through the general system; such as carrots. These have a direct bearing upon the application of that assimilated for the optic forces.

6/25/40
F. 55 yrs.
ANEMIA **2287-1**

Then, as to the diet, we would add more of the foods that carry vitamins B and B-1, with also G and M—which would be all of those vegetables that are yellow in nature—not only in color but in nature. Eat plenty of carrots, both cooked and raw.

Once each day one meal should consist principally of carrots. When cooked carrots are used, better that they be cooked with peas and a small quantity of diced potatoes.

11/21/43
COLD: CONGESTION **F. 59 yrs.**
ACIDITY **462-18**

Don't overeat, don't eat too much of vegetables or of pastries or of meats, but keep them well balanced. Have a great deal of carrots mixed with gelatin. These are good for the body. They will aid in all portions of the sensory system, especially in the eyes, the ears, and the drainages through the antrum and the soft tissue of the head; for these supply elements that keep these portions of the body bettered.

5/30/29
F. 31 yrs.
CONSTIPATION **1713-17**

Q. What should the body do to overcome constipation?

A. A great deal of vegetables, especially those that give iron, as carrots.

3/21/39
M. 9 yrs.
DIABETES: TENDENCIES **415-7**

Evenings—Vegetables—preferably those that grow above the ground, though carrots may be taken in moderation.

7/28/39
DEBILITATION: GENERAL **M. 27 yrs.**
ASSIMILATIONS: ELIMINATIONS: INCOORDINATION **1970-2**

Use plenty of carrots, both raw and cooked, but these cooked in their OWN juices (as in Patapar paper) and never those that have had any kind of preservatives on same.

9/1/39
M. 49 yrs.
PARKINSON'S DISEASE **1989-1**

Be mindful of the diet—there are plenty of vitamins. Have plenty of green vegetables. Plenty of carrots cooked in their own juices, saving the salts or the water in which such are cooked as a part of the diet.

4/29/42
F. 37 yrs.
GLAUCOMA **630-3**

The condition to aid, then, is the DIET—AND that which IS a stimuli to the glandular forces AND the forces of body where assimilations are carried on.

Each day have plenty or quantities of carrots, raw and cooked.

ASSIMILATIONS: ELIMINATIONS: INCOORDINATION **11/9/40**
CANCER: TENDENCIES **F. 61 yrs.**
ACIDITY & ALKALINITY **1697-2**

Q. What foods may be taken that will digest properly?

A. Any of those that are easily assimilated; that is, three times as much alkaline-reacting as acid-producing foods. This means the alkaline-REACTING, and not acid-producing. For instance, all the vegetables that are easily assimilated would be included; carrots cooked and raw, provided they are not sprayed with preservatives—these either canned or fresh.

10/20/32
BRONCHITIS: ELIMINATIONS: POOR **F. Adult**
ELIMINATIONS **4293-1**

Evenings—Well-cooked vegetables that grow *above* the ground; none that grow below the ground—none! Those that are of the activity as to make for tuberous forces and heavy starches (as all of these are) make for heaviness that is hard to eliminate. In the salad or green vegetables, carrots (which grow under the ground) may be used occasionally, but not too much of these.

5/31/44
F. 76 yrs.
ARTHRITIS **5175-1**

We would increase the amount of the vitamins which come and appear in carrots, for these natures will bring eliminations for the body.

7/12/35
BODY-BUILDING **F. 23 yrs.**
DIS-EASE: CONTAGION: PREVENTIVE **480-19**

Keep closer to the alkaline diets; using fruits, berries, vegetables particularly that carry iron, silicon, phosphorus and the like—and these as we have indicated.

Q. Are inoculations against contagious diseases necessary for me before sailing in September?

A. As we find, only where the requirements are such as to *demand* same would this be adhered to at all. So far as the body-physical condition is concerned, the adherence to the use of carrots *every* day at a meal or as a portion of the meal will insure against any contagious infectious forces with which the body may be in contact.

Q. Can immunization against them be set up in any other manner than by inoculations?

A. As indicated, if an alkalinity is maintained in the system—especially with carrots, these in the blood supply will maintain such a condition as to immunize a person.

11/3/43
M. 54 yrs.
GLANDS: ADRENALS: THYROID: GLAUCOMA **3276-1**

To be sure, have plenty of vegetables, especially such as carrots. A great deal of these combined with gelatin and gelatin preparations would be well. These we would include in the diet.

9/18/43
M. 22 yrs.
TUBERCULOSIS **3222-1**

Do have all the leafy vegetables the body can absorb—as foods are changed. Not too much of the pod or tuberous vegetables, though carrots should be taken. These are very good.

10/20/41
F. 64 yrs.
ARTHRITIS **1512-3**

Do not take too much of turnips nor of other root vegetables, such as potatoes of any kind, rutabagas or any of those natures. The only root vegetable that should be taken plentifully is carrots.

10/6/43
DEBILITATION: GENERAL **F. 31 yrs.**
BODY-BUILDING **3267-1**

In the diet, do keep body-building foods; including at least once each day plenty of carrots, raw and cooked; not necessarily at the same meal but alternate them. Prepare with other vegetables, but take plenty of carrots, but not with vinegar. These should be a portion of the diet regularly.

Doing these, we should bring the better conditions for this body.

2/23/25
M. 20 yrs.
BODY-BUILDING **77-2**

Q. What special foods should be given the body that would give to the mind and body strength, endurance and activity?

A. Green vegetable forces of every character, especially those of the tuberous nature. Of course some portions of them cooked, the greater number eaten raw. Carrots, those of that nature.

3/18/32
F. 38 yrs.
ADHESIONS: BLOOD-BUILDING **5515-1**

Evenings—Cooked vegetables . . . those that are of the blood-building in the vegetables—as of cooked carrots.

8/31/41
ARTHRITIS: PREVENTIVE **F. 51 yrs.**
BODY: GENERAL **1158-31**

Q. For balanced diet, what quantities should I take per week of carrots?

A. This should be a carrot a day, and you will find you will have better conditions in your teeth and in the digestive forces. Yet to make this so specific might become a hardship, but the character of preparation may be changed—and this becomes rather a needed supply.

3/18/44
ELIMINATIONS: INCOORDINATION **F. 28 yrs.**
EYES **3233-2**

Q. Is there any improvement in the condition of eyes?

A. As indicated there is improvement in the general health and in the eyes.

Q. Should the same diet be continued?

A. We would continue with the same diet, changing only as the spring vegetables come; keeping close to those that have been given that contribute to the activity of vision. Carrots in every form, prepared frequently with gelatin and in other manners that have been indicated.

3/21/39
F. 49 yrs.
RELAXATION **1158-21**

Q. Raw carrots?

A. Once or twice a day if so desired, about three days a week.

4/17/44
F. 36 yrs.
MULTIPLE SCLEROSIS **5031-1**

Have more of the vegetables growing under the ground than those growing above the ground, for this body; such as the tuberous natures—as carrots; all characters of vegetables that are grown under the ground. To be sure some leafy vegetables should be taken, but have at least 3 of those under the ground to one of those on the top of the ground, for this body.

4/14/43
M. 5 yrs.
CHILDREN: ABNORMAL **2963-1**

As to the foods—keep a normal, balanced diet; not an oversupply of any particular vitamins, but plenty of the iodine-producing or iodine-giving foods—as carrots.

12/2/40
DEBILITATION: GENERAL **F. 60 yrs.**
APPETITE: DIGESTION: INDIGESTION: NERVOUS **538-66**

Q. Any special foods at mealtime advised?

A. All of those that carry a great deal of iron and silicon, and things of that nature; that is, all of those that grow under the ground through the winter—as carrots.

1/10/41
APPENDICITIS: TENDENCIES **M. 33 yrs.**
ULCERS: DUODENAL **481-4**

Plenty of carrots—grated preferably, if taken raw—but take them both raw and cooked and used with whatever character of dressing is desired.

9/28/41
CONSTIPATION **M. 8 yrs.**
ASSIMILATIONS: POOR **2595-1**

Evenings—Take cooked carrots, but cooked in their own juices (as in Patapar paper), with a little of mashed potatoes, with a little broth. For this meal preferably have vegetables that are well cooked together, and the broth of the vegetables taken with same. These are the foods to be stressed in the diet.

10/20/43
GLAUCOMA **M. 46 yrs.**
HYPERTENSION **3305-1**

We may apply food values that may aid in staying the condition; that is, extra quantities of B-1 and (niacin) and those foods in excess—such as carrots and foods that are rich in those added principles that are active in the body forces pertaining to the optic centers or nerve centers.

Keep those foods that will carry such properties as indicated, adding in supplementary form the A, D and B.

ACIDITY: EYES **1/28/44**
ANEMIA **F. 63 yrs.**
ASSIMILATIONS: ELIMINATIONS: INCOORDINATION **3607-1**

In the diet do use a great deal of raw vegetables.

Q. What can be done for my eyes?

A. Do these things and we will get rid of this acid throughout the system and relieve the stress upon the kidneys, which will help the eyes. Eat lots of carrots, raw and cooked.

12/31/34
F. 22 yrs.
ELIMINATIONS: INCOORDINATION **480-13**

Q. How are my teeth, and should any be extracted?

A. Only local attention, as we find, is particularly needed at this time; especially if there is included plenty of calcium either in the treatments of same or in the diets—which is included specifically, of course, in carrots.

12/8/39
M. 32 yrs.
PINWORMS **1597-2**

As to the diet, following the three-day apple diet, let there be more of vegetables, and the supplying forces as will create iron, silicon and the like for the system. Hence we would include a great deal of carrots.

4/19/41
F. 51 yrs.
ASSIMILATIONS **1158-30**

Q. Shall I supplement with additional vitamin B tablets?

A. We find that if this vitamin is supplied in the diet it will be better than taking an overquantity of vitamin B, which would be the case if the tablets were taken as a supplement. With the Adiron taken, that is to aid in assimilation, it would be better to supplement the vitamin B in the diet, with such as carrots cooked and raw. These taken, as we find, with beef and fowl, should carry sufficient vitamins.

10/8/36
ANEMIA **F. 54 yrs.**
ARTHRITIS: TOXEMIA **1269-1**

Carrots, all of these that grow under the ground may be part of the diet. Those cooked, or the vegetables in the evening—as body, as roughage for the body.

10/17/34
F. 40 yrs.
HYPOCHONDRIA **1000-2**

In the matter of the diets . . . those of the phosphorous nature, and of those that carry these properties as are necessary—the creation with the chlorine foods carry the gold in its combination—follow these closely.

Q. What foods contain gold, silicon and phosphorus?

A. These are contained more in those of the carrots. Much of these depend upon where the vegetation is grown, as to the character of forces that are carried in same.

7/18/40
F. 39 yrs.
ASSIMILATIONS: ELIMINATIONS: INCOORDINATION **2309-1**

Take plenty of food values that carry vitamins B-1 and G. These are found especially in carrots (cooked or raw—and we would have them both ways often). These should be in the diet almost daily. Give these combined in different forms.

6/17/41
NERVOUS TENSION **F. 26 yrs.**
RHEUMATISM **2517-1**

THE BLOOD SUPPLY indicates an unbalanced condition in the chemical reactions, and a lack—in the beginning—of the vitamin or vital forces as might be best adapted to the body—B-1 and F, or B-2.

These produced a nervous reaction, or a lack of nerve vitamin forces. Thus, with the disturbances to the sympathetic system, the high nerve tension or nerve exhaustion that followed, there was a still greater reduction in the chemical forces of the body.

As to the diet throughout the period—keep close to those foods that will supply the greater quantity of B-1 vitamin.

Noons—Let at least a part of this meal consist of raw vegetables, which should include carrots—raw and grated. Also have plenty of cooked carrots, but cook them in their own juices (as in Patapar paper) and eat the juices with them.

10/11/43
F. 26 yrs.
ARTHRITIS **3285-1**

We should have easily assimilated foods, but those very high in the adding of B-Complex, or the vitamin B—as in carrots These should be a part of the diet daily with plenty of seafoods (not fresh water fish).

12/12/31
F. 46 yrs.
ULCERS: STOMACH **482-3**

In the evening meals, those of the well-cooked vegetables, but only those of the leafy nature—or that grow in pods; not the bulb nature. No carrots, nothing of that nature. The *tops* of these may be taken, and may be eaten, but not the bulb nature.

6/29/42
F. 25 yrs.
ANEMIA **2376-2**

Do have one meal each day consisting principally of raw vegetables; not all of the meal, but the greater portion.

Eat few of those vegetables, other than the carrots, that grow under the ground. Use mostly those above the ground—these well cooked.

6/6/40
ASSIMILATIONS: POOR **F. 19 yrs.**
ANEMIA **2277-1**

Eat all of the vegetables that are YELLOW in color. Especially carrots, both raw and cooked—these should be a portion of the diet each day.

10/17/34
M. Adult
ANEMIA **698-1**

In the diet, keep much of that which will add more phosphorus and gold to the system; as we will find in certain of the vegetables—as carrots and the like. These should be a portion of the diet each day; not that it would be these *only*—but keep more of an alkaline diet. No heavy or red meats.

Do this, and we will bring for this body a much nearer normal and *strengthened* condition.

8/27/40
F. 40 yrs.
ATHLETE'S FOOT: ECZEMA **2332-1**

Have plenty of vegetables, especially carrots.

APPLES: ELIMINATIONS **12/30/40**
ASSIMILATIONS: POOR **M 52 yrs**
COOKING UTENSILS: ALUMINUM: NOT RECOMMENDED **2423-1**

As to the diet after the first cleansing with the apples—we would have plenty of carrots—raw as well as cooked. For this body, do not eat foods prepared in aluminum at all; for, from the natural conditions and the supercharges of acids, the body will be allergic to the effects from aluminum on foods.

SPINE: SUBLUXATIONS **9/25/37**
MINERALS **F. 35 yrs.**
903-25

There is first an unbalancing of the elements in the activities of the system—or lack of sufficient calcium for the full activity of body-building.

Hence there should be the use of the food values that carry such in such measures as may be assimilated by the body. Those as we find in carrots especially should be a portion of the diet.

11/1/30
F. 21 yrs.
EPILEPSY **543-4**

Q. Are too many plants which come from under the ground being taken into system?

A. Take as little of these as may be taken, yet some may be used occasionally for that of the *weight* or body of food values in the system.

Q. Which ones should be taken from diet, and which ones may be taken?

A. Carrots may be preserved.

ASSIMILATIONS: POOR **8/19/35**
CANCER **F. 80 yrs.**
975-1

Noons—Preferably only the juices of, or very finely grated raw vegetables; such as carrots. These may be taken with or without the salad dressing. Or this may be altered at times to the juices only of *cooked* vegetables.

BABY CARE **9/4/41**
ELIMINATIONS **F. 2-1/2 yrs.**
1521-5

There needs to be those considerations for more of the foods carrying the vitamins B and D, rather than these taken separately.

We find that these would be obtained in the correct proportions, at least two to three times each week, of carrots—grated, or carrot juice, carrot salad or the like.

Q. Any suggestions to help increase or make eliminations more normal?

A. The changing in the diet, with vegetables of the form and prepared in the manner indicated, will aid in this direction. This is much preferable to taking or giving laxatives, or eliminants. The fresh vegetables.

5/25/42
M. 58 yrs.
NEURASTHENIA **816-13**

Add all of those vegetables that are yellow in their nature. Carrots cooked AND raw should be taken daily. These will aid in stimulating. Not that these should be the things alone taken, but these should form portions of the diet daily—some parts of these, see?

ANEMIA: TENDENCIES **10/2/43**
ASSIMILATIONS: ELIMINATIONS: INCOORDINATION **F. 37 yrs.**
KIDNEYS **1695-2**

Then take at least once each day the vitamin B-1. Do not take A.

Do take D and G, but these more in the foods than supplementing in the combinations. These will bring better forces to the body; that is, in the food values take plenty of carrots.

9/29/36
F. 33 yrs.
540-7

PREGNANCY

There should be those precautions that there be plenty of calcium in the system for developing of bone and muscle tissue. Most of this, of course, may be had from those vegetables that carry calcium and silicon and iron in the ways and manners that may be assimilated—as we would find from carrots. These as we find will make for developments and produce assimilations better for the body.

i)—Carrots—Raw

8/10/43
F. 44 yrs.
3148-1

CHILDBIRTH: AFTEREFFECTS
ELIMINATIONS

Also it would help to keep better eliminations for the body regularly. These may be controlled best, as we find, for this particular body by the diet. So include often in the diet carrots and the like. These may be grated or cut very fine and used with mayonnaise or an oil dressing; not to "burn out" with same as some might do, but change them as to their usage, and we shall find it will change the general elimination and increase the strengthening of the body, relieving those tensions that cause pressures to the head and to the secondary nervous system of the body.

Q. Should any particular foods be avoided or stressed in the diet?

A. Stress the raw foods as indicated, especially beets, carrots. Avoid macaroni, and white potatoes. That character of food should be avoided.

6/19/44
F. 46 yrs.
3051-6

ELIMINATIONS: POOR

Q. What is the best diet for this body?

A. Now that which is a well-balanced diet. But often use the raw vegetables which are prepared with gelatin. Use these at least three times each week. Those which grow more above the ground than those which grow below the ground. Do include, when these are prepared, carrots with that portion especially close to the top. It may appear the harder and the less desirable but it carries the vital energies, stimulating the optic reactions between kidneys and the optics.

3/26/44
M. 39 yrs.
4017-1

ADHESIONS: LESIONS

The diet should consist of liquids and semi-liquids, principally. Do use a great deal of the body-building foods such as vegetable juices, as carrots. These may be prepared not only in a juicer, but oft prepared in a salad, very finely ground and using the juices with same prepared in gelatin, so that there will be these activities through the body.

12/11/40
F. 57 yrs.
DEBILITATION: GENERAL **2185-2**

At least three times a week grate a fresh raw carrot and eat it—either between meals or at the lunch hour. This will be a helpful force for the glandular system as well as the activities of the digestive system, the kidneys, and those tendencies for the accumulations that tend to segregate themselves.

3/23/40
F. 12 yrs.
EPILEPSY **2153-1**

Have plenty of the vitamins, especially of foods that carry B, B-1, A, C and D. Such would be included, of course, in plenty of raw vegetables—as carrots; these raw, you see, and grated very fine, or the juice extracted from same—not large quantities taken (of the juices) but a little bit each day.

2/5/42
F. 24 yrs.
INJURIES **2679-1**

Q. Should vitamin capsules be continued?

A. For the time being. But, as there is the more ability to assimilate vitamins from the food values, these are much preferable to the concentrated form. While these may be taken, and we would take them for at least ten days or two weeks longer, we find that AS the proper food values are obtained from the character of the diet these should be left off—for they may be overdone, to be sure, by not being assimilated. Hence the assimilation of the vitamins through the use of the proper food values is much preferable.

Q. Any raw foods especially to be recommended?

A. Especially carrots. Every day. Not all at once, but some of these at one meal every day.

10/7/43
M. 68 yrs.
NEPHRITIS: TENDENCIES **1112-9**

Change the diet somewhat. Eat plenty of raw carrots. These will aid the body in the regular diet and will make for much better conditions,

6/2/44
ARTHRITIS: TENDENCIES **F. 49 yrs.**
CIRCULATION: INCOORDINATION **2970-2**

In the matter of the diet do take more raw foods, especially carrots, and such foods and do include with these gelatin oft. These grated, ground, but do use the juices of same with gelatin. These, with the other corrections, will change conditions of eyes, throat and all of the organs of the sensory system; improve hearing, vision, vocal box, as well as taste and sense of vibrations about the body.

4/6/44
F. 62 yrs.
NERVE-BUILDING **4033-1**

Q. Please suggest foods to stress and foods to avoid in the diet.

A. In the diet there should be the stressing of those that are nerve-building. Vegetables that are raw, especially carrots should be prepared quite often—in fact, have some of these every day, but prepare most often with gelatin because of the activities that cause the better nerve forces.

3/31/43
ASSIMILATIONS: ELIMINATIONS: INCOORDINATION **F. 18 yrs.**
BODY-BUILDING **2947-1**

Keep the diet body-building. Plenty of vitamins A and D; plenty of B-1 and the B-Complex. Plenty of carrots in a salad and by themselves. These may be juiced or they may be taken in a salad with a dressing.

This is not to be all the diet, of course, but these should form a great part of the diet—just so often as not to become obnoxious to the body, altering in the manner of preparation.

Q. What causes pain in arms, shoulders and back, and what can be done for relief?

A. The lack of sufficient energies being supplied to the nerve forces and the stimulation of the nerve plexus calling for more activity. AND at times a pressure in the assimilating system.

Thus the needs of keeping good eliminations.

Q. How can she best overcome constipation?

A. By the diet; and, as indicated, these are taken into consideration.

9/29/32
F. Adult
OBESITY **4784-1**

Noons—A whole green vegetable salad, with a little of the oils, or mayonnaise that is made of oils, as dressing. Use as many as three to four or five vegetables, see? Those below the ground may be taken in the fresh vegetable salad at the noon meals; as carrots, but not in the evening meals with meats or green cooked vegetables.

7/30/41
M. 26 yrs.
ANESTHESIA: AFTEREFFECTS **1710-6**

Q. Please give further corrective diet.

A. As indicated, it is necessary in the present to add plenty of the elements found in raw carrots, and occasionally salads. Not that the body is to live off these entirely, to be sure, but these are to be in the diet often—two to three times a week as a part of some meal during the day. The general diet should be for body-building. Be sure that most of the foods carry especially vitamin B. These are best found in vegetables of the yellow variety.

Q. What should be done to relieve the discomfort in small of the back, apparently resulting from spinal injections?

A. This has been indicated, as to the use of the corrective gases that will relieve gas in stomach, as well as to the general character of foods that will work with same through the intestinal tract—if combined with the character of adjustments indicated.

10/27/43
ANEMIA: TENDENCIES **F. 53 yrs.**
ELIMINATIONS: POOR **3316-1**

Do have plenty of carrots. It would be well to prepare these with the gelatin, by juicing or scraping them. These should never be combined with any vinegar or acetic acid. To be sure, these would not be all the foods that should be taken, but have plenty of these vegetables. Use more of the leafy than the pod or bulbular nature. Vegetable juices, soups or broths will be well.

3/22/44
M. 79 yrs.
APPETITE: CATARACTS **3288-2**

Q. Is carrot juice freshly made as good as eating ground carrots in a gelatin salad?

A. As indicated, vary the manners in which these are prepared. All of the vegetables, including carrots, may be juiced at times. At others if they are ground and prepared with gelatin, it will be preferable. This is to prevent these from becoming obnoxious to the body.

11/18/30
F. 60 yrs.
ELIMINATIONS: POOR **505-1**

In the matter of diet—these, as we find, will be more of the well balanced that carry more of the irons in their reaction—as will be found in those of all the vegetable forces, as of carrots (raw). Also it will be found that little of the meats should be taken.

7/30/40
F. Adult
OBESITY **2315-1**

Each meal should be preceeded by the grape juice—thirty minutes before eating.

Noons—Either cooked vegetable juices as in soups or the like, or an altogether raw salad consisting of such as carrots and the like. These when taken raw should be grated, or may be taken with the raw juices from these vegetables indicated—the juice extracted by use of a juicer, see?

8/24/44
F. 58 yrs.
ASTHENIA **5394-1**

In building up the body with foods, preferably have a great deal of raw vegetables for this body—as carrots. Take raw, with dressing, and oft with gelatin. Do preserve the juices with them when these are prepared in this manner in the gelatin.

7/15/30
F. 55 yrs.
ACIDITY **760-16**

Carrots, raw, especially scraped. These may be taken, that is, the raw, with the soups or broths.

1/17/44
F. 44 yrs.
ANEMIA **3564-1**

Keep plenty of raw vegetables; as carrots. Not necessarily at any one period but some every day. Often prepare these with gelatin—about three times a week, for gelatin also is needed in the body. Grate them, slice them, dice them, changing their manner of preparation so as not to become objectionable.

6/8/40
M. 55 yrs.
ANEMIA **2373-1**

Especially have carrots, take these freely with the meals whenever practical. At least have some of these once or twice a day. Especially the juice from raw, fresh carrots would be good—better that the cooked carrots; or the raw carrots would be well.

BLINDNESS: TENDENCIES: GLAUCOMA **4/21/44**
DEBILITATION: GENERAL **F. 80 yrs.**
EYES **5059-1**

Supply energies in the body through a great deal more of raw vegetables rather than meats for this body. Do have the vegetables often such as carrots, especially carrots and these may be oft juiced as well as grated or chopped fine and prepared with gelatin. Not so as to become obnoxious to the body, but supply these elements often for the body. When the juicer is used, just drink the carrot juice. This is well.

12/30/42
M. 21 yrs.
BODY-BUILDING: LOCOMOTION: IMPAIRED **2873-1**

The food values should be those fully well balanced with calcium, iron, and especially the vitamins B-1 and the B-Complex. These are much preferable for the body.

At least three times each week, then, supply these from the foods rather than the reinforced vitamins (though these reinforcements may be desirable if there is the inability of the body to assimilate foods that carry excesses or the full quantity of such vital forces).

Noons—At least a portion of this meal should include carrots—raw. Arrange these differently so that they do not become abhorrent to the body; sometimes in their regular state, other times grated, other times prepared in juice form.

1/4/40
ATROPHY: NERVES **M. 32 yrs.**
NERVES: REBUILDING **849-47**

The DIET—this must be, as the rest, CONSISTENTLY, PERSISTENTLY, followed.

Take more of the vegetable forces that are life giving in their assimilation through the body; more carrots (raw). These should be combined to make the greater part of one meal each day; or they may be taken with EACH meal if it is the more preferable. They MUST BE TAKEN, if there will be better recuperative forces, or the supplying to the system of properties and energies that are to be the real HEALING forces!

For here alone (in the diet) will there be the coming of curative or healing powers. All the rest are for the PREPARATIONS of the body for the USAGE of energies in food values, which may be had from those foods indicated to be supplied.

6/9/27
F. 1 yr.
BABY CARE 608-1

Well for the body to cut teeth on carrots (raw, see?)—these may be given, just so chunks are not cut off and swallowed too much.

10/23/43
F. 60 yrs.
ELIMINATIONS 3314-1

Have plenty of raw vegetables, and we will have better eliminations and better conditions for the body. Do eat carrots a great deal. These should be scraped or cut very fine and eaten raw, as in gelatin or in such a way that the body does not tire of same. At times they may be grated and eaten with salad dressings if desired, and at times cooked. These add better circulation especially for eyes, face and nasal passages.

2/23/35
DERMATITIS M. Adult
BLOOD: HUMOR: MENU: PSORIASIS 840-1

Noons—Preferably raw fresh vegetables; none cooked at this meal. These would consist of carrots, that make for purifying of the *humor* in the lymph blood as this is absorbed by the lacteal ducts as it is digested. We would not take any quantities of soups or broths at this period.

3/1/41
F. Adult
ARTHRITIS: NEURITIS: TENDENCIES 838-3

DO have at least once a day with the meal a raw vegetable salad, especially with such as carrots. These should be a part of the diet to aid in better stimulation for that being accomplished by the properties to set up eliminations and to purify the system, and also to aid that accomplished from the osteopathic adjustments AND the relaxing with the Infra Red Light treatments.

This does not mean, of course, that these are to be the ONLY foods taken. We merely give a list of the DO'S and the DON'TS.

5/9/29
F. 64 yrs.
ACIDITY: ASSIMILATIONS: BLOOD-BUILDING 1377-3

Q. Am I eating anything I should not?

A. These, in the diet, may be alternated some to better advantage. When the body finds that a portion of the raw diet works in a manner as to produce the tendency to feel full, *change* them from evening to morning meals. The scraped carrots will be well for the evening and noon meal, with the other ingredients given.

7/30/41
M. 26 yrs.
ANESTHESIA: AFTEREFFECTS 1710-6

Q. Please give further corrective diet.

A. As indicated, it is necessary in the present to add plenty of the elements found in raw carrots, and occasionally salads. Not that the body is to live off these entirely, to be sure, but these are to be in the diet often—two to three times a week as a part of some meal during the day. The general diet should be for body-building. Be sure that most of the foods carry especially vitamin B. These are best found in vegetables of the yellow variety.

9/3/41
GLANDS: THYROID **F. 33 yrs.**
BODY-BUILDING **2582-1**

Be mindful that there are the diets that carry full quantities of the vitamins that aid in the strength and body-building. These will be found in carrots and all forms of the raw vegetables. These should be a considerable part of the body's diet.

3/1/41
F. Adult
ARTHRITIS: NEURITIS: TENDENCIES **838-3**

DO have at least once a day with the meal a raw vegetable salad, especially with such as carrots. These should be a part of the diet to aid in better stimulation for that being accomplished by the properties to set up eliminations and to purify the system.

3/23/44
TUMORS **F. 61 yrs.**
EYES **3803-1**

The rest will have more effect upon the clarifying of the vision, as will the x-ray treatments for these conditions, than particular foods at the present time. Later if more raw vegetables are added, especially carrots and every form of tuberous vegetables, these will aid better in bringing better conditions for the body.

10/20/43
ASSIMILATIONS: POOR **F. 73 yrs.**
BODY-BUILDING **3304-1**

Keep to the body-building forces in the diet. Plenty of raw vegetables, such as carrots. These supply silicon, as well as that needed in other energies to replenish the body.

10/17/27
M. 8 mos.
BABY CARE **5520-2**

In tomatoes there is found the three necessary vitamins for growth and for *development*. The same is seen in carrots—save these are not *balanced* in the same ratio as in tomatoes—but *these* may be given in the raw state where the teeth are beginning to make their appearance. With same kept very *cold* is excellent for the child to teethe or to cut through, rubbing or using same against the gums. Only see that sufficient of the chunks or pieces are removed, so as not to cause too great a strain on the esophagus or swallowing. These will be found, though, to be good—for only a very little may be gummed or scraped away by the teeth as seen here.

Q. Should he have any cooked vegetable juices? If so, *how soon?*

A. As given, any of these as have been outlined are very good. We would *not* cook the carrots.

Q. Is there anything he can chew to make his teeth hurry through?
A. Carrots!

HAY FEVER
COMBINATIONS: EYES: VITAMINS

5/25/44
F. 55 yrs.
5148-1

Q. What will help the eyesight?

A. These we have been administering, but if gelatin will be taken with raw foods rather often (that is, prepare raw vegetables such as carrots often with same, but do not lose the juice from the carrots; grate them, eat them raw), we will help the vision.

BODY-BUILDING

3/29/40
F. 50 yrs.
1158-23

Noons—Special reference to all vegetables that are of the yellow variety stressed in the diet. This would include carrots.

8)—Cauliflower

RELAXATION

3/21/39
F. 49 yrs.
1158-21

Q. Raw cauliflower?
A. This about twice a week should be sufficient.

9)—Celery

GLANDS: INCOORDINATION

1/25/33
F. 44 yrs.
757-3

Noons—Preferably a whole *green* vegetable diet, consisting of such as celery, or any of those that make for the weight—as well as a balance of the diets that produce the *cleansing* effects throughout the system, see?

Evenings—Vegetables *well* cooked, but be sure that for each vegetable used that grows under the ground there are *two* used that grow *above* the ground, either in leafy vegetables or the pod vegetables, see?

ANEMIA: TENDENCIES
ASSIMILATIONS: ELIMINATIONS: INCOORDINATION
KIDNEYS

10/2/43
M. 37 yrs.
1695-2

Then take at least once each day the vitamin B-1. Do not take A.

Do take D and G, but these more in the foods than supplementing in the combinations. These will bring better forces to the body; that is, in the food values take plenty of celery.

ATROPHY: NERVES
NERVES: REBUILDING

1/4/40
M. 32 yrs.
849-47

The DIET—this must be, as the rest, CONSISTENTLY, PERSISTENTLY, followed.

Take more of the vegetable forces that are life giving in their assimilation through the body; more celery. These should be combined to make the greater part of one meal each day; or they may be taken with EACH meal if it is the more preferable. They MUST BE TAKEN, if there will be better recuperative forces, or the supplying to the system of properties and energies that are to be the real HEALING forces!

For here alone (in the diet) will there be the coming of curative or healing powers. All the rest are for the PREPARATIONS of the body for the USAGE of energies in food values, which may be had from those foods indicated to be supplied.

8/19/35
F. 80 yrs.
975-1

ASSIMILATIONS: POOR
CANCER

Noons—Preferably only the juices of, or very finely grated raw vegetables; such as celery. These may be taken with or without the salad dressing. Or this may be altered at times to the juices only of the *cooked* vegetables; or there may be had two or more vegetables combined to make for balancing of the elements in the body that are necessary, carrying silicon and iron that are as resistive forces and aids in the blood supply to eradicate these disturbing forces in the system.

6/4/26
M. 54 yrs.
4769-2

BLOOD-BUILDING

Let the diet be vegetable foods of that that grows *above* the ground. All that of the pod nature, see? Celery, and those of that nature. Not any tuberous nature.

7/22/31
F. 28 yrs.
3842-1

ASSIMILATIONS: DEBILITATION: GENERAL
BLOOD-BUILDING

We would give a diet that is easily assimilated. Let the diet be that as is nerve- and blood-building. And vegetables, as plenty of celery and the leafy vegetables.

12/30/42
M. 21 yrs.
2873-1

BODY-BUILDING: LOCOMOTION: IMPAIRED

The food values should be those fully well balanced with calcium, iron, and especially the vitamins B-1 and the B-Complex. These are much preferable for the body.

At least three times each week, then, supply these from the foods rather than the reinforced vitamins (though these reinforcements may be desirable if there is the inability of the body to assimilate foods that carry excesses or the full quantity of such vital forces).

Noons—At least a portion of this meal should include celery. Arrange differently so that they do not become abhorrent to the body; sometimes in the regular state, other times grated, other times prepared in juice form. Then have soups, broths or the like, and these should include celery.

4/28/42
F. 7 yrs.
EYES **2004-4**

Q. What further treatment should be applied for her eye condition?

A. A gentle massage given of evenings would be very well . . . And give the body PLENTY of celery. Have some of these in the meal each day.

4/21/44
BLINDNESS: TENDENCIES: GLAUCOMA **F. 80 yrs.**
DEBILITATION: GENERAL **5059-1**

Supply energies in the body through a great deal more of raw vegetables rather than meats for this body. Do have the vegetables often such as celery. Not so as to become obnoxious to the body, but supply these elements often for the body.

5/30/24
M. Adult
ASTHMA **4740-2**

To give then the relief to this body, first we would not eat meats, save fish or fowl and that not of too large quantities, using a great deal of celery or articles of the vegetable kingdom as those.

6/25/40
F. 55 yrs.
ANEMIA **2287-1**

Then, as to the diet, we would add more of the foods that carry vitamins B and B-1, with also G and M—which would be all of those vegetables that are yellow in nature—not only in color but in nature.

Once each day one meal should consist principally of celery and the like.

1/17/44
F. 44 yrs.
ANEMIA **3564-1**

Keep plenty of raw vegetables; as celery. Not necessarily at any one period but some every day. Often prepare these with gelatin—about three times a week, for gelatin also is needed in the body. Grate them, slice them, dice them, changing their manner of preparation so as not to become objectionable.

11/21/43
COLD: CONGESTION **M. 59 yrs.**
ACIDITY **462-18**

Don't overeat, don't have too much of vegetables or of pastries or of meats, but keep them well balanced. Have a great deal of celery mixed with gelatin. These are good for the body. They will aid in all portions of the sensory system, especially in the eyes, the ears, and the drainages through the antrum and the soft tissue of head; for these supply elements that keep these portions of the body bettered.

4/26/43
F. 32 yrs.
ACIDITY **1688-10**

Take celery especially. A small quantity of celery should be eaten each day; this, of course, raw—not in soups, not with the combination of cheeses or the like on same.

5/30/29
F. 31 yrs.
CONSTIPATION **1713-17**

Q. What should the body do to overcome constipation?

A. A great deal of vegetables, especially those that give iron, as celery, and those natures.

12/28/43
F. 75 yrs.
CANCER: SKIN **3532-1**

In the diet often have raw vegetables, especially celery, and all of the vegetables that may be well combined in a salad. These at times prepared with gelatin will be well to give strength to the muscular forces of the body.

8/24/44
F. 58 yrs.
ASTHENIA **5394-1**

In building up the body with foods, preferably have a great deal of raw vegetables for this body—as celery. Take raw, with dressing, and oft with gelatin. Do preserve the juices with them when these are prepared in this manner in the gelatin.

8/10/43
CHILDBIRTH: AFTEREFFECTS **F. 44 yrs.**
ELIMINATIONS **3148-1**

Also it would help to keep better eliminations for the body regularly. These may be controlled best, as we find, for this particular body by the diet. So include often in the diet celery. These may be grated or cut very fine and used with mayonnaise or an oil dressing; not to "burn out" with same as some might do, but change them as to their usage, and we shall find it will change the general elimination and increase the strengthening of the body, relieving those tensions that cause pressures to the head and to the secondary nervous system of the body.

4/17/31
DEBILITATION: GENERAL **M. 19 yrs.**
CHOREA **1225-1**

Noon—We would give those that carry more of the silicon, lime, salts—*these,* as we find, will be in the *green* vegetables. These in the form of salads, with any of the dressings that may make the salad the more palatable, including in these plenty of celery—and *all* of the green vegetables.

5/31/44
F. 76 yrs.
ARTHRITIS **5175-1**

We would increase the amount of the vitamins which come and appear in celery, for these natures will bring eliminations for the body.

7/12/35
BODY-BUILDING **F. 23 yrs.**
DIS-EASE: CONTAGION: PREVENTIVE **480-19**

Keep closer to the alkaline diets; using vegetables particularly that carry iron, silicon, phosphorus and the like—and these as we have indicated.

Q. Are inoculations against contagious diseases necessary for me before sailing in September?

A. As we find, only where the requirements are such as to *demand* same would this be adhered to at all. So far as the body-physical condition is concerned, the adherence to the use of celery *every* day at a meal or as a portion of the meal will insure against any contagious infectious forces with which the body may be in contact.

Q. Can immunization against them be set up in any other manner than by inoculations?

A. As indicated, if an alkalinity is maintained in the system—especially with celery, these in the blood supply will maintain such a condition as to immunize a person.

11/3/43
M. 54 yrs.
GLANDS: ADRENALS: THYROID: GLAUCOMA **3276-1**

To be sure, have plenty of vegetables, especially such as celery. A great deal of these combined with gelatin and gelatin preparations would be well. These we would include in the diet.

9/12/37
BLOOD: COAGULATION: POOR **F. 62 yrs.**
ACIDITY & ALKALINITY **1411-2**

Noons—Use green vegetables, raw, or salads, or sandwiches provided these are preferably of the celery.

9/29/32
F. Adult
OBESITY **4784-1**

Noons—A whole green vegetable salad, with a little of the oils, or mayonnaise that is made of oils, as dressing. Use as many as three to four or five vegetables, see? Those below the ground may be taken in the fresh vegetable salad at the noon meals; as celery, or the like, but not in the evening meals with meats or green cooked vegetables.

2/23/25
ASSIMILATIONS: ELIMINATIONS: INCOORDINATION **M. 46 yrs.**
BODY-BUILDING **3190-2**

Q. What special foods would give to the mind and body great strength, endurance and activity?

A. All of the vegetables, especially those of celery and of the like nature. Celery.

Q. What should the body do to reach its normal weight?

A. Keep the system in that as we have given, so we will bring the conditions necessary for rebuilding in system, for as we find, the body has reached that condition in the general system where the glands of body, the tissue in the arterial system, must be stimulated to give the correct incentives. This we will find through properties as given, and correct living.

NERVOUS SYSTEM: INCOORDINATION **5/19/30**
NEUROSIS **M. 50 yrs.**
NERVE-BUILDING **5475-2**

Q. Outline proper diet for body.

A. That as will give to the nerve system more of the *energy* as is necessary. That is, those of the vegetables that are nerve-building. Those that do not carry too much of the value of just weight, but that carry more *with* same that as is *assimilated* in system. As may be illustrated in this: In those of the green vegetables, those of the celery; these do not carry so much dross, but are *mostly* all assimilated, see?

4/1/31
APOPLEXY **M. 52 yrs.**
NERVE-BUILDING **3747-1**

The diets will be along those lines that make for nerve-*building*. Plenty of the green foods—as celery.

4/6/44
F. 62 yrs.
NERVE-BUILDING **4033-1**

Q. Please suggest foods to stress and foods to avoid in the diet.

A. In the diet there should be the stressing of those that are nerve-building. Vegetables that are raw, especially such as celery.

2/23/35
DERMATITIS **M. Adult**
BLOOD: HUMOR: MENU: PSORIASIS **840-1**

Noons—Preferably raw fresh vegetables; none cooked at this meal. These would consist of celery or the like that make for purifying of the *humor* in the lymph blood as this is absorbed by the lacteal ducts as it is digested. We would not take any quantities of soups or broths at this period.

4/19/21
M. Adult
BLOOD-BUILDING **4867-1**

To clarify the bloodstream and to take on more vitamins will be found rather in the vegetable diet, that especially of celery and such as that. Of course, others may be taken in moderation, but principally such as these given.

3/1/41
F. Adult
ARTHRITIS: NEURITIS: TENDENCIES **838-3**

DO have at least once a day with the meal a raw vegetable salad, especially with such as celery. These should be a part of the diet to aid in better stimulation for that being accomplished by the properties to set up eliminations and to purify the system, and also to aid that accomplished from the osteopathic adjustments AND the relaxing with the Infra Red Light treatments.

This does not mean, of course, that these are to be the ONLY foods taken. We merely give a list of the DO'S and the DON'TS.

12/15/27
M. 30 yrs.
ASTHENIA **4605-1**

As for the diet, let that be principally of that as almost pre-digested foods—though as much of raw vegetables as may be well taken, carrying plenty of iron and of salts; such as celery . . .

Do not take sedatives so much, though soda—plain bicarbonate of soda—may be taken in small quantities for same, *provided* the foods taken carry sufficient iron and salt and salts, or vegetable and fruit salts.

2/15/39
F. 52 yrs.
NEURASTHENIA **920-13**

And when the celery is selected, use the green portion rather than that which has been bleached. These portions have from twenty to forty percent more of the vitamins necessary for the sustaining of the better health, than those portions that are bleached by being covered or being forced into such a state.

9/25/42
APPENDIX: INTESTINES: COLON: PLETHORA **F. 32 yrs.**
NEURASTHENIA **2501-12**

Q. What can be done for extreme nervousness?

A. Taking or having in the diet plenty of celery juices, celery soups, celery raw, celery cooked. These would aid very much for this body.

3/21/39
F. 49 yrs.
RELAXATION **1158-21**

Q. Raw celery?

A. This should be taken with other foods, rather than by itself, two or three times a week.

2/23/25
M. 20 yrs.
BODY-BUILDING **77-2**

Q. What special foods should be given the body that would give to the mind and body strength, endurance and activity?

A. Green vegetable forces of every character, especially those of the tuberous nature. Of course some portions of them are cooked, the greater number eaten raw. Celery, those of that nature.

2/5/42
F. 24 yrs.
INJURIES **2679-1**

Q. Should vitamin capsules be continued?

A. The assimilation of the vitamins through the use of the proper food values is much preferable.

Q. Any raw foods especially to be recommended?

A. Especially celery. Every day. Not all at once, but some at one meal every day.

10/20/43
ASSIMILATIONS: POOR **F. 73 yrs.**
BODY-BUILDING **3304-1**

Keep to the body-building forces in the diet. Plenty of raw vegetables, such as celery. These supply silicon, as well as that needed in other energies to replenish the body.

5/29/30
M. 28 yrs.
BLOOD-BUILDING **102-2**

Take those that are not just *fat*-building, but *nerve*-building, and those that carry some, as may be termed, *just fodder* in the system; as will be seen in those of lots of celery, and such—that are taken as *green* vegetables.

3/23/40
F. 12 yrs.
EPILEPSY **2153-1**

Have plenty of the vitamins, especially of foods that carry B, B-1, A, C and D. Such would be included, of course, in plenty of raw vegetables—as celery. These raw, you see, and grated very fine, or the juice extracted from same—not large quantities taken (of the juices) but a little bit each day.

7/26/40
F. 12 yrs.
EPILEPSY **2153-1**

Noons—let the principal portion consist of celery, with some fruit juices or vegetable juices, or soup.

3/26/44
M. 39 yrs.
ADHESIONS: LESIONS **4017-1**

The diet should consist of liquids and semi-liquids, principally. Do use a great deal of the body-building foods such as vegetable juices; as celery. These may be prepared not only in a juicer, but oft prepared in a salad, very finely ground and using the juices with same prepared in gelatin, so that there will be these activities through the body.

3/28/44
M. 41 yrs.
ACIDITY & ALKALINITY **4008-1**

Q. Is there any combination of foods that could be truthfully called Brain Foods, Nerve Foods, Muscle Foods?

A. Those that are body-building; those that are nerve-building and those that supply certain elements. Vegetables that carry certain chemicals, as celery are especially nerve-building and supply the vitamins called the B and B-Complex, or B combinations.

12/8/39
M. 32 yrs.
PINWORMS **1597-2**

As to the diet, following the three-day apple diet, let there be more of vegetables, and the supplying forces as will create iron, silicon and the like for the system. Hence we would include a great deal of celery.

11/28/22
F. Adult
ANEMIA **4439-1**

Use whole wheat bread and vegetables that carry a high percentage of carbons such as celery.

6/9/27
F. 1 yr.
BABY CARE **608-1**

Q. What foods may be given the child besides the Mellin's Food?

A. Any foods that are of easy digestion. Celery—raw may be given, as much as eaten by the developing child, see? Not prepared in any special way and manner, but as may be taken in small quantity by the one using same.

1/30/28
F. Adult
ELIMINATIONS: POOR: TOXEMIA **81-2**

It would be necessary to meet the needs of the assimilation and of elimination of the blood and nerves center but one of those factors to chiefly consider is the diet. This would be found in chiefly the green vegetables and of those cooked vegetables that carry an amount of iron and such as found in the green vegetables such as celery, and all such vegetables.

10/17/34
F. 40 yrs.
HYPOCHONDRIA **1000-2**

In the matter of the diets . . . those of the phosphorus nature, and of those that carry these properties as are necessary—the creation with the chlorine foods carry the gold in its combination—follow these closely.

Q. What foods contain gold, silicon and phosphorus?

A. These are contained more in those of the celery—all such. Much of these depend on where the vegetation is grown, as to the character of forces that are carried in same.

7/22/31
ASSIMILATIONS: DEBILITATION: GENERAL **F. 28 yrs.**
BLOOD-BUILDING **3842-1**

We would give a diet that is easily assimilated. Let the diet be that as is nerve- and blood-building. And vegetables, as plenty of celery and the leafy vegetables.

1/12/40
F. 27 yrs.
NEURASTHENIA **2076-1**

Throughout this period the diet should consist more of the forces as in vitamin B-1. Plenty of celery. These especially should be taken daily, either in a raw salad or cooked, or the juices extracted in a juicer and taken in small quantities.

7/28/43
ANEMIA **F. 56 yrs.**
GENERAL: MULTIPLE SCLEROSIS **3118-1**

In the diet—keep to those things that heal within and without. A great deal of celery. These, of course, are to be used in sufficient quantity to satisfy the appetite but not to make them become as something disliked. So prepare them in many different forms.

10/11/43
F. 26 yrs.
ARTHRITIS **3285-1**

We should have easily assimilated foods, but those very high in the adding of B-Complex, or the vitamin B—as in celery. These should be a part of the diet daily with plenty of seafoods (not fresh water fish).

4/29/42
F. 37 yrs.
GLAUCOMA **630-3**

The condition to aid, then, is the DIET—AND that which IS a stimuli to the glandular forces AND the forces of body where assimilations are carried on.

Each day have plenty of quantities of celery.

2/17/39
M. 48 yrs.
BLOOD: COAGULATION: POOR **1787-3**

Be sure there is plenty of celery, as a part of the diet. This will enable the blood supply to be so improved as to make better coagulation when such would be necessary.

10)—Corn (A Grain)

10/5/36
F. 42 yrs.
CIRCULATION: POOR **1016-1**

Q. Any other advice as to diet?

A. As indicated from the slowed circulation, and the tendencies at times for the acidity, those things that pertain more to the alkaline-reacting diet would be the better. Rather would we give those things that the body should be warned against, and then most everything else may be taken . . . if it is taken in moderation, and *when* there is the *desire!* As there is the desire for food, whether it is the regular mealtime or at others, it would be best for *this* body to eat! If it desires to eat this or that, eat it! but do not mix it with other foods! Beware of certain food values in combination, as rice and corn at the same meal. Do not include too much of these, or scarcely any of these in the diet.

5/20/39
F. Adult

ANEMIA: ELIMINATIONS 1779-3

These as we find we would take, now, rather in periods—not merely as a routine; for these will aid not only in building resistance through portions of the system where there is the greater need of the more perfect circulation but will enable the digestive system to assimilate more of the iron as well as silicon for the system. These are necessary elements.

Hence we will find that the fresh vegetables—especially such as corn will be especially good as a part of the diet, regularly.

7/15/41
F. 61 yrs.

DEBILITATION: GENERAL 2535-1

In the matter of diet—take more of those foods that carry greater quantity of vitamin B-1—such as found in those foods that are yellow in color. Thus, yellow corn—these should form not the whole but a great deal of the diet.

3/15/37

BLOOD: HUMOR F. 56 yrs.

TOXEMIA 569-25

Q. What cooked vegetables may be taken?

A. Canned corn in minute quantities may be taken; that is, once or twice a week and not large quantities then.

11/29/40
F. 31 yrs.

ANEMIA 2414-1

Have plenty of all characters of foods that carry vitamins B-1 and G. As in corn or corn meal, using only the yellow variety. These will be found to be MOST beneficial, most agreeable, and easily digested.

7/23/43

ARTHRITIS F. 59 yrs.

ACIDITY 3110-1

Some proteins should be taken, but these should be included in the vegetables—in the manner in which they are prepared. Use more of the leafy variety than those of the bulbular or seed nature. Take a great deal of corn. These especially should be often a part of the diet.

12/28/38
F. 21 yrs.

HAY FEVER 1771-1

As to the diet—keep at least an eighty percent alkaline-producing diet to a twenty percent acid-producing. The plain foods are much preferable for the body; or, as would be expressed in some sections, plenty of corn and hominy would be well for the body—if it is prepared properly.

6/25/34
M. Adult

ASTHMA 595-1

Be mindful with the diet, that there are not those things that will tend to make for irritation to the respiratory system or the bronchi itself; that is, never too much of the tuberous nature of vegetables, and no hog meat—save there may be taken a little crisp bacon of mornings at times. More of the leafy vegetables, and not too much of those that are of the too great quantity of starch; though corn may be taken in moderation, especially the roasting ears if they are *boiled*—not fried, but boiled! Then the corn may be cut off the cob and prepared in that manner for the body, or it may be eaten off the cob. But the mastication of the food for this body should be the greater principle. Chew any mouthful of food at least fourteen times.

And this will bring very great relief to the body.

11)—Eggplant

3/15/37
BLOOD: HUMOR **F. 56 yrs.**
TOXEMIA **569-25**

The eggplant to be sure will assist. These should be taken about once a week, and with the effluvia as produced by their activities and other eliminating properties that are to be a portion of the activity, will work well together if they are taken about this often.

10/21/32
ELEPHANTIASIS: TENDENCIES **F. 18 yrs.**
ARTHRITIS: GLANDS: INCOORDINATION **951-1**

Supply an overabundant amount of those foods that carry iron, iodine and phosphorus in the system.

The evening meal may be of well-balanced vegetables that are of the leafy nature, and that carry more of those properties as given. We will find much in eggplant (no cabbage of any nature, either cold or cooked).

10/17/34
F. 40 yrs.
HYPOCHONDRIA **1000-2**

In the matter of the diets . . . those of the phosphorus nature, and of those that carry these properties as are necessary—the creation with the chlorine foods carry the gold in its combination—follow these closely.

Q. What foods contain gold, silicon and phosphorus?

A. These are contained more in those of the vegetable eggplants at times—parts of those depend on where they are grown—much of these depend upon where the vegetation is grown, as to the character of forces that are carried in same.

12)—Kale

3/21/39
M. 9 yrs.
DIABETES: TENDENCIES **415-7**

Evenings—Vegetables—preferably those that grow above the ground. Kale, these should be a part of the diet. No fried foods at any of the meals.

3/9/37
F. 71 yrs.
ARTHRITIS 1224-2

The vegetables would be cooked preferably in Patapar paper, served in their own juices—or serve them with same, see? Hence not any of the dried seeds or beans or the like would be included, but rather the fresh vegetables—plenty of kale well cooked in their *own* juices.

1/10/41
M. 60 yrs.
ELIMINATIONS: INCOORDINATION 1963-2

None of vegetables that are of the pod variety. Those of the natures that grow UNDER the ground are preferable, but plenty also of the leafy variety such as kale. These, too, should be prepared in their own juices—or in Patapar paper.

10/27/41
F. 31 yrs.
DERMATITIS: CIRCULATION: POOR 1688-8

Q. Are vegetables such as kale, etc., good for me now?

A. Good if these are well cooked, but not in a lot of grease. These should be cooked in their own juices and the juice taken as well as the vegetable. For, the effective or more healthful portions of kale is in the water that comes from same by cooking.

3/22/32
F. 42 yrs.
COLITIS 404-2

Q. Why cannot this body eat a cooked green vegetable, such as kale?

A. It may. Well these be added in the system—so that they will act with the gastric juices.

13)—Lentils

3/18/32
F. 38 yrs.
ADHESIONS: BLOOD-BUILDING 5515-1

Evenings—Cooked vegetables . . . those that are of the blood building in the vegetables—as of lentils.

12/2/37
F. 5 yrs.
COLD: COMMON 1490-1

In the matter of the diets, keep these well balanced in the body, blood and nerve building. Especially vegetables of the bulbous nature as lentils and the like.

10/4/35
ANEMIA M. 41 yrs.
DEBILITATION: GENERAL 1014-1

Vegetables, especially lentils. These should be the principal foods for the evening meals. Not too much, but satisfy the appetite.

12/30/42
M. 21 yrs.
BODY-BUILDING: LOCOMOTION: IMPAIRED **2873-1**

The food values should be those fully well balanced with calcium, iron, and especially the vitamins B-1 and the B-Complex. These are much preferable for the body.

At least three times each week, then, supply these from the foods rather than the reinforced vitamins (though these reinforcements may be desirable if there is the inability of the body to assimilate foods that carry excesses or the full quantity of such vital forces).

To be sure, these are not all the foods that are to be taken:

Noons—Have soups, broths or the like, and these should include mixed vegetables—but not too much of the dried vegetables; and lentils or such.

5/30/24
M. Adult
ASTHMA **4740-2**

Lentils, that character of foods may be eaten. Not much sweets but those that add nutriment to the system, without overtaxing the digestive organs in elimination.

10/11/37
DIABETES: TENDENCIES **M. 67 yrs,**
ACIDITY **1454-1**

Hence we would have the stimulating foods such as lentils in their combinations.

5/30/29
F. 31 yrs.
CONSTIPATION **1713-17**

A great deal of vegetables, especially those that give iron, as lentils.

3/25/30
ACIDITY & ALKALINITY **F. 45 yrs.**
DIGESTION: INDIGESTION **5625-1**

In the noon day those of the vegetables that care for the blood and nerve building, and that will produce not an overactivity but as a counter-*irritant* of activity in the kidneys, which will reduce the stimuli in the circulation in the hepatics. These we will find in those of the vegetable forces that grow especially in pods, as lentils. These also may be added in a consistent manner with those of the non-acid or of the alkaline-*producing* conditions for the system.

3/21/39
M. 9 yrs.
DIABETES: TENDENCIES **415-7**

Evenings—Vegetables—preferably those that grow above the ground. Lentils, these should be a part of the diet. No fried foods at any of the meals.

8/13/38
F. 45 yrs.
ARTHRITIS **1659-1**

As to diet, this should carry a great deal of the salts of vegetables AND fruits—rather than meats. Never any fried foods at any time. The vegetables should be cooked in their OWN juices—that is, in Patapar paper. The juices that come from same shall be well mixed with the vegetables themselves, so that the body gets the benefit of those; such as lentils—with their salts as come from same—after being well washed and cooked in the Patapar paper, but DO NOT put meat or anything of the kind in same. Season only with a little butter and sufficient salt or pepper to satisfy the appetite or to be palatable to the taste of the body.

6/3/41
DEBILITATION: GENERAL **M. 25 yrs.**
APPENDICITIS **1970-1**

(Do not begin this diet, of course, until after the period of the grape poultices and the grape diet.) Vegetables may then be taken, if cooked in their OWN salts, or their OWN juices—and eat the juices with same; cooking all in Patapar paper. Such as lentils.

9/1/39
M. 49 yrs.
PARKINSON'S DISEASE **1989-1**

Be mindful of the diet—that there are plenty of vitamins. Have plenty of green vegetables—as lentils—these cooked in their own salts (as in Patapar paper) saving the salts or the water in which such are cooked as a part of the diet.

11/18/30
F. 60 yrs.
ELIMINATIONS: POOR **505-1**

In the matter of diet—these, as we find, will be more of the well balanced that carry more of the irons in their reaction—as will be found in those of all the vegetable forces, as of lentils. Also, it will be found that little of the meats should be taken.

4/1/31
APOPLEXY **M. 52 yrs.**
NERVE-BUILDING **3747-1**

The diets will be along those lines that make for nerve *building.* Plenty of lentils, and such may be taken.

3/28/44
M. 41 yrs.
ACIDITY & ALKALINITY **4008-1**

Q. Is there any combination of foods that could be truthfully called Brain Foods, Nerve Foods, Muscle Foods?

A. Those that are body building; those that are nerve building and those that supply certain elements. Those foods that grow under the ground of certain characters, as well as lentils supply certain sulphurs as well as other elements that are needed in the body for better chemical balance.

7/22/31
ASSIMILATIONS: DEBILITATION: GENERAL **F. 28 yrs.**
BLOOD-BUILDING **3842-1**

We would give a diet that is easily assimilated. Let the diet be that as is nerve and blood building. And vegetables, lentils, and the like.

1/26/35
F. 59 yrs.
INJURIES **3823-2**

Evenings—A well-balanced vegetable diet. Fresh lentils may be a part of the diet, provided they are prepared in their *own* sauce—as cooked in Patapar paper, so that all the juices and vitamins may be retained in same.

2/23/25
M. 20 yrs.
BODY-BUILDING **77-2**

Q. What special foods should be given the body that would give to the mind and body strength, endurance and activity?

A. Green vegetable forces of every character, especially those of the tuberous nature. Of course, some portions of them are cooked, the greater number eaten raw. Lentils—those of that nature.

14)—Lettuce

1/5/36
F. 46 yrs.
COLITIS: TENDENCIES **404-6**

Q. Should plenty of lettuce be eaten?

A. Plenty of lettuce should always be eaten by most *every* body; for this supplies an effluvium in the bloodstream itself that is a destructive force to *most* of those influences that attack the bloodstream. It's a purifier.

5/29/30
M. 28 yrs.
BLOOD-BUILDING **102-2**

Take those that are not just *fat* building, but *nerve* building, and those that carry some, as may be termed, *just fodder* in the system; as will be seen in those of lots of lettuce, and especially of the lettuce that *does not* head.

9/2/29
CHILDREN: ABNORMAL **M. 7 yrs.**
NERVOUS SYSTEMS: INCOORDINATION **758-2**

Those that are a stimuli for the nerve system are lettuce—lettuce especially . . .

9/25/37
SPINE: SUBLUXATIONS **F. 35 yrs.**
MINERALS **903-25**

There is first an unbalancing of the elements in the activities of the system—or lack of sufficient calcium for the full activity of body building.

Hence there should be the use of the food values that carry such in such measures as may be assimilated by the body. Those as we find in lettuce especially should be a portion of the diet.

10/20/43
ASSIMILATIONS: POOR **F. 73 yrs.**
BODY-BUILDING **3304-1**

Keep to the body-building forces in the diet. Plenty of raw vegetables, such as lettuce. These supply silicon, as well as that needed in other energies to replenish the body.

ANEMIA: TENDENCIES **10/2/43**
ASSIMILATIONS: ELIMINATIONS: INCOORDINATION **F. 37 yrs.**
KIDNEYS **1695-2**

Then take at least once each day the vitamin B-1. Do not take A.

Do take D and G, but these more in the foods than supplementing in the combinations. These will bring better forces to the body; that is, in the food values take plenty of lettuce.

1/25/33
F. 44 yrs.
GLANDS: INCOORDINATION **757-3**

Noons—Preferably a whole *green* vegetable diet, consisting of such as lettuce, or any of those that make for the weight—as well as a balance of the diets that produce the *cleansing* effects throughout the system, see?

Evenings—Vegetables *well* cooked, but be sure that for each vegetable used that grows under the ground there are *two* used that grow *above* the ground, either in leafy vegetables or the pod vegetables, see?

7/27/39
F. 27 yrs.
DEBILITATION: GENERAL **480-52**

Keep a general upbuilding in the diet, by the body-building influences. Have plenty of lettuce, cole or raw cabbage with same occasionally.

These as we find should bring much better results and experiences for the body.

1/4/40
ATROPHY: NERVES **M. 32 yrs.**
NERVES: REBUILDING **849-47**

The DIET—this must be, as the rest, CONSISTENTLY, PERSISTENTLY, followed.

Take more of the vegetable forces that are life giving in their assimilation through the body; more lettuce. These should be combined to make the greater part of one meal each day; or they may be taken with EACH meal if it is the more preferable. They MUST BE TAKEN, if there will be better recuperative forces, or the supplying to the system of properties and energies that are to be the real HEALING forces!

For here alone (in the diet) will there be the coming of curative or healing powers. All the rest are for the PREPARATIONS of the body for the USAGE of energies in food values, which may be had from those foods indicated to be supplied.

8/19/35
ASSIMILATIONS: POOR **F. 80 yrs.**
CANCER **975-1**

Noons—Preferably only the juices of, or very finely grated raw vegetables, such as lettuce. These may be taken with or without the salad dressing. Or this may be altered at times to the juices only of the *cooked* vegetables; or there may be had two or more vegetables combined to make for balancing of the elements in the body that are necessary, carrying silicon and iron that are as resistive forces and aids in the blood supply to eradicate these disturbing forces in the system.

6/4/26
M. 54 yrs.
BLOOD-BUILDING **4769-2**

Let the diet be vegetable foods of that that grows *above* the ground. All that of the pod nature, see? Lettuce, and those of that nature. Not any tuberous nature.

12/30/42
M. 21 yrs.
BODY-BUILDING: LOCOMOTION: IMPAIRED **2873-1**

The food values should be those fully well balanced with calcium, iron, and especially the vitamins B-1 and the B-Complex. These are much preferable for the body.

At least three times each week, then, supply these from the foods rather than the reinforced vitamins (though these reinforcements may be desirable if there is the inability of the body to assimilate foods that carry excesses or the full quantity of such vital forces).

Noons—At least a portion of this meal should include lettuce. Arrange it differently so it does not become abhorrent to the body; sometimes in the regular state, other times grated, other times prepared in juice form.

4/28/42
F. 7 yrs.
EYES **2004-4**

Q. What further treatment should be applied for her eye condition?

A. A gentle massage given of evenings would be very well . . . And give the body PLENTY of lettuce. Have some of these in the meal each day.

BLINDNESS: TENDENCIES: GLAUCOMA **4/21/44**
DEBILITATION: GENERAL **F. 80 yrs.**
EYES **5059-1**

Supply energies in the body through a great deal more of raw vegetables rather than meats for this body. Do have the vegetables often such as lettuce. Not so as to become obnoxious to the body, but supply these elements often for the body.

6/25/40
F. 55 yrs.
ANEMIA **2287-1**

Then, as to the diet, we would add more of the foods that carry vitamins B and B-1, with also G and M—which would be all of those vegetables that are yellow in nature—not only in color but in nature.

Once each day one meal should consist principally of lettuce.

1/17/44
F. 44 yrs.
ANEMIA **3564-1**

Keep plenty of raw vegetables; as lettuce. Not necessarily at any one period but some every day. Often prepare these with gelatin—about three times a week, for gelatin also is needed in the body. Grate them, slice them, dice them, changing their manner of preparation so as not to become objectionable.

11/21/43
COLD: CONGESTION **F. 59 yrs.**
ACIDITY **462-18**

Don't overeat, don't have too much of vegetables or of pastries or of meats, but keep them well balanced. Have a great deal of lettuce, mixed with gelatin. These are good for the body. They will aid in all portions of the sensory system, especially in the eyes, the ears, and the drainages through the antrum and the soft tissue of head; for these supply elements that keep these portions of the body bettered.

5/30/29
F. 31 yrs.
CONSTIPATION **1713-17**

A great deal of vegetables, especially those that give iron, as lettuce.

2/17/39
M. 48 yrs.
BLOOD: COAGULATION: POOR **1787-3**

Be sure there is plenty of green or leaf lettuce taken as a part of the diet. This will enable the blood supply to be so improved as to make better coagulation when such would be necessary.

12/17/31
F. Adult
ACIDITY & ALKALINITY: PSORIASIS **5557-1**

At another period of the day let's have a great deal of the leafy and green vegetables such as lettuce and preferably that that does not head—for this body; more soporiferous than that of the iceberg.

5/19/30
NERVOUS SYSTEMS: INCOORDINATION: NEUROSIS **M. 50 yrs.**
NERVE-BUILDING **5475-2**

Q. Outline proper diet for body.

A. That as will give to the nerve system more of the *energy* as is necessary. That is, those of the vegetables that are nerve building. Those that do not carry too much of the value of just weight, but that carry more *with* same that as is *assimilated* in system. As may be illustrated in this: In those of the green vegetables, those of the lettuce—*head,* especially—for were the other character taken much by the body it would produce too much drowsiness.

8/24/44
F. 58 yrs.
ASTHENIA **5394-1**

In building up the body with foods, preferably have a great deal of raw vegetables for this body—as lettuce. Take raw, with dressing, and oft with gelatin. Do preserve the juices with them when these are prepared in this manner in the gelatin.

7/10/30
BLOOD-BUILDING **M. 65 yrs.**
ASSIMILATIONS **4806-1**

We would be mindful of the diet, that there are those of the full rebuilding—especially of those that build for the blood supply.

Then we would have, in the noon meal, those preferably of the vegetables that are raw, in part—and there may be added some seafoods, with oils as dressings for same. Plenty of lettuce, and such, in this meal.

5/31/44
F. 76 yrs.
ARTHRITIS **5175-1**

We would increase the amount of the vitamins which come and appear in lettuce, for these natures will bring eliminations for the body.

7/12/35
BODY-BUILDING **F. 23 yrs.**
DIS-EASE: CONTAGION: PREVENTIVE **480-19**

The diet should be more body-building; that is, less acid foods and more of the alkaline-reacting will be the better in these directions. Those food values carrying an easy assimilation of iron, silicon, and those elements or chemicals—as most all forms of vegetables that grow under the ground, most of the vegetables of a leafy nature. These should form a greater part of the regular diet in the present—and in the preparation for those activities to come later, whether in relationships in the physical manner or those in the mental forces that are necessary in such activities.

Keep closer to the alkaline diets; using vegetables particularly that carry iron, silicon, phosphorus and the like—and these as we have indicated.

Q. Are inoculations against contagious diseases necessary for me before sailing in September?

A. As we find, only where the requirements are such as to *demand* same would this be adhered to at all. So far as the body-physical condition is concerned, the adherence to the use of lettuce *every* day at a meal or as a portion of the meal will insure against any contagious infectious forces with which the body may be in contact.

Q. Can immunization against them be set up in any other manner than by inoculations?

A. As indicated, if an alkalinity is maintained in the system—especially with lettuce. These in the blood supply will maintain such a condition as to immunize a person.

4/29/42
F. 37 yrs.
GLAUCOMA 630-3

The condition to aid, then, is the DIET—AND that which IS a stimuli to the glandular forces AND the forces of body where assimilations are carried on.

Each day have plenty or quantities of lettuce.

11/3/43
M. 54 yrs.
GLANDS: ADRENALS: THYROID: GLAUCOMA 3276-1

To be sure, have plenty of vegetables, especially such as lettuce. A great deal of these combined with gelatin and gelatin preparations would be well. These we would include in the diet.

9/12/37
BLOOD: COAGULATION: POOR M. 62 yrs.
ACIDITY & ALKALINITY 1411-2

Noons—Use green vegetables, raw, or salads, or sandwiches provided these are preferably of the lettuce.

4/6/44
F. 62 yrs.
NERVE-BUILDING 4033-1

Q. Please suggest foods to stress and foods to avoid in the diet.

A. In the diet there should be the stressing of those that are nerve building. Vegetables that are raw, especially such as lettuce.

2/23/35
DERMATITIS M. Adult
BLOOD: HUMOR: MENU: PSORIASIS 840-1

Noons—Preferably raw fresh vegetables; none cooked at this meal. These would consist of lettuce, or the like, that make for purifying of the *humor* in the lymph blood as this is absorbed by the lacteal ducts as it is digested. We would not take any quantities of soups or broths at this period.

4/23/30
APOPLEXY: AFTEREFFECTS F. Adult
BLOOD-BUILDING 5667-1

We would be mindful of the diet, that it consists of much that grows *above* the ground, as of the lettuce, and such *green* vegetables. Any of the salads that carry large quantities of iron. Now this, apparently, would be the creating of blood, but blood of a character is needed, when the pressure is already abnormal.

3/18/32
F. 38 yrs.
ADHESIONS: BLOOD-BUILDING 5515-1

Evenings—Cooked vegetables . . . those that are of the blood building in the vegetables—as of lettuce. Not a great deal of any foods.

4/19/21
M. Adult
BLOOD-BUILDING 4867-1

To clarify the blood stream and to take on more vitamins will be found rather in the vegetable diet, that especially of lettuce, and such as that. Of course, others may be taken in moderation, but principally such as these given.

3/1/41
F. Adult
ARTHRITIS: NEURITIS: TENDENCIES 838-3

DO have at least once a day with the meal a raw vegetable salad, especially with such as lettuce. These should be a part of the diet to aid in better stimulation—for that being accomplished by the properties to set up eliminations and to purify the system, and also to aid that accomplished from the osteopathic adjustments AND the relaxing with the Infra Red Light treatments.

This does not mean, of course, that these are to be the ONLY foods taken. We merely give a list of the DO'S and the DON'TS.

12/15/27
M. 30 yrs.
ASTHENIA 4605-1

As for the diet, let that be principally of that as almost pre-digested foods—though as much of raw vegetables as may be well taken, carrying plenty of iron and of salts; such as lettuce.

7/28/43
F. 56 yrs.
ANEMIA 3118-1

In the diet—keep to those things that heal within and without. A great deal of lettuce. These, of course, are to be used in sufficient quantity to satisfy the appetite but not to make any of them become as something disliked.

2/15/39
F. 52 yrs.
NEURASTHENIA 920-13

And when lettuce is selected, use the green portion rather than that which has been bleached. These portions have from twenty to forty percent more of the vitamins necessary for the sustaining of the better health, than those portions that are bleached by being covered or being forced into such a state.

12/18/30
M. 24 yrs.
BACILLOSIS: POLIOMYELITIS 135-1

Noon—More of the vegetables that are *raw.* These may be made into salads with salad dressings, especially with as much of the olive oil as is palatable and that will be assimilated with the character of foods. This would include lettuce, and all of those that may be used as such.

2/5/42
F. 24 yrs.
INJURIES 2679-1

Q. Should vitamin capsules be continued?

A. The assimilation of the vitamins through the use of the proper food values is much preferable.
Q. Any raw foods especially to be remembered?
A. Especially lettuce. Every day. Not all at once, but some at one meal every day.

3/23/40
F. 12 yrs.
EPILEPSY **2153-1**
Have plenty of the vitamins, especially of foods that carry B, B-1, A, C and D. Such would be included, of course; in plenty of raw vegetables—as lettuce; these raw, you see, and grated very fine, or the juice extracted from same—not large quantities taken (of the juices) but a little bit each day.

7/26/40
F. 12 yrs.
EPILEPSY **2153-2**
Noons—Let the principal portion consist of lettuce with some fruit juices or vegetable juices, or soup.

3/26/44
M. 39 yrs.
ADHESIONS: LESIONS **4017-1**
The diet should consist of liquids and semi-liquids, principally. Do use a great deal of the body-building foods such as vegetable juices; as lettuce. These may be prepared not only in a juicer, but oft prepared in a salad, very finely ground and using the juices with same prepared in gelatin, so that there will be these activities through the body.

4/7/37
F. 29 yrs.
COLD: CONGESTION: AFTEREFFECTS **808-6**
Q. Is my present diet correct?
A. As indicated it is very good, though there may be a little change to the fresh vegetables. Lettuce may be taken, either green, cooked, or in whatever way is most palatable for the body.

3/28/44
M. 41 yrs.
ACIDITY & ALKALINITY **4008-1**
Q. Is there any combination of foods that could be truthfully called Brain Foods, Nerve Foods, Muscle Foods?
A. Those that are body building; those that are nerve building and those that supply certain elements. Vegetables that carry certain chemicals, as lettuce are especially nerve building and supply the vitamins called the B and B-complex, or B combinations.

12/8/39
M. 32 yrs.
PINWORMS **1597-2**
As to the diet, following the three-day apple diet, let there be more of vegetables, and the supplying forces as will create iron, silicon and the like for

the system. Hence we would include a great deal of lettuce.

6/9/27
F. 1 yr.
BABY CARE **608-1**

Lettuce, raw may be given, as much as eaten by the developing child, see? Not prepared in any special way and manner, but as may be taken in small quantity by the one using same.

10/17/34
F. 40 yrs.
HYPOCHONDRIA **1000-2**

In the matter of the diet . . . those of the phosphorus nature, and of those that carry these properties as are necessary—the creation with the chlorine foods carry the gold in its combination—follow these closely.

Q. What foods contain gold, silicon and phosphorus?

A. These are contained more in those of the lettuce. Much of these depend on where the vegetation is grown, as to the character of forces that are carried in same.

7/22/31
ASSIMILATIONS: DEBILITATION: GENERAL **F. 28 yrs.**
BLOOD-BUILDING **3842-1**

We would give a diet that is easily assimilated. Let the diet be that as is nerve and blood building. And vegetables, lettuce and the like.

8/10/43
CHILDBIRTH: AFTEREFFECTS **F 44 yrs.**
ELIMINATIONS **3148-1**

Also it would help to keep better eliminations for the body regularly. These may be controlled best, as we find, for this particular body by the diet. So include often in the diet lettuce. These may be grated or cut very fine and used with mayonnaise or an oil dressing; not to "burn out" with same as some might do, but change them as to their usage, and we shall find it will change the general elimination and increase the strengthening of the body, relieving those tensions that cause pressures to the head and to the secondary nervous system of the body.

1/12/40
F. 27 yrs.
NEURASTHENIA **2076-1**

Throughout this period the diet should consist more of the forces as in vitamin B-1; plenty of lettuce. These especially should be taken daily, either in a raw salad or cooked, or the juices extracted in a juicer and taken in small quantities.

10/11/43
F. 26 yrs.
ARTHRITIS **3285-1**

We would have easily assimilated foods, but those very high in the adding of B Complex, or the vitamin B—as in lettuce. These should be a part of the diet daily with plenty of seafoods (not fresh water fish).

i)—Lettuce and Cabbage

1/9/35
M. 1 yr.
WORMS **786-1**

As we find with this body, the affectations are from the activity of not the stomach but intestinal infections—from a form of worms, that make for the irritations, for the lack of appetite and at other times an overappetite; at times the belching up of foods and the spitting up, restlessness at night, the inability for the body to be as active and tendency for the cold and congestion through the system. These are the conditions as we find that affect the body; these make for the quick pulsations at times, a little rise of temperature that comes at times, irritation in the throat, the irritation in the mucous membranes of the nostrils and face, the overactivity at times of the kidneys, the effect produced upon the eliminations, and especially a peculiar color and odor that is indicated from the stool.

In meeting these conditions for this body, as we find, we would first give that for a whole day the body should be fed only—with some malted milk, or the like—green lettuce and green cabbage. Then in the evening of that same day we would give, under the direction of a physician only, a small dose of calomel and santonin; about four grains of the calomel with about one and one-half grains of the santonin.

These we would follow in the next day with very small broken doses of Fletcher's Castoria, to make for the settling of the stomach and for the toning of the digestive system. Give about a quarter to half a teaspoonful every half hour until there has been indicated the activity from the system of the Castoria by the change in the temperature and the quietness to the body, see?

Q. How may you get a child of this age to eat green lettuce and green cabbage?

A. It'll have to be cut up and seasoned, and taken. It won't take a large quantity, but it is the effect of these that we need for the activity of the calomel and santonin to have its effect upon the infesting forces of the body.

15)—Mustard Greens

3/8/35
F. 37 yrs.
ARTHRITIS **631-6**

Noons—Preferably the entirely green raw vegetables, such as raw mustard. These may be taken with whole wheat wafers with a mayonnaise or salad dressing.

1/17/44
F. 44 yrs.
ANEMIA **3564-1**

Keep plenty of raw vegetables; as mustard. Not necessarily at any one period but some every day. Often prepare these with gelatin—about three times a week, for gelatin also is needed in the body. Grate them, slice them, dice them, changing their manner of preparation so as not to become objectionable.

1/25/33
F. 44 yrs.
GLANDS: INCOORDINATION **757-3**

Noons—Preferably a whole *green* vegetable diet, any of those that make for the weight as well as a balance of the diets that produce the *cleansing* effects throughout the system, see? Mustard greens—*any* of these. And there may be used with these a French dressing or mayonnaise, to make them more palatable.

7/30/41
M. 26 yrs.
ANESTHESIA: AFTEREFFECTS **1710-6**

Q. Please give further corrective diet.

A. As indicated, it is necessary in the present to add plenty of the elements found in salads. Not that the body is to live off these entirely, to be sure, but these are to be in the diet often—two to three times a week as a part of some meal during the day. The general diet should be for body-building. Be sure that most of the foods carry especially vitamin B. These are best found in mustard and the like.

8/19/35
ASSIMILATIONS: POOR **F. 80 yrs.**
CANCER **975-1**

Noons—Preferably only the juices of, or very finely grated raw vegetables; such as mustard or the like. These may be taken with or without the salad dressing. Or this may be altered at times to the juices only of the *cooked* vegetables; or there may be had two or more vegetables combined to make for balancing of the elements in the body that are necessary, carrying silicon and iron that are as resistive forces and aids in the blood supply to eradicate these disturbing forces in the system.

1/10/41
M. 60 yrs.
ELIMINATIONS: INCOORDINATION **1963-2**

None of vegetables that are of the pod variety. Those of the natures that grow UNDER the ground are preferable, but plenty also of the leafy variety, such as mustards and the like. These, too, should be prepared in their own juices—or in Patapar paper.

6/3/41
DEBILITATION: GENERAL **M. 25 yrs.**
APPENDICITIS **1970-1**

(Do not begin this diet, of course, until after the period of the grape poultices and the grape diet.) Vegetables may bo then taken, if cooked in their OWN salts, or their OWN juices—and eat the juices with same; cooking all in Patapar paper. Such as mustard.

7/30/41
M. 26 yrs.
ANESTHESIA: AFTEREFFECTS **1710-6**

The general diet should be for body-building. Be sure that most of the foods carry especially vitamin B. These are best found in vegetables of the yellow variety, as well as in mustard and the like.

4/18/35
ANEMIA **M. Adult**
MENU: ASSIMILATIONS: POOR **898-1**

The evening meal should consist of the vegetables, especially such as mustard, all the leafy vegetables and all the bulbular nature save the white potatoes.

Keep these consistently, persistently; we will gain weight, we will put off this dullness, this tendency for catching cold, this weakness throughout the whole system; and bring the body—in six to eight months—to its normal weight of about a hundred and fifty pounds.

2/23/35
DERMATITIS **M. Adult**
BLOOD: HUMOR: MENU: PSORIASIS **840-1**

Noons—Preferably raw fresh vegetables; none cooked at this meal. These would consist of mustard, or the like, that make for purifying of the *humor* in the lymph blood as this is absorbed by the lacteal ducts as it is digested. We would not take any quantities of soups or broths at this period.

5/6/43
F. 37 yrs.
OBESITY **2988-1**

But do take, at least once each day . . . mustard and such greens as are taken raw. These may be taken with oil or with any salad dressing to suit the taste.

8/23/27
DIABETES: TENDENCIES **M. 26 yrs.**
ELIMINATIONS: INCOORDINATION **4145-1**

Q. Does this body have any habits indulged in excessively?

A. Too much of those as is seen in the *manner* of eating, and in that of the imbibing of those conditions that produce too much reaction from alcoholic condition *in* the system. Not as the excess of alcohol as consumed, but excess of alcohol as produced by the way and manner of eating, and by the indulging in those conditions that produce alcoholic reaction in the system itself.

The diet shall be those principally of vegetables, and especially of greens—mustard—all of those properties as carry much iron.

8/13/38
F. 45 yrs.
ARTHRITIS **1659-1**

As to diet, this should carry a great deal of the salts of vegetables AND fruits—rather than meats. Never any fried foods at any time. The vegetables would be cooked in their OWN juices—that is, in Patapar paper. The juices that come from same shall be well mixed with the vegetables themselves, so that the body gets the benefit of those; such as mustard—with their salts as come from same—after being well washed and cooked in the Patapar paper, but DO NOT put meat or anything of the kind in same. Season only with a little butter and sufficient salt or pepper to satisfy the appetite or to be palatable to the taste of the body.

7/30/41
M. 26 yrs.
ANESTHESIA: BODY-BUILDING **1710-6**

The general diet should be for body-building. Be sure that most of the foods that carry especially vitamin B. These are found in vegetables of the yellow variety, as well as in mustard and the like.

16)—Okra

4/8/38
F. 48 yrs.
ANEMIA **694-4**

In the diet, too often the inclinations have been for not sufficient of the body-building forces. Hence as we find, all those foods carrying quantities of gluten as okra, as well as those natures as from any of the forms of gelatins or the combinations of same—should be a portion of the diet.

Q. Do I need a tonic containing iron? If so, please prescribe.

A. As we find, the glutens as with the foods indicated should be sufficient. In the present there are too many poisons in the system for a tonic to be assimilated properly. However, after the flushing of the system, a tonic would be most beneficial.

6/20/39
M. 32 yrs.
ARTHRITIS **849-37**

At least once every day try—at least—to eat some okra. This is well also to keep that necessary for the very activities as will come with the general system.

6/12/39
F. 40 yrs.
ANEMIA **1387-2**

Through the summer periods include a great deal of gumbo, or okra.

8/15/38
DIARRHEA **F. 52 yrs.**
BODY-BUILDING **560-8**

In the matter of the diets, keep those that are body-building. Plenty of okra once or twice a day, with beef juices—these would supply gluten as well as the necessary forces for the better coagulation in the activities of the lymph and the circulatory forces in the blood supply.

10/7/40
F. 23 yrs.
ANEMIA **2376-1**

Have plenty of okra whenever possible, even though it is canned, but not that which has vinegar in same. These and such characters, provided they are not fried, should be a portion of the diet—though, to be sure, not all of the diet.

7/23/43
ARTHRITIS **F. 59 yrs.**
ACIDITY **3110-1**

Use more of the leafy variety than those of the bulbular or seed nature. Take a great deal of okra. These especially should be often a part of the diet.

8/10/43
CHILDBIRTH: AFTEREFFECTS **F. 44 yrs.**
ELIMINATIONS **3148-1**

Also it would help to keep better eliminations for the body regularly. These may be controlled best, as we find, for this particular body by the diet. So include often in the diet okra. We shall find it will change the general elimination and increase the strengthening of the body, relieving those tensions that cause pressures to the head and to the secondary nervous system of the body.

11/6/35
M. 24 yrs.
BODY-BUILDING **533-7**

In the diets keep those things that will agree, yet we will find it will be necessary to change; but that are body-building. Vegetables especially such as okra will supply the necessary influences, of course, with other things.

10/17/34
M. Adult
ANEMIA **698-1**

In the diet, keep much of that which will add more phosphorus and gold to the system; as we will find in certain of the vegetables—as okra, and the like. These should be a portion of the diet each day; not that it would be these *only*—but keep more of an alkaline diet.

8/27/40
F. 40 yrs.
ATHLETE'S FOOT: ECZEMA **2332-1**

Have plenty of vegetables, especially okra and the like.

17)—Onions: General

5/20/38
F. 68 yrs.
TOXEMIA **1593-1**

Onions boiled are very well for the body. These (the onions OR the artichoke) may be taken at the noon meal with the raw vegetables, or they may be a portion of the evening meal when leafy vegetables, well cooked, rather than those of the tuberous nature, would be taken. Have the proportion of at least five vegetables above the ground to one under the ground; and three of the leafy nature to two of the pod nature that grow above the ground. This does not mean that all of these varieties are to be had at one meal, but rather these proportions should be kept in the diet throughout.

ANEMIA: TENDENCIES **10/2/43**
ASSIMILATIONS: ELIMINATIONS: INCOORDINATION **F. 37 yrs.**
KIDNEYS **1695-2**

Then take at least once each day the vitamins B-1. Do not take A.

Do take D and G, but these more in the foods than supplementing in the combinations. These will bring better forces to the body; that is, in the food values take plenty of onions.

7/27/39
F. 27 yrs.
DEBILITATION: GENERAL **480-52**

Keep a general upbuilding in the diet, by the body-building influences. Plenty of onions, raw as well as cooked.

These as we find should bring much better results and experiences for the body.

8/19/35
ASSIMILATIONS: POOR **F. 80 yrs.**
CANCER **975-1**

Noons—Preferably only the juices of, or very finely grated raw vegetables; such as onions. Or this may be altered at times to the juices only of the *cooked* vegetable.

DEBILITATION: GENERAL **1/12/44**
GLAUCOMA **F. 58 yrs.**
EYES **3552-1**

And then in the general diet add a great deal of vegetables that have a direct bearing upon the optic forces through the general system; such as onions. These have a direct bearing upon the application of that assimilated for the optic forces.

3/9/37
F. 71 yrs.
ARTHRITIS **1224-2**

The vegetables would be cooked preferably in Patapar paper, served in their own juices—or serve them with same, see? Hence not any of the dried seeds or beans or the like would be included, but rather the fresh vegetables—plenty of onions well cooked in their *own* juices.

5/19/30
NERVOUS SYSTEMS: INCOORDINATION: NEUROSIS **F. 50 yrs.**
NERVE-BUILDING **5475-2**

Q. Outline proper diet for body.

A. That as will give to the nerve system more of the *energy* as is necessary. That is, those of the vegetables that are nerve building. Those that do not carry too much of the value of just weight, but that carry more *with* same that as is *assimilated* in system. As may be illustrated in this: In those of the green vegetables, those of the onion are *mostly* all assimilated, see?

9/2/29
CHILDREN: ABNORMAL **M. 7 yrs.**
NERVOUS SYSTEMS: INCOORDINATION **758-2**

Those that are a stimuli for the nerve system are onions—cooked, not raw—but the *juices* of same, in moderation . . .

8/31/41
ARTHRITIS: PREVENTIVE **F. 51 yrs.**
BODY: GENERAL **1158-31**

Q. Onions?

A. About twice or three times a week; cooked, and—if agreeable—raw once or twice.

10/20/34
ACIDITY: LESIONS **F. 48 yrs.**
ACIDITY **703-1**

Have at least three of the leafy vegetables to one below the ground, or with the leafy vegetables there may be one or two of the bulbous nature. Onions may be considered among these (but eat these only well-cooked, not raw).

7/25/36
F. 32 yrs.
KIDNEYS: PREGNANCY **540-6**

Keep a well-balance between the diets for sufficient calcium and lime; as in onions. Things of that nature carry these in such quantities that they may be easily assimilated. So let the foods that are prepared occasionally have more and more of these.

11/6/35
M. 24 yrs.
BODY-BUILDING **533-7**

In the diets keep those things that will agree, yet we will find it will be necessary to change; but that are body-building. Vegetables especially such as onions (boiled) will supply the necessary influence, of course with other things.

5/6/43
F. 37 yrs.
OBESITY **2988-1**

Little of pod vegetables; or as of onions, or the like.

4/19/41
F. 51 yrs.
ASSIMILATIONS **1158-30**

Q. Shall I supplement with additional vitamin B tablets?

A. We find that if this vitamin is supplied in the diet it will be better than taking an overquantity of vitamin B, which would be the case if the tablets were taken as a supplement. With the Adiron taken, that is to aid in assimilation, it would be better to supplement the vitamin B in the diet, with such as onions cooked and raw. These taken, as we find, with beef and fowl, should carry sufficient vitamins.

7/18/40
F. 39 yrs.
ASSIMILATIONS: ELIMINATIONS: INCOORDINATION 2309-1

Take plenty of food values that carry vitamin B-1 and G. No fried foods at any time. Plenty of boiled onions. These should be a part of the diet once or twice a week.

i)—Onions—Raw

3/26/44
M. 39 yrs.
ADHESIONS: LESIONS 4017-1

The diet should consist of liquids and semi-liquids, principally. Do use a great deal of the body-building foods such as vegetable juices; as onions. These may be prepared not only in a juicer, but oft prepared in a salad, very finely ground and using the juices with same prepared in gelatin, so that there will be these activities through the body.

2/23/35
M. Adult
BLOOD: HUMOR: MENU: PSORIASIS 840-1

Noons—Preferably raw fresh vegetables; none cooked at this meal. These would consist of onions, or the like (not cucumbers) that make for purifying of the *humor* in the lymph blood as this is absorbed by the lacteal ducts as it is digested. We would not take any quantities of soups or broths at this period.

3/8/35
F. 37 yrs.
ARTHRITIS 631-6

Noons—Preferably the entirely green raw vegetables, such as onions or onion tops. These may be taken with whole wheat wafers with a mayonnaise or salad dressing.

1/17/44
F. 44 yrs.
ANEMIA 3564-1

Keep plenty of raw vegetables; onions. Not necessarily at any one period but some every day. Often prepare these with gelatin—about three times a week, for gelatin also is needed in the body. Grate them, slice them, dice them, changing their manner of preparation so as not to become objectionable.

ALLERGIES: METALS: ECZEMA 12/29/43
DERMATITIS M. 32 yrs.
ECZEMA 3422-1

Do include in the diet during those periods a great deal of raw vegetables, especially onions and the like.

18)—Parsnips

8/31/41
ARTHRITIS: PREVENTIVE **F. 51 yrs.**
BODY: GENERAL **1158-31**

Q. What are the best sources of calcium in foods?

A. Vegetables such as parsnips, and all of those that grow under the ground.

1/10/41
M. 60 yrs.
ELIMINATIONS: INCOORDINATION **1963-2**

Q. What weight is best for body?

A. That which is natural or normal weight by the general exercise. Do not attempt to take those things to cause reduction at the present, other than in the diet outlined. Use parsnips; these may be taken in moderation. But beware of dried beans or peas or things of that nature.

11/29/39
ELIMINATIONS: INCOORDINATION **F. 40 yrs.**
ANEMIA **2050-1**

In the matter of the diets through these periods—we will find that those foods combining a greater quantity of vitamin B-1 (thiamine) would be especially most beneficial to the body, as they will aid in eliminating those disturbances through the whole of the system, especially as related to the conditions carried in the bloodstream itself.

In parsnips, and such we will find the greater quantity, or the active forces from this vitamin needed by this particular body.

2/23/25
ASSIMILATIONS: ELIMINATIONS: INCOORDINATION **M. 46 yrs.**
BODY-BUILDING **3190-2**

Q. What special foods would give to the mind and body great strength, endurance and activity?

A. All of the vegetables, especially those of parsnips and of the like nature. Parsnips.

Q. What should the body do to reach its normal weight?

A. Keep the system in that as we have given, so we will bring the conditions necessary for rebuilding in system for as we find, the body has reached that condition in the general system, where the glands of body, the tissue in the arterial system, must be stimulated to give the correct incentives. This we will find through properties as given, and correct living.

10/11/37
DIABETES: TENDENCIES **M. 67 yrs.**
ACIDITY **1454-1**

Hence we would have the stimulating foods such as parsnips, or leafy vegetables these in their combinations.

10/29/43
F. 36 yrs.
3331-1

ASTHMA
ASTHMA: ELIMINATIONS

Beware of rutabaga, but parsnips are very good.

6/9/27
F. 1 yr.
608-1

BABY CARE

Well for the body to cut teeth on parsnips (raw, see?) these may be given, just so chunks are not cut off and swallowed too much.

12/2/40
F. 60 yrs.
538-66

DEBILITATION: GENERAL
APPETITE: DIGESTION: INDIGESTION: NERVOUS

Q. Any special foods at mealtime advised?

A. All of those that carry a great deal of iron and silicon, and things of that nature; that is all of those that grow under the ground through the winter—as parsnips and the like, see?

6/9/44
M. 12 yrs.
5192-1

ASTHMA

Q. What causes the deep ridges in thumbnail and what treatments should be followed?

A. These are the activities of the glandular force, and the addition of those foods which carry large quantities of calcium will make for bettered conditions in this direction. Eat parsnips, in their regular season.

19)—Peas: General

3/18/32
F. 38 yrs.
5515-1

ADHESIONS: BLOOD-BUILDING

Evenings—Cooked vegetables . . . those that are of the blood building in the vegetables—as of peas. Not a great deal of any foods.

1/25/33
F. 44 yrs.
757-3

GLANDS: INCOORDINATION

Noons—Preferably a whole *green* vegetable diet; any of those that make for the weight as well as a balance of the diets that produce the *cleansing* effects throughout the system, see? Raw foods—peas that have been cooked, but not wholly cooked, see? And there may be used with these a French dressing or mayonnaise, to make them more palatable.

7/27/39
F. 27 yrs.
480-52

DEBILITATION: GENERAL

Keep a general upbuilding in the diet, by the body-building influences. Plenty of all forms of the bulbular vegetables—peas and the like.

These as we find should bring much better results and experiences for the body.

12/2/37
F. 5 yrs.
COLD: COMMON **1490-1**

In the matter of the diets, keep these well balanced in the body, blood and nerve building.

Especially vegetables of the bulbous nature as peas.

6/4/26
M. 54 yrs.
BLOOD-BUILDING **4769-2**

Let the diet be vegetable foods of that that grows *above* the ground. All that of the pod nature, see? Peas and those of that nature. Not any tuberous nature.

3/25/30
ACIDITY & ALKALINITY **F. 45 yrs.**
DIGESTION: INDIGESTION **5625-1**

In the noon day those of the vegetables that care for the blood and nerve building, and that will produce not an overactivity but as a counter-*irritant* of activity in the kidneys, which will reduce the stimuli in the circulation in the hepatics. These we will find in those of the vegetable forces that grow especially in pods, as peas, and such. These also may be added in a consistent manner with those of the non-acid or of the alkaline-*producing* conditions for the system.

3/17/38
F. 52 yrs.
CANCER **601-29**

In the matter of the diet—as has been indicated—whatever may be given is very well, provided such as the bulbous nature—as dried peas or the like—are not used as a portion of the diet.

Q. Please itemize foods that allay inflammatory conditions?

A. As just indicated, most any of the foods desired may be taken except those of the bulbous natures as indicated.

3/21/39
M. 9 yrs.
DIABETES: TENDENCIES **415-7**

Evenings—Vegetables—preferably those that grow above the ground. Peas, these should be a part of the diet. No fried foods at any of the meals.

ANEMIA **12/8/36**
ASSIMILATIONS: POOR **F. Adult**
TOXEMIA **1303-1**

Peas—either black or green or English—may be taken with bread—for these form a different reaction.

8/13/38
F. 45 yrs.
ARTHRITIS **1659-1**

As to diet, this should carry a great deal of the salts of vegetables AND fruits—rather than meats. Never any fried foods at any time. The vegetables would be cooked in their OWN juices—that is, in Patapar paper. The juices that come from same shall be well mixed with the vegetables themselves, so that the body gets the benefit of those; such as peas—with their salts as come from same—after being well washed and cooked in the Patapar paper, but DO NOT put meat or anything of the kind in same. Season only with a little butter and sufficient salt or pepper to satisfy the appetite or to be palatable to the taste of the body.

9/1/39
M. 49 yrs.
PARKINSON'S DISEASE **1989-1**

Be mindful of the diet—that there are plenty of vitamins; have plenty of green vegetables—as peas—these cooked in their own salts (as in Patapar paper) saving the salts or the water in which such are cooked as a part of the diet.

8/12/40
F. 33 yrs.
ANEMIA: DIGESTION: INDIGESTION **2320-1**

Have peas—well cooked, but in their own juices (as in Patapar paper). Not large quantities of these ever, but take a little at least three times each day—that is, each meal consisting of some.

ASSIMILATIONS: ELIMINATIONS: INCOORDINATION **11/9/40**
CANCER: TENDENCIES **F. 61 yrs.**
ACIDITY & ALKALINITY **1697-2**

Q. What foods may be taken that will digest properly?

A. Any of those that are easily assimilated; that is, three times as much alkaline-reacting as acid-producing foods. This means the alkaline-REACTING, and not acid-producing. For instance, all the vegetables that are easily assimilated would be included: peas—provided they are not sprayed with preservatives—these either canned or fresh.

4/1/31
APOPLEXY **M. 52 yrs.**
NERVE-BUILDING **3747-1**

The diets will be along those lines that make for nerve *building*. Plenty of peas and such may be taken.

8/27/40
F. 40 yrs.
ATHLETE'S FOOT: ECZEMA **2332-1**

Little of the beans that are dried—as peas or the like, or the bulbular foods.

10/20/34
ACIDITY: LESIONS **F. 48 yrs.**
ACIDITY **703-1**

Have at least three of the leafy vegetables to one below the ground, or with the leafy vegetables there may be one or two of the bulbous nature—as peas.

10/5/38
DEBILITATION: GENERAL **F. 40 yrs**
OBESITY: TENDENCIES **1657-2**

Have more of the vegetables—the leafy variety would be preferable to those of the bulbular nature or such as peas or the like (that is, the dried, see?).

1/26/35
F. 59 yrs.
INJURIES **3823-2**

Evenings—A well-balanced vegetable diet. Fresh peas may be a part of the diet, provided it is prepared in its *own* source—as cooked in Patapar paper, so that all the juices and vitamins may be retained in same.

2/23/25
M. 20 yrs.
BODY-BUILDING **77-2**

Q. What special foods should be given the body that would give to the mind and body strength, endurance and activity?

A. Green vegetable forces of every character, especially those of the tuberous nature. Of course some portions of them are cooked, the greater number eaten raw. Peas—those of that nature.

7/22/31
ASSIMILATIONS: DEBILITATION: GENERAL **F. 28 yrs.**
BLOOD-BUILDING **3842-1**

We would give a diet that is easily assimilated. Let the diet be that as is nerve and blood building. And vegetables, peas, and the like.

i)—Peas—Green

DEBILITATION: GENERAL **1/12/44**
GLAUCOMA **F. 58 yrs.**
EYES **3552-1**

And then in the general diet add a great deal of vegetables that have a direct bearing upon the optic forces through the general system; such as green peas. These have a direct bearing upon the application of that assimilated for the optic forces.

20)—Peppers—Green

1/5/36
F. 46 yrs.
COLITIS: TENDENCIES **404-6**

Q. What is the food value of raw green peppers?

A. They are better in combination than by themselves. Their tendency is for an activity to the pylorus; not the activity in the pylorus itself, but more in the activity from the flow of the pylorus to the churning effect upon the duodenum in its digestion. Hence it is an activity for *digestive* forces.

Peppers, then, taken with green cabbage, lettuce, are very good for this body; taken in moderation.

4/26/35
F. 53 yrs.
GLANDS: INCOORDINATION **906-1**

Be mindful that there is at least *one* meal each day taken of *raw* green vegetables; this doesn't mean green in color only but those that are raw and fresh, not stale vegetables. These may include such as pepper.

21)—Poke (A Weed)

4/29/43
F. 45 yrs.
MENOPAUSE **2985-1**

In the diet, keep away from too much of starches. In this period, especially, we would take much of the foods that act as clarifiers or purifiers to the blood supply; such as poke salad. We do not mean pork meat, but poke salad . . . the plant. Cook the very tender leaves, allow to come almost to a boil and pour off the first water, then put in fresh, clear, cold water, and cook a few minutes. This taken about twice each week for three to four weeks will make a great deal of change in these periods of irritation from the superficial circulation. If three to four stalks of the Irish Potato tops are put with the poke salad, it will be most beneficial.

12/11/37
F. 43 yrs.
CONSTIPATION **1446-3**

Q. Should I continue with the same diet?

A. Continue near the same diet. Of course, as the seasons change it is well—would be excellent for this body, as soon as it is practical to have wild GREENS; including poke. This is not meat (pork), but is POKE—the NEW buds as greens, see?

10/29/43
F. 36 yrs.
ASTHMA: ELIMINATIONS **3331-1**

To include all forms of leafy greens—as poke—as this is very tender, but be careful how it is prepared. Put the tender poke leaves in plain water and allow to come almost to a boil, pour off the water or drain and then the leaves can be mixed with any other greens. The activity of these would be purifying, in such a way that will be found in few other such greens or vegetables.

4/1/43
POLIOMYELITIS **F. 11 yrs.**
BLOOD-BUILDING **2948-1**

At least three times a week have either carrots or beets, or beet tops, as a part of the diet. These should be cooked, even the beet tops—very soon cook with the tender shoots of poke; not, however, without the poke having been first prepared, but these are especially blood purifiers, adding to the body forces. Prepare the poke by first putting in cold water, letting it come almost to a boil; then drain, as through a colander—the water will be rather greenish. Then it may be cooked with the beet tops. And these are excellent, at least two to three times each week; as are the carrots. These may be cooked with fresh peas, and diced for the body, if desired.

12/28/43
F. 56 yrs.
CANCER **3515-1**

Eat very young poke—the tender shoots of the poke weed—to act as a purifier for the body. Prepare it in this manner: When cutting sufficient to make a small dish or salad, put in cold water and let come to a boil. Strain or drain off, as in a colander—or put in a colander and let all the juice drain off. Then prepare or cook the remaining leaves with other greens, especially such as lamb's tongue and wild mustard—about an equal quantity. This eaten once a week will purify the whole body.

22)—Potatoes: General

7/14/39
ACIDITY **M. 34 yrs.**
GLANDS: THYROID **1681-2**

Beware of too much of white bread or of white potatoes; though the skins of Irish potatoes and those portions close to same should be a part of the diet (rather than the bulk of the potato), for the salts from these will produce a better condition in the scalp and in those portions of the glandular system activity as related to the functions of the thyroid.

10/17/34
M. Adult
ANEMIA **698-1**

In the diet, keep much of that which will add more phosphorus and gold to the system; as we will find in certain of the vegetables—as the rind of Irish potatoes (not the pulp), and the like. These should be a portion of the diet each day; not that it would be these *only*—but keep more of an alkaline diet.

8/19/35
ASSIMILATIONS: POOR **F. 80 yrs.**
CANCER **975-1**

Q. What diet should be followed, with specific recommendations for breakfast, dinner and supper?

A. Those foods, as we find, that are body building, but that carry very little of the tuberous growths. No Irish potatoes. None of those things that make for the bulbous nature in the system; for each of these carries a chemical reaction that does not make for activity with the system. Hence we would give *this* as an outline, though, to be sure, there may be changes at times for these things would naturally become of such a rote as to be offensive to the body if they were continued in this manner alone.

Q. What foods should be avoided?

A. As indicated, those of the tuberous nature—potatoes and the like.

7/15/30
F. 55 yrs.
ACIDITY **760-16**

The potato, provided same is baked—*not* boiled in grease, though some butter, but very little, may be added to same, but eat rather the peel and that close to same—little or none of that in center, unless those of the yam variety is taken.

10/14/35
M. 17 yrs.
GLANDS: INCOORDINATION: HYPOTHYROIDISM **1078-1**

In the matter of the diet, remove too much of starches. But the skins of the Irish potatoes and that close to same carry salts that will go well with the activities of *all* the glands, and thus be most beneficial.

5/30/29
F. 31 yrs.
CONSTIPATION **1713-17**

Q. Are potatoes good for the body?

A. Potatoes not so well as those vegetables *above* the ground, and of the other natures as have been given. Potatoes in small quantities and prepared with the jacket on, and the jackets eaten also, are very good, if not an overquantity is taken, and be sure to eat the jacket.

11/30/37
F. 34 yrs.
ACIDITY & ALKALINITY **1300-2**

As we find, we would keep close to an alkaline diet, rather than an excess acid-producing diet. Hence, leaving out such excess acid-producing foods, most anything else may be taken.

Do NOT eat fried foods of ANY kind, especially never fried—French fried potatoes. Mashed potatoes may be taken occasionally, or especially those prepared with the jackets—if the jacket is eaten rather than the pulp, for this is very well for the body.

4/2/39
F. 38 yrs.
CHOLECYSTITIS **1857-1**

When potatoes are eaten, use only that portion close to the skin (and the skin itself), rather than too much of the bulk of same.

4/29/38
F. 77 yrs.
TOXEMIA **1586-1**

Evenings—Do not take fried foods morning, noon OR evening! especially not fried potatoes. The vegetables should be cooked in their OWN salts, and these juices preserved—NOT thrown away! The broths or juices from the cooking of any of the vegetables in their own broths (or cooked in Patapar paper) may be saved and taken as a portion of the noon meal, or as a change from the diet outlined for the noon meal. Do not cook the vegetables with meats to season them; only use a little butter, with pepper or salt or such.

3/15/44
F. 26 yrs.
PARALYSIS **3694-1**

Add all of the foods that carry silicon and the salts that may revibrate with the applications of the gold to the nerve centers for assimilation; as foods of the tuberous nature of every character—the potatoes. These should be parts of the foods for the body. Have at least five vegetables grown below the ground to one grown above the ground, or in that proportion.

9/12/37
BLOOD: COAGULATION: POOR **F. 62 yrs.**
ACIDITY & ALKALINITY **1411-2**

When the body is under stress or strain by being tired, overactive, and then would eat heavy foods these would produce acidity. The same would be true if there were fried foods such as fried potatoes eaten when there is a little cold or the body has gotten exceedingly cold or damp, these would produce (if fried) an acid, and become hard upon the system; while the same taken as mashed or as roasted with other foods would react differently.

7/19/43
F. 33 yrs.
ARTHRITIS **3134-1**

The body should not take white potatoes. These should be barred from the diet.

12/3/35
F. 51 yrs.
OBESITY: TENDENCIES **1073-1**

As to the matter of the diets, these become naturally with the general conditions of the body, a necessary element or influence.

Do not eat white bread nor potatoes; though the skins of Irish potatoes—whether roasted or boiled or baked—are well for the body; for the salts that are in same close to the peel will supply starch *and* carbohydrates in a manner that the activities of the Vitamins A and D are in such proportions as to build strength and vitality in the structural portions, and in the tendons and the muscular forces, such as to build resistance—and not build fat.

4/19/21
M. Adult
BLOOD-BUILDING **4867-1**

To clarify the blood stream and to take on more vitamins will be found rather in the vegetable diet, that especially of potatoes and such as that. Of course, others may be taken in moderation, but principally such as these given.

10/20/24
ACIDITY: LESIONS **F. 48 yrs.**
ACIDITY **703-1**

Q. What diet?

A. Eat a good deal of potato peeling—that is, like the baked Irish potato—but not any quantity of the pulp.

10/6/42
F. 25 yrs.
ANEMIA **2376-3**

For this particular body, however, take the Irish potato rather often, but eat the jackets with the potato—whether roasted or boiled, eat the peel with it, and you will keep a better activity through the glandular forces, that will keep a better balance in the system.

2/23/28
F. 21 mos.
TOXEMIA **608-4**

Potatoes, only those that are mashed or prepared in the shell itself, see? or roasted—none that has grease with same, save butter.

7/22/31
ACIDITY **F. 28 yrs.**
ASSIMILATIONS: ELIMINATIONS: INCOORDINATION **2261-1**

The pulp of potatoes, whether those of Irish potatoes or yams. The skins, or those close to the skin may be taken—but no fried meats. No fried vegetables—nothing *fried* should be taken by the body—see?

4/17/44
F. 36 yrs.
MULTIPLE SCLEROSIS **5031-1**

Have more of the vegetables growing under the ground than those growing above the ground, for this body; such as the tuberous natures—potatoes, all characters of vegetables that are grown under the ground. To be sure some leafy vegetables should be taken, but have at least 3 of those under the ground to one of those on the top of the ground, for this body.

10/23/36
BLOOD: HUMOR **F. 35 yrs.**
OBESITY **1276-1**

Do not combine potatoes with rice or spaghetti or white bread, or if either or any one of these is taken *do not* eat meat at that meal!

8/11/36
ANEMIA **F. Adult**
CIRCULATION: INCOORDINATION **1247-1**

We would also be mindful that no white breads, no great quantities of potatoes are taken; though the potato jackets may be taken provided these are roasted.

3/27/35
F. 52 yrs.
ACIDITY & ALKALINITY **805-2**

Q. What can I do to avoid losing so much weight? Outline the proper diet.

A. Those foods, now, that are the body-building; as starches and proteins, if these are taken without other food values that make for the combinations that produce distress or disorder; that is, not quantities of starches and proteins combined, you see, but these taken one at one meal and one at another will be most helpful. As potatoes, whether white or the yam activity with butter, should not be taken with fats or meats; but using these as a portion of one meal with *fruits* or vegetables is well. When meats are taken, use mutton, fowl or the like, and do not have heavy starches with same—but preferably fruits or vegetables.

3/21/37
F. 26 yrs.
CIRCULATION: POOR **23-3**

In the matter of the diet, keep same well balanced as to an alkaline and an acid reaction. Do not combine at the same meals potatoes, white bread, spaghetti or macaroni. Do not combine any two of these in the same meal. Eat rather potatoes in the jacket and the peel rather than the pulp; the salts of these are most beneficial to the very activities of the body.

Q. Any other advice for the body at this time?

A. Keep in that of constructive thought; because, to be sure, the thoughts of the body act upon the emotions as well as the assimilating forces. Poisons are accumulated or produced by anger or by resentment or animosity. Keep sweet!

2/23/25
M. 20 yrs.
BODY-BUILDING **77-2**

Q. What special foods should be given the body that would give to the mind and body strength, endurance and activity?

A. Green vegetable forces of every character, especially those of the tuberous nature. Of course, some portions of them cooked, the greater number eaten raw. Potatoes, forces of that character.

11/8/34
DEBILITATION: GENERAL **F. 12 yrs.**
BODY-BUILDING **632-6**

In the diet, beware of too much starches of *any* kind; that is, do *not* include potatoes. However, *roast* potatoes with the jackets would be all right, if there would be eaten only the jackets and the small portion that adheres to the jacket—for this portion of the potato carries properties that are *not* acid-producing and not too great an amount of starch; but do not eat the bulk of the potato!

8/12/37
F. 36 yrs.
1422-1

LACERATIONS: STOMACH

No food that makes for a quantity of alcohol in its activity in the system. Beware of potatoes in any form . . .

1/28/44
F. 63 yrs.
3607-1

ACIDITY: EYES
ANEMIA
ASSIMILATIONS: ELIMINATIONS: INCOORDINATION

In the diet, do not eat white potatoes.

Q. What can be done for my eyes?

A. Do these things and we will get rid of this acid throughout the system and relieve the stress upon the kidneys, which will help the eyes.

10/30/37
M. 48 yrs.
470-19

DIABETES: TENDENCIES

When white potatoes are taken, take them with the jackets and eat that close to the jacket AND the jacket preferably to the greater portion of the pulp. These are not to be excluded; neither would cheese or macaroni be excluded.

2/20/38
F. 40 yrs.
1540-1

OBESITY

Potatoes should not be a portion of the diet save occasionally, once or twice a week—and even then we would only eat the jacket and that close to same, rather than too much of the pulp or bulk.

2/13/37
F. 17 yrs.
1339-1

OBESITY

No potatoes with meats. No starches that have the greases should be taken at the same time with meats.

2/21/34
M. 20 yrs.
521-1

EPILEPSY

Evenings—Vegetables at this meal may include any of those that are well-cooked in their *own* sauce, or their *own* liquid, not adding waters nor seasoning until after they are cooked. And have three that grow *above* the ground to one that grows below the ground, but may include the tops and the roots of such; as fresh Irish potatoes, *when* such below the ground are prepared. Not at all times, but that the vitamin forces of these may carry the necessary elements for creating a balance in the system that has long been lacking in sufficient of the phosphorus, silicon, iron and iodine. Hence all the vegetables that carry these properties should be included in the meals from day to day; for they are more easily assimilated by the body or system from vegetable matter than from any other source or character.

12/31/34
F. 22 yrs.
ELIMINATIONS: INCOORDINATIONS 480-13

Q. How are my teeth, and should any be extracted?

A. Only local attention, as we find, is particularly needed at this time; especially if there is included plenty of calcium either in the treatments of same or in the diets—which is included, specifically, of course, in the jackets of Irish potatoes, and the like,

2/27/35
M. 26 yrs.
EPILEPSY 567-7

Never include much starches as from potatoes or from any of the starchy elements, for these tend to make for a slowing up of the conditions in the system.

1/7/37
CIRCULATION: POOR F. 44 yrs.
ELIMINATIONS: POOR 1315-6

Leave off potatoes of any kind at *any* time, and especially no fried potatoes ever!

9/27/39
BRONCHITIS: TENDENCIES M. 38 yrs.
ACIDITY 1956-2

Be careful of the diet, that there is not too much of the foods that are acid-producing—that is, too great a quantity of potatoes and never white potatoes at the same meal with white bread.

12/12/31
F. 46 yrs.
ULCERS: STOMACH 482-3

In the evening meals, those of the well-cooked vegetables, but only those of the leafy nature—or that grow in pods; not the bulb nature. No potatoes, nothing of that nature. The tops of these may be taken, and may be eaten, but not the bulb nature.

3/20/35
M. Adult
ASTHMA 861-1

Beware of white bread. Do not use these in the diet, or too many of white or sweet potatoes; these make for the accumulations of starches that are hard upon such a condition.

5/6/43
F. 37 yrs.
OBESITY 2988-1

Have little of pod vegetables or as of white potatoes, or even yams.

i)—Potato Peelings

4/17/44
F. 34 yrs.
ASSIMILATIONS: ELIMINATIONS: INCOORDINATION 2072-14

Q. What foods or treatments are especially good for bringing more of the luster—reds, coppers, and golds—back into the hair?

A. Nothing better than the peelings of Irish potatoes or the juices from same. Don't just put the peelings in water and cook them, because most of the necessary properties will go out, but put them in Patapar paper to cook them.

2/27/42
EYES: COLOR BLINDNESS M. 25 yrs.
CIRCULATION: INCOORDINATION 820-2

Do not use large quantities of potatoes, though the peelings of same may be taken at all times—they are strengthening, carrying those influences and forces that are active with the glands of the system.

5/19/30
NERVOUS SYSTEMS: INCOORDINATION: NEUROSIS M. 50 yrs.
NERVE-BUILDING 5475-2

Q. Outline proper diet for body.

A. That as will give to the nerve system more of the *energy* as is necessary. That is, those of the vegetables that are nerve building. Those that do not carry too much of the value of just weight, but that carry more *with* same that as is assimilated in system. As may be illustrated in this: In potatoes of any character, better were the body to eat the peel than for the other portion.

3/22/38
F. 29 yrs.
MINERALS: CALCIUM: TEETH 1523-3

Q. What foods are acid-forming for this body?

A. All of those that are combining fats with sugars. Starches naturally are inclined for acid reaction. But a normal diet is about twenty percent acid- to eighty percent alkaline-producing.

Q. Suggest diet beneficial to preserving teeth.

A. Potato peelings are particularly given to preserving the teeth; anything that carries quantities of calcium or aids to the thyroids in its production would be beneficial so it is not overbalanced, see?

10/23/39
M. 20 yrs.
ASSIMILATIONS: POOR 984-3

Q. Please give a good hair tonic.

A. To eat potato peelings, too, is good; or the juice or soup of same.

Q. Not the potato itself?

A. We are speaking of the care for the hair! If you like potatoes, eat 'em!

9/5/42
F. 33 yrs.
HAIR: COLOR RESTORER 2582-2

Q. What would you advise to prevent my hair from turning gray?

A. Use the juice of potato peelings at least three times a week. Cook the Irish potato peelings in a little water (with a top on the container, of course), and drink the juice from same.

Use on the hair, after the cleansing, a little white Vaseline. This will keep the hair from turning gray.

4/25/40
ACIDITY **F. Adult**
DEBILITATION: GENERAL **2179-1**

The skins of the Irish or white potatoes—and that very close to the same—are very good; for the salts in these are well for the body. Even if the potato peels are cooked a long time in water and the juice or soup or broth from same taken; it would be excellent.

9/25/43
F. 45 yrs.
HAIR: COLOR RESTORER **3051-3**

Q. Will canichrome tablets I take restore color to hair?

A. NO! If the juice of potato peelings is taken regularly (two or three times a week) it will keep the hair nearer to its normal color than all other forms of chemical preparations.

Q. How eliminate dryness to hair and skin?

A. Just as given, when there is a perfect condition in the scalp, in the activities of the thyroid, by keeping a correct balance, the oil, the dryness, the color will be normal for the body. Don't try to make something abnormal for self that should be this or that condition.

5/26/44
F. 56 yrs.
HAIR: TEXTURE **5197-1**

Q. How can I improve texture of hair?

A. Better be glad that you have it, but the peelings of Irish potato boiled and taken once a day will improve the texture of the hair. This will require a long period of about 6 months. Two ounces of this fresh juice a day.

8/27/43
M. 31 yrs.
ELIMINATIONS: POOR: BALDNESS **2301-5**

Q. To prevent falling hair?

A. Don't worry too much about this. The drinking of the soup made from Irish potato peels will also be helpful. Stew the peels from three or four potatoes in a little water and drink about twice a week.

1/3/35
INJURIES: ACCIDENTS: AFTEREFFECTS **M. 29 yrs.**
HAIR: COLOR RESTORER **416-5**

Q. What can I do, if anything, about my hair turning gray so prematurely?

A. With those shocks to the nervous system there has been changed a great deal of the pigment, or the flow of the activities. If you would prevent the hair from turning gray, let at least two meals each day be taken of the peeling of Irish potatoes—it'll turn it to its normal color again! They may be cooked, yes.

5/1/36
F. 54 yrs.
GLANDS: THYROID **906-2**

Q. What causes the condition with nails and what should be done for it?

A. This arises from the lack of proper balance in the activities of the glands that produce the necessary forces or influences for this portion of the system itself. For the body takes from the food values, by the activity of the glandular forces, for the creating of various elements. For the nails—or the cuticle itself is not the same characterization (though it may be taken from the same food forces) as that of the lymph or that of the blood; yet it is a lack of a functioning then of a gland.

With this balance in the digestive forces created, by creating a better assimilation, these parts of the body will be aided. And we find that the use or the eating of the potato *peel* will add those elements that will produce an activity; not of such disturbances as to overbalance them, but through the thyroids—as to make these conditions better.

3/25/39
PRESCRIPTIONS: POTATO PEELINGS, IRISH **F. 50 yrs.**
TEETH: ENAMEL-BUILDING **1000-22**

Q. The enamel on my front teeth seems to be wearing away. Is there any special treatment for this, or is there a special diet?

A. A diet that will carry more of enamel-building foods would be well; or calcium foods—as well as the SKINS of Irish potatoes; not so much the bulk of the potato but the peel.

6/1/39
DERMATITIS: GLANDS **F. 52 yrs.**
GLANDS: HAIR **1904-1**

Then as to the diet: Add to the diet the Irish potato PEEL, but not the pulp a great deal. It would be better if the nice potatoes are cleansed, peeled and only the PEELINGS cooked and eaten! Throw the other part away, or give it to the chickens, or distribute it in some other manner besides eating it!

5/22/42
M. 40 yrs.
CIRCULATION: INCOORDINATION **412-14**

Q. Can anything be done to prevent hair from falling out?

A. The improvement of the general health will help this more than anything, though this is an inherent condition. As we find, it may be particularly aided if a good massage is given occasionally with any good antiseptic. And drink the juice or soup as would be made from Irish potato peelings. Do this two or three times a week.

Q. Can anything be done to prevent it from turning gray?

A. The same conditions.

Q. Is this a lack in my system or natural for age?

A. As indicated, it is an inherent condition as well as a general debilitation—through the general health, as from those deficiencies outlined.

23)—Radishes

ALLERGIES: METALS: ECZEMA **12/29/43**
DERMATITIS **M. 32 yrs.**
ECZEMA **3422-1**

As we find, from these vibrations, there are those effects from metallic substance that, because of certain elements in the blood supply, produce a very disagreeable and a very aggravating rash—wherever portions of the body become damp; forming into a running sore, or weeping eczema.

Do include in the diet during those periods a great deal of raw vegetables. Radishes are also well, provided they are cut or grated or scraped. Taken in such a manner these release elements that are not released even in digestion, when taken whole.

1/25/33
F. 44 yrs.
GLANDS: INCOORDINATION **757-3**

Noons—Preferably a whole *green* vegetable diet, consisting of such as radishes, or any of those that make for the weight—as well as a balance of the diets that produce the *cleansing* effects throughout the system, see?

8/19/35
ASSIMILATIONS: POOR **F. 80 yrs.**
CANCER **975-1**

Noons—Preferably only the juices of, or very finely grated raw vegetables; such as radishes. These may be taken with or without the salad dressing. Or this may be altered at times to the juices only of the *cooked* vegetables; or there may be had two or more vegetables combined to make for balancing of the elements in the body that are necessary, carrying silicon and iron that are as resistive forces and aids in the blood supply to eradicate these disturbing forces in the system.

1/17/44
F. 44 yrs.
ANEMIA **3564-1**

Keep plenty of raw vegetables; as radishes and the like. Not necessarily at any one period but some every day. Often prepare these with gelatin—about three times a week, for gelatin also is needed in the body. Grate them, slice them, dice them, changing their manner of preparation so as not to become objectionable.

5/30/29
F. 31 yrs.
CONSTIPATION **1713- 17**

A great deal of vegetables, especially those that give iron, as radishes.

5/19/30
NERVOUS SYSTEMS: INCOORDINATION: NEUROSIS **M. 50 yrs.**
NERVE-BUILDING **5475-2**

Q. Outline proper diet for body.

A. That as will give to the nerve system more of the *energy* as is necessary. That is, those of the vegetables that are nerve-building. Those that do not carry too much of the value of just weight, but that carry more *with* same that as is *assimilated* in system. As may be illustrated in this: In those of the green vegetables, those of the radish are *mostly* all assimilated, see?

3/26/44
M. 39 yrs.
ADHESIONS: LESIONS **4017-1**

The diet should consist of liquids and semi-liquids, principally. Do use a great deal of the body-building foods such as vegetable juices; as radishes. These may be prepared not only in a juicer, but oft prepared in a salad, very finely ground and using the juices with same prepared in gelatin, so that there will be these activities through the body.

24)—Rutabaga (Swedish Turnip)

4/17/44
F. 36 yrs.
MULTIPLE SCLEROSIS **5031-1**

Rutabaga, all such are well for this body; not in too large quantities, but they form the salts and the character of vitamins in the right combinations to make for the strengthening of this body.

1/4/36
F. 22 yrs.
BLOOD-BUILDING: MINERALS: CALCIUM DEFICIENCY **578-5**

Q. Please give in full a blood-building diet for my body.

A. Those as indicated that have a quantity or an excess of the calcium, and those that will make for a balance in the iodines with the potassiums of the system itself.

Rutabaga, and such natures are those that carry the vitamins necessary for body-building with *this* body.

9/1/39
M. 49 yrs.
PARKINSON'S DISEASE **1989-1**

Be mindful of the diet—that there are plenty of vitamins. Have plenty of green vegetables. Plenty of rutabaga. All of these should be included, but they should be cooked in their own juices, saving the salts or the water in which such are cooked as a part of the diet.

4/18/35
M. Adult
MENU: ASSIMILATIONS: POOR **898-1**

The evening meal should consist of the vegetables, especially such as rutabaga, all the leafy vegetables and all the bulbular nature save the white potatoes.

Keep these consistently, persistently; we will gain weight, we will put off this dullness, this tendency for catching cold, this weakness throughout the whole system; and bring the body—in six to eight months—to its normal weight of about a hundred and fifty pounds.

2/27/42
F. 52 yrs.
COLD: CONGESTION **404-10**

Q. What vegetables are especially good for my body, considering the condition of kidneys?

A. Rutabaga, cooked.

25)—Salsify (Oyster Plant)

9/25/37
SPINE: SUBLUXATIONS **F. 35 yrs.**
MINERALS: CALCIUM **903-25**

There is first an unbalancing of the elements in the activities of the system—or lack of sufficient calcium for the full activity of body-building.

Hence there should be the use of the food values that carry such in such measures as may be assimilated by the body. Those as we find in the oyster plant and those of such natures especially should be a portion of the diet.

12/2/40
DEBILITATION: GENERAL **F. 60 yrs.**
APPETITE: DIGESTION: INDIGESTION: NERVOUS **538-66**

Q. Any special foods at mealtime advised?

A. All of those that carry a great deal of iron and silicon, and things of that nature; that is—all of those that grow under the ground through the winter—as oyster plant—all of these are beneficial.

1/20/33
F. 18 yrs.
GLANDS: INCOORDINATION **951-2**

Have green vegetables. Also those foods that carry sufficient elements of gold and phosphorus which are found partially from the characterization of vegetable forces—as in the oyster plant, especially in those of *that* nature.

12/30/42
M. 21 yrs.
BODY-BUILDING: LOCOMOTION: IMPAIRED **2873-1**

The food values should be those fully well balanced with calcium, iron, and especially the vitamins B-1 and the B-Complex. These are much preferable for the body.

At least three times each week, then, supply these from the foods rather than the reinforced vitamins (though these reinforcements may be desirable if there is the inability of the body to assimilate foods that carry excesses or the full quantity of such vital forces).

To be sure, these are not all the foods that are to be taken:

Noons—Have soups, broths or the like, and these should include the oyster plant.

1/4/36
F. 22 yrs.
BLOOD-BUILDING: MINERALS: CALCIUM DEFICIENCY **578-5**

Q. Please give in full a blood-building diet for my body.

A. Those as indicated that have a quantity or an excess of the calcium, and those that will make for a balance in the iodines with the potassium of the system itself.

Salsify, and such natures are those that carry the vitamins necessary for body-building with *this* body.

5/30/24
M. Adult
4740-2

ASTHMA

To give then the relief to this body, first we would not eat meats, save fish or fowl and that not of too large quantities, using a great deal of salsify, or articles of the vegetable kingdom as those.

8/29/41
F. 25 yrs.
2579-1

COMBINATIONS: OBESITY

Also have plenty of those foods such as salsify or oyster plant, especially—that carry those characters of salts that tend to eliminate these hardening centers in the tendons of the body.

3/21/39
M. 9 yrs.
415-7

DIABETES: TENDENCIES

Evenings—Vegetables—preferably those that grow above the ground, though salsify and such natures may be taken in moderation.

1/10/41
M. 60 yrs.
1963-2

ELIMINATION: INCOORDINATION

Q. What weight is best for body?

A. That which is the natural or normal weight by the general exercise. Do not attempt to take those things to cause reduction at the present, other than in the diet outlined. Use the oyster plant; these may be taken in moderation. But beware of dried beans or peas or things of that nature.

9/1/39
M. 49 yrs.
1989-1

PARKINSON'S DISEASE

Be mindful of the diet—that there are plenty of vitamins. Have plenty of green vegetables. Plenty of oyster plant. All of these should be included, but they should be cooked in their own juices, saving the salts or the water in which such are cooked as a part of the diet.

10/21/32
F. 18 yrs.
951-1

ELEPHANTIASIS: TENDENCIES
ARTHRITIS: GLANDS: INCOORDINATION

One meal each day we would supply principally of nature's sugars, nature's laxatives—any of the active principles in such. A great deal of those forces may be found in salsify.

3/15/44
F. 26 yrs.
PARALYSIS **3694-1**

Add all of the foods that carry silicon and the salts that may revibrate with the applications of the gold to the nerve centers for assimilation; as foods of the tuberous nature of every character—the oyster plant. These should be parts of the foods for the body. Have at least five vegetables grown below the ground to one grown above the ground, or in that proportion.

9/18/43
M. 22 yrs.
TUBERCULOSIS **3222-1**

Do have all the leafy vegetables the body can absorb—as foods are changed. Not too much of the pod or tuberous vegetables, though the oyster plant should be taken. These are very good.

10/20/41
F. 64 yrs.
ARTHRITIS **1512-3**

All forms of vegetables, but as much of the leafy nature as practical. Do not take too much of turnips nor of other root vegetables, such as potatoes of any kind, rutabagas or any of those natures. The oyster plant as a root vegetable, however, is not so bad.

2/23/25
ASSIMILATIONS: ELIMINATIONS: INCOORDINATION **M. 46 yrs.**
BODY-BUILDING **3190-2**

Q. What special foods would give to the mind and body great strength, endurance and activity?

A. All of the vegetable, especially those of salsify.

Q. What should the body do to reach its normal weight?

A. Keep the system in that as we have given, so we will bring the conditions necessary for rebuilding in system, for as we find, the body has reached that condition in the general system where the glands of body, the tissue in the arterial system, must be stimulated to give the correct incentives. This we will find through properties as given, and correct living.

3/18/32
F. 38 yrs.
ADHESIONS: BLOOD-BUILDING **5515-1**

Evenings—Cooked vegetables . . . those that are of the blood-building in the vegetables—as of salsify. Not a great deal of any foods.

8/13/36
M. 40 yrs.
CANCER **1242-2**

Q. Where and in what form can salsify be procured at this season of the year?

A. Very soon it may be procured regularly. Or it may be procured through the Libby-McNeil [?] & Libby, as preserved or canned.

12/9/36
ARTHRITIS: TENDENCIES F. 63 yrs.
BODY-BUILDING 1302-1

In the matter of the diets: here we need body-building foods but those that tend to be more alkaline-producing than acid. For the natural inclinations of disturbed conditions in a body are to produce acidity through the bloodstream. Hence we need to revivify same by the use of much of those that produce more of the enzymes, more of the hormones for the blood supply; yet not overburdening the body with those unless the balance in the vitamin forces is carried.

Hence as we will find, not heavy foods or fried foods ever, nor combinations where there are quantities of starches or quantities of starches with sweets taken at the same time. The leafy vegetables preferably to the tuberous, though certain tuberous ones are necessary. The oyster plant, these prepared with not too much butter—but a little cream. These especially carry elements that are the more easily assimilated by the body.

8/15/38
F. 52 yrs.
BODY-BUILDING 560-8

In the matter of the diets, keep those that are body-building. Plenty of oyster plant once or twice a day, such natures as these would be well—with beef juices—these would supply gluten as well as the necessary forces for the better coagulation in the activities of the lymph and the circulatory forces in the blood supply.

11/1/30
F. 21 yrs.
EPILEPSY 543-4

Q. Are too many plants which come from under the ground being taken into system?

A. Take as little of these as may be taken, yet some may be used occasionally for that of the *weight* or body of food values in the system.

Q. Which ones should be taken from diet, and which ones may be taken?

A. Salsify may be preserved, as also may be those of the nature that are of that character.

6/9/44
M. 12 yrs.
ASTHMA 5192-1

Q. What causes the deep ridges in thumbnail and what treatments should be followed?

A. These are the activities of the glandular force, and the addition of those foods which carry large quantities of calcium will make for bettered conditions in this direction. Eat oyster plant, in their regular season.

12/31/34
F. 22 yrs.
ELIMINATIONS: INCOORDINATION 480-13

Q. How are my teeth, and should any be extracted?

A. Only local attention, as we find, is particularly needed at this time; especially if there is included plenty of calcium either in the treatments of same or in the diets—which is included specifically, of course, in salsify.

12/8/39
M. 32 yrs.
PINWORMS **1597-2**

As to the diet, following the three-day apple diet, let there be more of vegetables, and the supplying forces as will create iron, silicon and the like for the system. Hence we would include a great deal of oyster plant, and the like.

11/28/22
F. Adult
ANEMIA **4439-1**

Use whole wheat bread and vegetables that carry a high percentage of carbons such as salsify.

9/29/36
F. 33 yrs.
PREGNANCY **540-7**

There should be those precautions that there be plenty of calcium in the system for developing of bone and muscle tissue. Most of this, of course, may be had from those vegetables that carry calcium and silicon and iron in the ways and manners that may be assimilated—as we would find from salsify especially.

10/8/36
ANEMIA **F. 54 yrs.**
ARTHRITIS: TOXEMIA **1269-1**

Noons—Preferably a combination of meat juices *or* vegetable juices, but do not put the two together!

The oyster plant, all that grow under the ground may be a part of the diet. These cooked, or the vegetables in the evening—as roughage for the body.

10/17/34
M. Adult
ANEMIA **698-1**

In the diet, keep much of that which will add more phosphorus and gold to the system; as we will find in certain of the vegetables—as salsify, and the like. These should be a portion of the diet each day; not that it would be these *only*—but keep more of an alkaline diet.

11/6/35
GLANDS: THYROID: HYPOTHYROIDISM **F. 63 yrs.**
MINERALS **1049-1**

In the matter of the diet, this would be rather important. Occasionally use a great deal of those things that carry quantities of iodine, for this the body requires. But for this body it will be most soluble from vegetables; salsify and the like.

8/5/29
F. 43 yrs.
MENU: NEURASTHENIA **2713-1**

Pod vegetables are very good, but particularly those of the root nature as . . . salsify.

4/17/44
F. 36 yrs.
MULTIPLE SCLEROSIS **5031-1**

Have more of the vegetables growing under the ground than those growing above the ground, for this body; such as the tuberous natures—the oyster plant; all characters of vegetables that are grown under the ground. To be sure some leafy vegetables should be taken, but have at least 3 of those under the ground to one of those on the top of the ground, for this body.

4/1/31
APOPLEXY **M. 52 yrs.**
NERVE-BUILDING **3747-1**

The diets will be along those lines that make for nerve-*building*. Plenty of the green foods—as salsify.

11/16/36
BLOOD: COAGULATION: POOR **F. 41 yrs.**
BODY-BUILDING **1100-8**

In the diet include those foods that are blood- and body-building, that carry iron in such manners as may be assimilated by the body. Those activities from the properties in the oyster plant (salsify) and things of such natures are the better in carrying these properties to the system.

Q. How can the bodily resistance be kept up, especially during the winter months?

A. By following those suggestions that have just been indicated, we find we may build resistances for this body, through the periods of sudden changes or distresses that may come from sudden changes to the bodily temperature.

26)—Soybeans

12/30/42
M. 21 yrs.
BODY-BUILDING: LOCOMOTION: IMPAIRED **2873-1**

The food values should be those fully well balanced with calcium, iron, and especially the vitamins B-1 and the B-Complex. These are much preferable for the body.

At least three times each week, then, supply these from the foods rather than the reinforced vitamins (though these reinforcements may be desirable if there is the inability of the body to assimilate foods that carry excesses or the full quantity of such vital forces).

To be sure, these are not all the foods that are to be taken:

Noons—Have soups, broths or the like, and these should include mixed vegetables—but not too much of the dried vegetables; though soybeans can be used at times.

27)—Spinach

10/17/27
M. 8 mos.
BABY CARE **5520-2**

As is seen, another *well*-balanced food for the child is spinach that is well cooked, with no oil or grease save butter, and this mashed until almost only the strained portions are given. This will furnish another vitamin, an iron that is excellent for the blood, especially for *this* condition existent with this child.

1/25/33
F. 44 yrs.
GLANDS: INCOORDINATION **757-3**

Noons—Preferably a whole *green* vegetable diet, any of those that make for the weight—as well as a balance of the diets that produce the *cleansing* effects throughout the system, see? Raw spinach. And there may be used with these a French dressing or mayonnaise, to make them more palatable.

4/23/30
APOPLEXY: AFTEREFFECTS **F. Adult**
BLOOD-BUILDING **5667-1**

We would be mindful of the diet that it consist of much that grows *above* the ground, as the spinach, and such *gree*n vegetables. Any of the salads that carry large quantities of iron. Now this, apparently, would be the creating of blood, but blood of a character is needed, when the pressure is already abnormal.

12/2/37
F. 5 yrs.
COLD: COMMON **1490-1**

In the matter of the diets, keep these well balanced in the body, blood and nerve-building.

NOT spinach, for this body!

8/19/35
ASSIMILATIONS: POOR **F. 80 yrs.**
CANCER **975-1**

Noons—preferably only the juices of, or very finely grated raw vegetables; such as spinach. These may be taken with or without the salad dressing. Or this may be altered at times to the juices only of the *cooked* vegetables.

10/4/35
ANEMIA **M. 41 yrs.**
DEBILITATION: GENERAL **1014-1**

Evenings—Vegetables, especially spinach. These should be the principal foods for the evening meals. Not too much, but satisfy the appetite.

5/30/29
F. 31 yrs.
CONSTIPATION **1713-17**

A great deal of vegetables, especially those that give iron, as spinach.

3/21/39
M. 9 yrs.
415-7

DIABETES: TENDENCIES

Evenings—Vegetables—preferably those that grow above the ground. Spinach, these should be a part of the diet. No fried foods at any of the meals.

1/10/41
M. 60 yrs.
1963-2

ELIMINATIONS: INCOORDINATION

None of vegetables that are of the pod variety. Those of the natures that grow UNDER the ground are preferable, but plenty also of the leafy variety, such as spinach. These, too, should be prepared in their own juices—or in Patapar paper.

9/1/39
M. 49 yrs.
1989-1

PARKINSON'S DISEASE

Be mindful of the diet—that there are plenty of vitamins. Have plenty of green vegetables, as spinach, all of these cooked in their own salts (as in Patapar paper), saving the salts or the water in which such are cooked as a part of the diet.

3/8/35
F. 37 yrs.
631-6

ARTHRITIS

Noons—Preferably the entirely green raw vegetables, such as the raw spinach. These may be taken with whole wheat wafers with a mayonnaise or salad dressing.

11/18/30
F. 60 yrs.
505-1

ELIMINATIONS: POOR

In the matter of diet—these, as we find, will be more of the well balanced that carry more of the irons in their reaction—as will be found in those of all the vegetable forces, as of spinach. Also it will be found that little of the meats should be taken.

11/12/35
M. 50 yrs.
1055-1

ADHESIONS: LESIONS

In the diets, be mindful that we keep those things that add iron, silicon, and gold in the system. It may be necessary later to change some of these, but in the present let the diet consist greatly of vegetables that are of the leafy nature; as spinach, but *not* with grease in same. These should be cooked in their own juices. Preferably cook each in Patapar paper, or in a fireless or waterless cooker. These are preferable, but *not* in aluminum.

8/5/29
F. 43 yrs.
2713-1

MENU: NEURASTHENIA

Q. Would you specify the necessary diet?

A. It's been given! As an outline for such, it was given in that it should carry more of the iodines. Vegetables that grow above the ground, as spinach. At least each day have a vegetable that is raw.

3/31/43
ASSIMILATIONS: ELIMINATIONS: INCOORDINATION **F. 18 yrs.**
BODY-BUILDING **2947-1**

Keep the diet body-building. Plenty of vitamins A and D; plenty of B-1 and the B-Complex. Plenty of spinach—though the spinach would be best taken raw as a salad with a dressing.

This is not to be all the diet, of course, but these should form a great part of the diet—just so often as not to become obnoxious to the body; altering in the manner of preparation.

4/18/35
ANEMIA **M. Adult**
MENU: ASSIMILATIONS: POOR **898-1**

The evening meal should consist of the vegetables, especially such as spinach, all the leafy vegetables and all the bulbular nature save the white potatoes.

2/23/35
DERMATITIS **M. Adult**
BLOOD: HUMOR: MENU: PSORIASIS **840-1**

Noons—Preferably raw fresh vegetables; none cooked at this meal. These would consist of spinach, or the like that make for purifying of the *humor* in the lymph blood as this is absorbed by the lacteal ducts as it is digested. We would not take any quantities of soups or broths at this period.

4/19/21
M. Adult
BLOOD-BUILDING **4867-1**

To clarify the bloodstream and to take on more vitamins will be found rather in the vegetable diet, that especially of spinach, and such diet as that. Of course, others may be taken in moderation, but principally such as these given.

2/15/39
F. 52 yrs.
NEURASTHENIA **920-13**

And when the spinach is selected, use the green portion rather than that which has been bleached. These portions have from twenty to forty percent more of the vitamins necessary for the sustaining of the better health, than those portions that are bleached by being covered or being forced into such a state.

3/21/39
F. 49 yrs.
RELAXATION **1158-21**

Q. Spinach and other leafy vegetables?

A. Once, twice or three times a week.

6/16/40
F. 64 yrs.
ARTHRITIS **2282-1**

Q. Regarding my health, and the arthritis condition, is it indicated as to what I should do for relief?

A. Keep down the acids in the system. Keep away from too much flesh in the diet; having more of NATURE'S foods; as spinach, as well as these in bulk for food.

3/23/40
F. 12 yrs.
EPILEPSY **2153-1**

Have plenty of the vitamins, especially of foods that carry B, B-1, A, C and D. Such would be included, of course, in plenty of raw vegetables—as spinach; these raw, you see, and grated very fine, or the juice extracted from same—not large quantities taken (of the juices) but a little bit each day.

4/7/37
F. 29 yrs.
COLD: CONGESTION: AFTEREFFECTS **808-6**

Q. Is my present diet correct?

A. As indicated it is very good, though there may be a little change to the fresh vegetables. Spinach may be taken, either green, cooked, or in whatever way is most palatable for the body.

1/30/28
F. Adult
ELIMINATIONS: POOR: TOXEMIA **81-2**

It would be necessary to meet the needs of the assimilation and of elimination of the blood and nerves center but one of those factors to chiefly consider is the diet. This would be found in chiefly the green vegetables and of those cooked vegetables that carry an amount of iron and such as found in the green vegetables such as spinach and all such vegetables.

7/22/31
ASSIMILATIONS: DEBILITATION: GENERAL **F. 28 yrs.**
BLOOD-BUILDING **3842-1**

We would give a diet that is easily assimilated. Let the diet be that as is nerve- and blood-building. And vegetables, spinach, and the like.

8/23/27
DIABETES: TENDENCIES **M. 26 yrs.**
ELIMINATIONS: INCOORDINATION **4145-1**

Q. Does this body have any habits indulged in excessively?

A. Too much of those as is seen in the *manner* of eating, and in that of the imbibing of those conditions that produce too much reaction from alcoholic condition *in* the system. Not as the excess of alcohol as consumed, but excess of alcohol as produced by the way and manner of eating, and by the indulging in those conditions that produce alcoholic reaction in the system itself.

The diet shall be those principally of vegetables, and especially of greens—spinach—all of those properties as carry much iron.

28)—Squash

9/4/41
BABY CARE **F. 2-1/2 yrs.**
ELIMINATIONS **1521-5**

There needs to be those considerations for more of the foods carrying the vitamins B and D, rather than these taken separately.

We find that these would be obtained in the correct proportions, at least two to three times each week, of yellow squash and the like.

Q. Any suggestions to help increase or make eliminations more normal?

A. The changing in the diet, with vegetables of the form and prepared in the manner indicated, will aid in this direction. This is much preferable to taking or giving laxatives, or eliminants. The fresh vegetables.

8/31/41
ARTHRITIS: PREVENTIVE **F. 51 yrs.**
BODY: GENERAL **1158-31**

Q. Yellow squash?

A. This as often as practical through the regular season. Include pumpkins a little bit later, because these are a good source of many of the needed vitamins.

6/20/40
M. 34 yrs.
BODY-BUILDING **1861-5**

As to the general health—there should be plenty of the food values that are nerve- and blood- and tissue-building. Have plenty of the vitamins, especially that may be had from THESE combined in the diet:

Through the summer have plenty of yellow neck squash, plenty of all characters of the vegetables—ESPECIALLY those that are yellow in color.

Not that the body is to be abnormal in these directions, but these things carry the character of vitamins necessary for this body.

Of course, take *every* form of food that carries the general body-building influences through the system.

6/3/41
DEBILITATION: GENERAL **M. 25 yrs.**
APPENDICITIS **1970-1**

(Do not begin this diet, of course, until after the period of the grape poultices and the grape diet.) Vegetables may then be taken, if cooked in their OWN salts, or their OWN juices—and eat the juices with same; cooking all in Patapar paper. Such as onions with squash and the like.

6/6/40
ASSIMILATIONS: POOR **F. 19 yrs.**
ANEMIA **2277-1**

Then the diet: Eat all of the vegetables that are especially YELLOW in color; as squash (only the yellow character).

10/20/34
ACIDITY: LESIONS **F. 48 yrs.**
ACIDITY **703-1**

Have at least three of the leafy vegetables to one below the ground, or with the leafy vegetables there may be one or two of the bulbous nature—as squash.

7/25/36
F. 32 yrs.
KIDNEYS: PREGNANCY **540-6**

Keep a well-balance between the diets for sufficient calcium and lime; as in squash. Things of that nature carry these in such quantities that they may be easily assimilated. So let the foods that are prepared occasionally have more and more of these.

8/27/40
M. 39 yrs.
VITAMINS: DEFICIENT **826-13**

Have every form of vegetable that carries the yellow coloring matter. These are products that carry the vitamin B in quantities of a helpful nature; also most of these carry G.

It is only necessary that there be the consideration of the proper foods; especially such as squash. These in the varied forms or manners as may be prepared would be most helpful.

11/6/35
M. 24 yrs.
BODY-BUILDING **533-7**

In the diets keep those things that will agree, yet we will find it will be necessary to change; but that are body-building. Vegetables especially such as squash will supply the necessary influence, of course with other things.

3/28/44
M. 41 yrs.
ACIDITY & ALKALINITY **4008-1**

Do not eat fried foods, for this particular body. Do have at least two vegetables that grow above the ground (whether they are such as squash or the like) to one that grows under the ground, or about the same combination as with the raw vegetables.

If man would consider same, even in an ordinary term, there are at least three of those that grow above the ground that man eats raw, to one under the ground that he eats raw. This applies to cooked foods also, meats or other foods.

6/27/41
F. 18 yrs.
ANEMIA **1207-2**

Have the regular foods; those that carry quantities, or an excess, of vitamin B-1 especially such as would be found in all foods that are yellow in nature or color. Eat plenty of yellow squash, and the like. There should be excesses of these in the diet, though—to be sure—other foods would be taken normally.

4/19/41
F. 51 yrs.
1158-30

ASSIMILATIONS

Q. Shall I supplement with additional vitamin B tablets?

A. We find that if this vitamin is supplied in the diet it will be better than taking an overquantity of vitamin B, which would be the case if the tablets were taken as a supplement. With the Adiron taken, that is to aid in assimilation, it would be better to supplement the vitamin B in the diet, with such as yellow squash. These taken, as we find, with beef and fowl, should carry sufficient vitamins.

10/17/34
M. Adult
698-1

ANEMIA

In the diet, keep much of that which will add more phosphorus and gold to the system; as we will find in certain of the vegetables—as squash, and the like. These should be a portion of the diet each day; not that it would be these *only*—but keep more of an alkaline diet.

3/29/40
F. 50 yrs.
1158-23

BODY-BUILDING

Now, as to the diet:

There has been the tendency to leave off those things that make for a better stimulation to the blood- and body-building forces.

This is merely an outline:

Noons—Special reference to all vegetables that are of the yellow variety stressed in the diet. This would include squash and the like; only the yellow neck squash, of course, or yellow squash that comes much later—but these can be obtained and might be a part of the diet.

7/18/40
F. 39 yrs.
2309-1

ASSIMILATIONS: ELIMINATIONS: INCOORDINATION

Take plenty of food values that carry vitamin B-1 and G. These are found especially in the yellow neck squash. These should be in the diet almost daily. Give these combined in different forms.

5/15/41
F. Adult
2500-1

ANEMIA: DEBILITATION: GENERAL

We would add B-1 in the foods. Also yellow neck squash, these are well for the body.

8/27/40
F. 40 yrs.
2332-1

ATHLETE'S FOOT: ECZEMA

Have plenty of vegetables, especially squash.

29)—Sweet Potatoes and Yams

2/27/37
COMBINATIONS: ASSIMILATIONS **F. Adult**
ELIMINATIONS: INCOORDINATION **1342-1**

Roasted yams or sweet potatoes are very good if plenty of butter is taken with same.

6/6/40
ASSIMILATIONS: POOR **F. 19 yrs.**
ANEMIA **2277-1**

Eat all of the vegetables that are especially YELLOW in color. The sweet potatoes or yams—only the yellow variety used.

5/20/38
F. 68 yrs.
TOXEMIA **1593-1**

Keep white potatoes AWAY FROM THIS BODY! Sweet potatoes or yams may be taken occasionally.

9/18/43
M. 22 yrs.
TUBERCULOSIS **3222-1**

Do have all the leafy vegetables the body can absorb—as foods are changed. Not too much of the pod or tuberous vegetables, though sweet potatoes should be taken. These are very good.

3/15/44
F. 26 yrs.
PARALYSIS **3694-1**

Add all of the foods that carry silicon and the salts that may revibrate with the applications of the gold to the nerve centers for assimilation; as foods of the tuberous nature of every character—the yams (sweet potatoes). These should be parts of the foods for the body. Have at least five vegetables grown below the ground to one grown above the ground, or in that proportion.

1/4/36
BLOOD-BUILDING: MINERALS **F. 22 yrs.**
CALCIUM DEFICIENCY **578-5**

Q. Please give in full a blood-building diet for my body.

A. Those as indicated that have a quantity or an excess of the calcium, and those that will make for a balance in the iodines with the potassiums of the system itself.

Sweet potatoes are those that carry the vitamins necessary for body-building with *this* body.

8/27/32
F. 72 yrs.
CIRRHOSIS OF LIVER **2092-1**

Evenings—Well-cooked vegetables, but preferably all those that grow *above* the ground, than those that grow *in* the ground; though the yam may be included rather than the white potato.

9/10/23
M. Adult
ELIMINATIONS: INCOORDINATION **4232-1**

Let the diet be not of meats, or of sweets, but of vegetable matter that grows above the ground, not of the tuberous nature, such as potatoes or yams—see?

4/20/40
F. 74 yrs.
ARTHRITIS **1224-3**

Evenings—The meal principally should consist of vegetables, but eliminate any form of potatoes; though yams or the like may be occasionally used.

10/8/36
ANEMIA **F. 54 yrs.**
ARTHRITIS: TOXEMIA **1269-1**

Noons—Preferably a combination of meat juices *or* vegetable juices, but do not put the two together!

Keep away from white bread and white potatoes! Yams, all of these that grow under the ground may be a part of the diet. Those cooked—the vegetables in the evening—as roughage for the body.

3/15/37
BLOOD: HUMOR **F. 56 yrs.**
TOXEMIA **569-25**

Q. What cooked vegetables may be taken?

A. Any of the leafy vegetables. Yams may be taken provided they have not been frozen, and these—of course—with butter.

2/27/42
F. 52 yrs.
COLD: CONGESTION **404-10**

Q. What vegetables are especially good for my body, considering the condition of kidneys?

A. Sweet potatoes—these cooked.

9/16/41
ELIMINATIONS: INCOORDINATION **F. 2 yrs.**
VITAMINS **2015-8**

Be mindful as to the diets; keeping plenty of the vitamins, especially B-1, A and G. These will be found principally in yellow yams.

30)—Tomatoes

10/4/35
DIABETES: TENDENCIES **M. 57 yrs.**
ACIDITY & ALKALINITY **584-5**

Q. What has been the effect on my system of eating so many tomatoes?

A. Quite a dissertation might be given as to the effect of tomatoes upon the human system. Of all the vegetables, tomatoes carry most of the vitamins in a well-balanced assimilative manner for the activities in the system. Yet if these are not cared for properly, they may become very destructive to a physical organism; that is, if they ripen after being pulled, or if there is the contamination with other influences.

In *this* particular body, as we find, the reactions from these have been not *always* the *best.* Neither has there been the normal reaction from the eating of same. For it tends to make for an irritation or humor. Nominally, though, these should form at least a portion of a meal three or four days out of every week; and they will be found to be *most* helpful.

The tomato is one vegetable that in most instances (because of the greater uniform activity) is preferable to be eaten after being canned, for it is then much more uniform.

The reaction in this body, then, has been to form an acid of its own; though the tomato is among those foods that may be taken as the *non*-acid forming. But these should be of the best in *every* instance where they are used.

Q. What brand of canned tomatoes is best?

A. Libby's are more *uniform* than most.

APPLES: ELIMINATIONS **12/30/40**
ASSIMILATIONS: POOR **M. 52 yrs.**
COOKING UTENSILS: ALUMINUM: NOT RECOMMENDED **2423-1**

For this body, do not eat foods prepared in aluminum at all; for, from the natural conditions and the supercharges of acids, the body will be allergic to the effects from aluminum on foods—especially tomatoes.

12/18/30
M. 24 yrs.
BACILLOSIS: POLIOMYELITIS **135-1**

Noon—Tomatoes, if they are *ripened on the vine;* otherwise, those that are canned *without* preservative—or especially benzoate of soda. (Do not use such as use that as preservative. These may be used, especially the juices of same. Any that are palatable, that are raw.

1/7/34
F. 21 yrs.
GLANDS: INCOORDINATION **480-3**

Lunch—Rather green vegetables entirely. Tomatoes may be used with either fruits or vegetables, see? or at the same meal with either.

7/17/43
M. 31 yrs.
ALLERGIES: METALS: ECZEMA **2518-3**

Q. What effect does . . . fresh tomatoes have on this condition?

A. Fresh tomatoes should not be harmful for the body.

1/4/36
8LOOD-BUILDING: MINERALS **F. 22 yrs.**
CALCIUM DEFICIENCY **578-5**

Tomatoes, and such natures are those that carry the vitamins necessary for body-building with *this* body.

12/31/40
M. 51 yrs.
ASTHMA **2424-1**

Have plenty of leafy vegetables rather than the dried. Tomatoes should be especially taken, but raw rather than cooked; that is, those canned and eaten just as they are when taken from the can are preferable, in most cases, to those that are shipped or fresh.

8/29/41
F. 25 yrs.
COMBINATIONS: OBESITY **2579-1**

There are certain foods to which the body is allergic. This will necessitate that they not be used with ANY of those foods that grow above the ground, but only those that grow under the ground; that is: tomatoes would be served at the same meal with potatoes, while taking them with corn, peas or beans would be harmful.

6/28/28
M. 21 yrs.
ARTHRITIS **849-4**

The diet will be those as have been outlined, abstaining from meats or butter, but as much of the vegetable forces as possible; especially tomatoes—these are *well* for the body, *properly* prepared. The fruit only when well ripened on the vine; not as gathered green and ripened afterward. That that is well ripened, seasoned with salt, pepper, and if vinegar is preferable—or sugar and vinegar—this would be well to use with same.

5/30/29
F. 31 yrs.
CONSTIPATION **1713-17**

Tomatoes are very good, provided they are fully ripe—*preferable* that these be taken in the juice, rather than the pulp of same.

5/1/38
F. Adult
ARTHRITIS **932-1**

Noons—Only raw green vegetables, as tomatoes (this doesn't sound like much for this type, yet it would be well if not too much is taken; one slice or one quarter will not be too much, provided it is cut well with), lettuce, *green* cabbage, celery, carrots, spinach, onions, radish, and the like. These *green, fresh, crisp;* never any of the wilted or withered, but use more *outside* leaves than inside of the vegetables or the salad leaves or the like. Such a salad may be taken with either oil or mayonnaise dressing.

6/9/27
F. 20 mos.
TOXEMIA **608-3**

Plenty of the juice of tomatoes, and canned tomatoes—not of the fresh—those that are canned without benzoate of soda; or in those of the California fruit company brands.

4/17/31
DEBILITATION: GENERAL **M. 19 yrs.**
CHOREA **1225-1**

Mornings—Tomatoes, tomato juice, those of *any* of the stewed fruits—see? fresh or those preserved, provided they are not preserved in or with benzoate of soda.

ASSIMILATIONS: ELIMINATIONS: INCOORDINATION **11/9/40**
CANCER: TENDENCIES **F. 61 yrs.**
ACIDITY & ALKALINITY **1697-2**

Q. What foods may be taken that will digest properly?

A. Any of those that are easily assimilated; that is, three times as much alkaline-reacting as acid-producing foods. This means the alkaline-REACTING, and not acid-producing. For instance, all the vegetables that are easily assimilated would be included, provided they are not sprayed with preservatives—these either canned or fresh. Canned tomatoes, if not canned with benzoate of soda, are preferable to the raw—to be sure—at this season of the year.

10/20/32
BRONCHITIS: ELIMINATIONS: POOR **F. Adult**
ELIMINATIONS **4293-1**

Evenings—Well-cooked vegetables that grow *above* the ground; none that grow below the ground—none! Tomatoes are especially good for the body, though these have been tabu by some who have given a diet for the body. Especially the tomato juices that are prepared or preserved are good, provided they are *not* preserved with any form of preservative matter such as benzoate of soda or similar preservatives; but such as Libby's or the like are of the nature that is helpful to the body.

8/5/29
F. 43 yrs.
MENU: NEURASTHENIA **2713-1**

At least each day have a vegetable that is raw. Many tomatoes are good for the body even though they apparently at times make a rash. These will disappear, if properly served and properly cared for in their preparation. The *juices* of tomatoes are well.

2/23/35
DERMATITIS **M. Adult**
BLOOD: HUMOR: MENU: PSORIASIS **840-1**

Noons—Preferably raw fresh vegetables; none cooked at this meal. These would consist of tomatoes, or the like that make for purifying of the *humor* in the lymph blood as this is absorbed by the lacteal ducts as it is digested. We would not take any quantities of soups or broths at this period.

4/19/21
M. Adult
BLOOD-BUILDING **4867-1**

To clarify the bloodstream and to take on more vitamins will be found rather in the vegetable diet, that especially of tomatoes and such diet as that. Of course, others may be taken in moderation, but principally such as these given.

10/17/27
M. 8 mos.
BABY CARE **5520-2**

Q. How long should the tomatoes be cooked before giving him the juice?

A. Don't cook 'em! for in tomatoes there is found the three *necessary* vitamins for growth and for *development.* Hence the good use that this is for the *development* of the child that has the tendency to be backward in starting, as it were, in growth. The same is seen in carrots—save these are not *balanced* in the same ratio as in tomatoes. With tomatoes, choose the well ripe, and strain or mash out the juice so that only the juice and little or none of the pulp or seed is taken. Very little necessary, but the necessary vitamins are taken in these two properties, especially for a growing child.

Q. Should he have any cooked vegetable juices? If so, *how soon?*

A. As given, any of these as have been outlined are very good. We would *not* cook the tomatoes.

12/15/27
M. 30 yrs.
ASTHENIA **4605-1**

As for the diet, let that be principally of that as almost pre-digested foods—though as much of raw vegetables as may be well taken, carrying plenty of iron and of salts.

Fruits may be taken in moderation—especially tomatoes.

9/2/29
CHILDREN: ABNORMAL **M. 7 yrs.**
NERVOUS SYSTEMS: INCOORDINATION **758-2**

Those that are a stimuli for the nerve system are tomatoes—the *juices* of same, and it will be found that those that are *canned without* the sodas will be *better* than those of the fresh variety, *unless* it be those that are *well* ripened on the vine, but those as taken and ripened by artificial forces—or by sun, without the vine—not well for the body.

ASSIMILATIONS: ELIMINATIONS: INCOORDINATION **2/18/28**
ASTHENIA **F. Adult**
TUMORS: TENDENCIES **4789-1**

As much of the tomato as the body will assimilate will be found well in keeping an equal balance in the vitamins for the system.

Do this as given and we will bring much better conditions for this body, preventing any accumulations in the form of tumor—as indicated in plethora condition existent in portions of the system—yet not well defined to that state where these may not be eliminated, were the proper precautions taken as given.

5/16/29
F. Adult
TOXEMIA **5571-1**

Tomatoes, sufficient amount of these—both of those that have been preserved (that is, canned) and of the fresh variety. These are good.

7/22/31
ACIDITY **F. 28 yrs.**
ASSIMILATIONS: ELIMINATIONS: INCOORDINATION **2261-1**

Those of tomatoes are especially good for the body, not overly ripe ones but full ripe—and those that ripen on the vine, rather than in the sun or in the air; or those that have been prepared properly, without benzoate of soda; this is one fruit that becomes better by being canned.

4/25/40
ACIDITY **F. Adult**
DEBILITATION: GENERAL **2179-1**

If tomatoes are used, those that are canned are preferable to those ripened after being taken from the vine.

1/7/37
CIRCULATION: POOR **F. 44 yrs.**
ELIMINATIONS: POOR **1315-6**

Do not take tomatoes either cooked or raw *with* other green cooked or raw vegetables; though tomatoes by themselves (preferably the canned) are very good as a portion of the noon meal, or an evening meal.

7/26/43
M. 2 yrs.
ELIMINATIONS: INCOORDINATION **3109-1**

Fruits such as tomatoes are tabu for the body.

10/20/43
ASSIMILATIONS: POOR **F. 73 yrs.**
BODY-BUILDING **3304-1**

Keep to the body-building forces in the diet. Plenty of raw vegetables, such as tomatoes and the like. These supply silicon, as well as that needed in other energies to replenish the body.

7/26/40
F. 12 yrs.
EPILEPSY **2153-2**

Noons—Let the principal portion consist of tomatoes (these in moderation), with some fruit juices or vegetable juices, or soup.

10/11/43
F. 26 yrs.
ARTHRITIS **3285-1**

We should have easily assimilated foods, but those very high in the adding of B-Complex, or the vitamin B—as in tomatoes. These should be a part of the diet daily with plenty of seafoods (not fresh water fish).

2/21/34
M. 20 yrs.
EPILEPSY **521-1**

Noons—Tomatoes, not in great quantities, for these—even with a salad—would preferably be canned, provided they are not such that carry preservatives in the preparation, unless they are *well* ripened on the vine and gathered fresh—*then* the fresh tomatoes may be taken, but not those that are ripened artificially or superficially.

At this meal there may also be had oils, as olive oil or the dressings that make such a meal more palatable.

6/24/41
ELIMINATIONS: INCOORDINATION **M. 29 yrs.**
ECZEMA **2518-1**

Never use spaghetti, for this body, with tomatoes and peppers. Spaghetti may be taken, but preferably with the meats.

7/28/43
ANEMIA **F. 56 yrs.**
GENERAL: MULTIPLE SCLEROSIS **3118-1**

In the diet—keep to those things that heal within and without. A great deal of tomatoes. These, of course, are to be used in sufficient quantity to satisfy the appetite but not to make them become as something disliked. So prepare them in many different forms.

7/10/30
M. 65 yrs.
BLOOD-BUILDING: MENU: ASSIMILATIONS **4806-1**

We would be mindful of the diet, that there are those of the full rebuilding—especially of those that build for the blood supply.

In the noon meal, those preferably of the vegetables that are raw, in part—and there may be added some seafoods, with oils as dressings for same. Plenty of tomatoes.

2/12/38
F. 61 yrs.
ARTHRITIS **1512-2**

Q. May I eat tomatoes?

A. These should be very little, not large quantities of these. A little would be very well, but not very much—and these occasionally.

8/27/40
F. 40 yrs.
ATHLETE'S FOOT: ECZEMA **2332-1**

Little of fruits; not much of the mixtures of the various acids; that is, NEVER combine peaches with tomatoes at the same meal—but either of these in moderation may be taken occasionally.

5/26/28
COLD: CONGESTION **M. 33 yrs.**
LIVER: KIDNEYS: INCOORDINATION **900-386**

Q. Would it be well for me to eat vegetables such as corn, tomatoes, and the like?

A. Corn and tomatoes are excellent. More of the vitamins are obtained in tomatoes than in any other *one* growing vegetable.

31)—Turnips: General

10/6/43
DEBILITATION: GENERAL **F. 31 yrs.**
BODY-BUILDING **3267-1**

In the diet, do keep body-building foods. Turnips also should be included whenever in season, the tops as well as the root itself.

Doing these, we should bring the better conditions for this body.

9/25/37
SPINE: SUBLUXATION5 **F. 35 yrs.**
MINERALS **903-25**

There is first an unbalancing of the elements in the activities of the system—or lack of sufficient calcium for the full activity of body-building.

Hence there should be the use of the food values that carry such in such measures as may be assimilated by the body. Those as we find in turnips especially should be a portion of the diet.

1/10/42
M. 12 yrs.
DIABETES: TENDENCIES **415-8**

Have plenty of those foods that carry some calcium, as turnips. The turnips may be cooked with a little pork or plain, and then seasoned.

2/21/34
M. 20 yrs.
EPILEPSY **521-1**

Evenings—Vegetables at this meal may include any of those that are well cooked in their *own* sauce, or their *own* liquid, not adding waters nor seasoning until after they are cooked. And have three that grow *above* the ground to one that grows below the ground, but may include the tops and the roots of such; as turnips, *when* such below the ground are prepared. Not at all times, but that the vitamin forces of these may carry the necessary elements for creating a balance in the system that has long been lacking in sufficient of the phosphorus, silicon, iron and iodine. Hence all the vegetables that carry these properties should be included in the meals from day to day; for they are more easily assimilated by the body or system from vegetable matter than from any other source or character.

1/4/36
BLOOD-BUILDING: MINERALS **F. 22 yrs.**
CALCIUM DEFICIENCY **578-5**

Q. Please give in full a blood-building diet for my body.

A. Those as indicated that have a quantity or an excess of the calcium, and those that will make for a balance in the iodines with the potassiums of the system itself.

Turnips are those that carry the vitamins necessary for body-building with *this* body.

5/30/24
M. Adult

ASTHMA **4740-2**

Turnips, that character of foods may be eaten. Not much sweets but those that add nutriment to the system, without overtaxing the digestive organs in elimination.

1/10/41
M. 60 yrs.

ELIMINATIONS: INCOORDINATION **1963-2**

Q. What weight is best for body?

A. That which is the natural or normal weight by the general exercise. Do not attempt to take those things to cause reduction at the present, other than in the diet outlined. Use turnips and such; these may be taken in moderation. But beware of dried beans or peas or things of that nature.

9/1/39
M. 49 yrs.

PARKINSON'S DISEASE **1989-1**

Be mindful of the diet—that there are plenty of vitamins. Have plenty of green vegetables. Plenty of turnips, cooked in their own juices, saving the salts or the water in which such are cooked as a part of the diet.

10/21/32

ELEPHANTIASIS: TENDENCIES **F. 18 yrs.**
ARTHRITIS: GLANDS: INCOORDINATION **951-1**

Supply an overabundant amount of those foods that carry iron, iodine and phosphorus in the system. Beware of any that would carry more of those that would add silicon in the system.

The evening meal may be of well-balanced vegetables that are of the leafy nature, and that carry more of those properties as given. We will find much in turnips.

3/15/44
F. 26 yrs.

PARALYSIS **3694-1**

Add all of the foods that carry silicon and the salts that may revibrate with the applications of the gold to the nerve centers for assimilation; as foods of the tuberous nature of every character—every form of turnip. These should be parts of the foods for the body. Have at least five vegetables grown below the ground to one grown above the ground, or in that proportion.

8/5/42
F. 37 yrs.

PREGNANCY **1505-4**

Q. What particularly in the diet should she avoid, to prevent this condition in the kidneys?

A. Any of those that tend to carry influences that are overactive on the kidneys. Not such as turnips or some of the vegetables that grow under the ground. Keep on top of the ground more now with all of the vegetables eaten.

8/31/41
ARTHRITIS: PREVENTIVE **F. 51 yrs.**
BODY: GENERAL **1158-31**

Q. What are the best sources of calcium in foods?

A. Vegetables such as turnips, and all of those that grow under the ground.

12/18/30
M. 24 yrs.
BACILLOSIS: POLIOMYELITIS **135-1**

Noon—More of the vegetables that are *raw.* These may be made into salads with salad dressings, especially with as much of the olive oil as is palatable and that will be assimilated with the character of foods. This would include turnips, and all of those that may be used as such.

4/17/44
F. 36 yrs.
MULTIPLE SCLEROSIS **5031-1**

Turnips, such are well for this body; not in too large quantities, but they form the salts and the character of vitamins in the right combinations to make for the strengthening of this body.

12/2/40
DEBILITATION: GENERAL **F. 60 yrs.**
APPETITE: DIGESTION: INDIGESTION: NERVOUS **538-66**

Q. Any special foods at mealtime advised?

A. All of those that carry a great deal of iron and silicon, and things of that nature; that is—turnips, turnip greens, all of those that grow under the ground through the winter . . . these are beneficial.

10/7/43
M. 68 yrs.
NEPHRITIS: TENDENCIES **1112-9**

Change the diet somewhat. Eat plenty of turnips. These will aid the body in the regular diet and will make for much better conditions.

2/23/25
M. 20 yrs.
BODY-BUILDING **77-2**

Q. What special foods should be given the body that would give to the mind and body strength, endurance and activity?

A. Green vegetable forces of every character, especially those of the tuberous nature. Of course some portions of them cooked, the greater number eaten raw: Turnips, those of that nature.

11/29/39
F. 40 yrs.
ELIMINATIONS: INCOORDINATION **2050-1**

In the matter of the diets through these periods—we will find that those foods combining a greater quantity of vitamin B-1 (thiamine) would be especially most beneficial to the body, as they will aid in eliminating those disturbances through the whole of the system, especially as related to the conditions carried in the bloodstream itself.

In turnips and such we will find the greater quantity, or the active forces from this vitamin needed by this particular body.

10/8/36
ANEMIA **F. 54 yrs.**
ARTHRITIS: TOXEMIA **1269-1**

Noons—preferably a combination of meat juices *or* vegetable juices, but do not put the two together!

Turnips, these that grow under the ground may be a part of the diet. Those cooked, or the vegetables in the evening—as roughage for the body.

11/6/35
GLANDS: THYROID: HYPOTHYROIDISM **F. 63 yrs.**
MINERALS **1049-1**

In the matter of the diet, this would be rather important. Occasionally use a great deal of those things that carry quantities of iodine, for this the body requires. But for this body it will be most soluble from vegetables; turnips and the like.

i)—Turnip Greens

12/12/31
F. 46 yrs.
ULCERS: STOMACH **482-3**

In the evening meals, those of the well-cooked vegetables, but only those of the leafy nature—or that grow in pods; not the bulb nature. No turnips, nothing of that nature. The *tops* of these may be taken, and may be eaten, but not the bulb nature.

7/15/30
F. 55 yrs.
ACIDITY **760-16**

Turnips, provided they are not with that of pork—for these would be unsavory. The tops are the better for the body.

10/27/41
F. 31 yrs.
DERMATITIS: CIRCULATION: POOR **1688-8**

Q. Are vegetables such as turnip greens good for me now?

A. Good if these are well cooked, but not in a lot of grease. These should be cooked in their own juices and the juice taken as well as the vegetable. For, the effective or more healthful portions of turnips is in the water that comes from same by cooking.

3/22/32
F. 42 yrs.
COLITIS **404-2**

Q. Why cannot this body eat a cooked green vegetable, such as turnip greens?

A. It may. Well these be added in the system—so that they will act with the gastric juices.

DIABETES: TENDENCIES 8/23/27 M. 26 yrs.
ELIMINATIONS: INCOORDINATION 4145-1

The diet shall be those principally of vegetables, and especially of greens—turnip greens—all of those properties as carry much iron.

32)—Water Cress

ANEMIA 1/17/44 F. 44 yrs. 3564-1

Keep plenty of raw vegetables; as water cress. Not necessarily at any one period but some every day. Often prepare these with gelatin—about three times a week, for gelatin also is needed in the body. Grate them, slice them, dice them, changing their manner of preparation so as not to become objectionable.

COLD: CONGESTION 11/21/43 M. 59 yrs.
ACIDITY 462-18

Don't overeat, don't have too much of vegetables or of pastries or of meats, but keep them well balanced. Have a great deal of water cress, mixed with gelatin. These are good for the body. They will aid in all portions of the sensory system, especially in the eyes, the ears, and the drainages through the antrum and the soft tissue of head; for these supply elements that keep these portions of the body bettered.

ARTHRITIS 7/23/43 F. 59 yrs.
ACIDITY 3110-1

Some proteins should be taken, but these should be included in the vegetables—in the manner in which they are prepared. Use more of the leafy variety than those of the bulbular or seed nature. Especially water cress, combined with green mustard and lettuce and celery, should also be in the diet.

ASSIMILATIONS: ELIMINATIONS: INCOORDINATION 10/29/43 F. 13 yrs.
HEADACHE: MIGRAINE 3326-1

Water cress, especially, should be taken—and these raw.

ARTHRITIS: TENDENCIES 6/14/43 F. 47 yrs. 585-11

Add to the diet a great deal of water cress and we will find it will change a great deal of these disturbances.

CANCER: SKIN 12/28/43 F. 75 yrs. 3532-1

In the diet often have raw vegetables, especially water cress and all of the vegetables that may be well combined in a salad. These at times prepared with gelatin will be well to give strength to the muscular forces of the body.

8/24/44
F. 58 yrs.
ASTHENIA **5394-1**

In building up the body with foods, preferably have a great deal of raw vegetables for this body—as water cress. Take raw, with dressing, and oft with gelatin. Do preserve the juices with them when these are prepared in this manner in the gelatin.

8/10/43
CHILDBIRTH: AFTEREFFECTS **F. 44 yrs.**
ELIMINATIONS **3149-1**

Also it would help to keep better eliminations for the body regularly. These may be controlled best, as we find, for this particular body by the diet. So include often in the diet water cress, the activities as to "Grasses" (so called). These may be grated or cut very fine and used with mayonnaise or an oil dressing; not to "burn out" with same as some might do, but change them as to their usage, and we shall find it will change the general elimination and increase the strengthening of the body, relieving those tensions that cause pressures to the head and to the secondary nervous system of the body.

Q. Should any particular foods be avoided or stressed in the diet?

A. Stress the raw foods as indicated, especially water cress.

5/31/44
F. 76 yrs.
ARTHRITIS **5175-1**

We would increase the amount of the vitamins which come and appear in water cress, for these natures will bring eliminations for the body.

10/27/43
ANEMIA: TENDENCIES **F. 53 yrs.**
ELIMINATION: POOR **3316-1**

Do have plenty of water cress. It would be well to prepare these with the gelatin, by juicing or scraping them. These should never be combined with any vinegar or acetic acid. To be sure, these would not be all the foods that should be taken, but have plenty of these vegetables. Use more of the leafy than the pod or bulbular nature. Vegetable juices, soups or broths will be well.

7/30/41
M. 26 yrs.
ANESTHESIA: AFTEREFFECTS **1710-6**

The general diet should be for body-building. Be sure that most of the foods carry especially vitamin B. These are best found in vegetables of the yellow variety, as well as in water cress.

11/3/43
M. 54 yrs.
GLANDS: ADRENALS: THYROID: GLAUCOMA **3276-1**

To be sure, have plenty of vegetables, especially such as water cress. A great deal of these combined with gelatin and gelatin preparations would be well. These we would include in the diet.

9/13/43
M. 41 yrs.
ARTHRITIS 3077-1

Liquids and semi-liquids for the present, beef juices. These will be the better, with the regular vegetables that are beneficial. Do include in these a great deal of water cress in the diet.

4/6/44
F. 62 yrs.
NERVE-BUILDING 4033-1

In the diet there should be the stressing of those that are nerve-building. Vegetables that are raw, especially such as water cress.

7/21/44
F. 60 yrs.
CANCER: LUNGS 5374-1

Water cress should be taken very often, as also the foods which are used as garnishes for dishes, as with steak or the like.

6/2/44
ARTHRITIS: TENDENCIES F. 49 yrs.
CIRCULATION: INCOORDINATION 2970-2

In the matter of the diet do take more raw foods, especially water cress and such foods and do include with these gelatin oft. These grated, ground, but do use the juices of same with gelatin. These, with the other corrections, will change conditions of eyes, throat and all of the organs of the sensory system; improve hearing, vision, vocal box, as well as taste and sense of vibrations about the body.

7/17/43
F. 69 yrs.
ARTHRITIS 3138-1

A small can of water cress, as it is prepared for usage in salads and the like. Do this daily for at least sixty days. You will find changes will be brought. This is not all that is to be taken, to be sure, but this should be a part of the diet each day. The elements here are to keep down the tendency for the flare in the bloodstream of those conditions that produce irritation and weakness.

7/17/43
ALLERGIES: METALS: ECZEMA M. 31 yrs.
ECZEMA 2518-3

Each day we would take internally a small can of water cress. This may be taken at two meals or at one meal, but take a small can each day.

7/28/43
ANEMIA F. 56 yrs.
MULTIPLE SCLEROSIS 3118-1

In the diet—keep to those things that heal within and without. Use plenty of water cress . . . These, of course, are to be used in sufficient quantity to satisfy the appetite but not to make any of them become as something disliked. So prepare them in many different forms.

7/30/41
M. 26 yrs.
ANESTHESIA: AFTEREFFECTS **1710-6**

Q. Please give further corrective diet.

A. As indicated, it is necessary in the present to add plenty of the elements found in salads. Not that the body is to live off these entirely, to be sure, but these are to be in the diet often—two to three times a week as a part of some meal during the day. The general diet should be for body-building. Be sure that most of the foods carry especially vitamin B. These are best found in vegetables of the yellow variety, as well as in water cress and the like.

10/9/43
ELIMINATIONS: POOR **F. 55 yrs.**
BODY-BUILDING **2992-2**

In the diet, keep strengthening foods; that is, plenty of seafoods, plenty of vegetables of the leafy variety, including water cress often.

4)—Vegetable Juices: General

6/16/40
F. 64 yrs.
ARTHRITIS **2282-1**

Q. Regarding my health, and the arthritis condition, is it indicated as to what I should do for relief?

A. Keep down the acids in the system. Keep away from too much flesh in the diet; having more of NATURE'S foods; as carrot, spinach, and celery juices, as well as these in bulk for food.

7/6/40
HEART: TOXEMIA **F. 65 yrs.**
APPETITE **1152-10**

Q. Are raw vegetable juices, plain and mixed, well for me to take?

A. These are very good provided they are the correct ones. Carrot juice, spinach juice, celery and lettuce juices are very well mixed. Beet juices should be cooked, not taken raw.

7/28/34
F. 54 yrs.
RHEUMATISM **133-4**

Noons—Not too much should be taken at this meal, and that only of vegetable juices. And the preferable way to prepare such juices would be through cooking the vegetables after tying them in Patapar paper; not putting them in water to boil, but cooking either in the Patapar paper or in a steam cooker, so that only the juices from the vegetables may be obtained—and no water added in the cooking at all. Then these juices should be combined and seasoned to the taste. This activity will build into the system the proper associations with that which has been indicated by the corrections in the spine and make for corrections in the activities throughout the digestive system.

1/9/35
M. 1 yr.
WORMS **786-1**

We would begin with a body-*building* diet.

Noons—A part of this meal should consist of the vegetable juices, as Gerber's—or they may be combined from fresh vegetable juices, but not where they have been cooked with greases. Better that these be the juices taken from vegetables prepared in a steam cooker or Patapar paper, then only seasoned for the strengthening forces that may make it palatable to the body. And a little fowl or wild game may be given at times to the body.

5/1/35
M. 1-1/2 yrs.
WORMS: PINWORMS: AFTEREFFECTS **786-2**

Gerber's vegetable juices are good for the body; these may be taken at times, or prepared with a little gluten in same—as with rice (this should be the brown or unpolished rice) or barley mixed with same at times.

9/29/34
M. Adult
ABRASIONS: TOXEMIA **675-1**

Noons—Preferably either a raw green vegetable salad—or all vegetable juices; not those juices that are cooked with meats, but the juices that are combined of themselves, cooked either in a heater or Patapar paper.

3/12/36
MUSCULAR DYSTROPHY **M. 43 yrs.**
INTESTINES: GAS **1127-1**

In the diet keep to those things that cause less and less of the gas to form in the digestive system, through a very depleted or very ineffective activity of a peristaltic movement. Hence use vegetable juices prepared in their own salts—these would be better for the body. Hence do not cook the vegetables together that are given the body, but separate—in Patapar paper; or serve each one separate, and it will be found to be more helpful, more beneficial to the body.

3/22/44
M. 79 yrs.
APPETITE: CATARACTS **3288-2**

Vary the juices. A combination of juices may be used from several vegetables; such as carrots, lettuce, celery, water cress, onion, radishes, all of these may be included. Change them so that the body does not grow tired of them. These, as we find, should bring better conditions and keep a better equilibrium for the body.

9/22/36
M. 75 yrs.
CANCER **1263-1**

In the matter of the diet, keep more to the liquids and semi-liquids. The juices of vegetables, combinations of these should be taken.

7/16/35
F. 64 yrs.
ARTHRITIS **950-1**

Mornings—Rather the juices of vegetables than citrus fruits; as a combination of spinach, cabbage, lettuce, celery, mustard, all cooked together in clear water—*boiled* heavily, strained off, seasoned and taken as a drink.

Q. Should nothing be taken for breakfast except the vegetable juices?

A. With the brown bread or a cereal drink.

Always the breads should be toasted, and of the whole wheat variety.

10/8/36
ANEMIA **F. 54 yrs.**
ARTHRITIS: TOXEMIA **1269-1**

Noons—Preferably a combination of meat juices *or* vegetable juices, but do not put the two together! There may be at times chicken broth with rice or barley, or there may be beef stock with combinations of vegetables, but *preferably* only vegetable juices *or* meat juices.

7/26/40
F. 12 yrs.
EPILEPSY **2153-2**

Refrain from any large quantities of sweets. Preferably have vegetables and vegetable juices as the principal portion of the diet.

1/24/35
M. Child
COLD: CONGESTION **738-2**

If there will be kept a more alkaline condition in the body, the better will be the general conditions and welfare. With the cold and congestion in the present, almost an entire liquid diet would be the better. Vegetable juices and some broths, with a strengthening in the beef juices (without the meat).

Q. What should be done for the fever?

A. It may be reduced by the use of the fluids, or the non-acid fluids in the food.

1/23/39
M. 32 yrs.
ASSIMILATIONS: POOR **1798-1**

Q. Should just the juices of vegetables be taken?

A. Other than this will be poison to the system! If you feed him every fifteen or thirty minutes, he can get powerful fat on it!

Q. Should any fruit juices be taken?

A. These may be given occasionally, to change from the others; but it will have to be careful with same.

As indicated, the vegetables of all characters cooked in their OWN juices—this doesn't mean boil with meat or water or anything else, but boil in their OWN juices, in Patapar paper!

11/7/33
DEBILITATION: GENERAL **M. Adult**
ANEMIA **432-1**

Noons, or the meals between the main meals of the day—would be vegetable juices that are strong in their activity toward supplying the elements that create for the body blood and nerve plasm (which are the iron and salts of vegetables and fruits that make for *replenishing* to the system).

10/23/43
F. 44 yrs.
ASTHMA **3046-2**

Q. Is there some food that I eat which aggravates my condition?

A. Any sweets will aggravate the condition, or too much starches. Vegetable juices, all of these are better for the body—whenever there are such symptoms or tendencies.

5/18/43
M. 63 yrs.
ARTHRITIS **3009-1**

Have a great deal of the juices, especially such as lettuce, celery, carrots, beets, radishes and the like. And include with the beets the beet tops—these cooked, you see. These should be taken often, the cooked beets and carrots. If these are adhered to, we will bring bettered conditions for this body.

6/20/40
M. 34 yrs.
BODY-BUILDING **1861-5**

As to the general health—there should be plenty of the food values that are nerve- and blood- and tissue-building. Have plenty of the vitamins, especially that may be had from THESE combined in the diet:

Each day take at least two ounces of raw carrot and spinach juice, or carrot and lettuce juice. These may be combined or taken separately.

3/29/40
F. 50 yrs.
BODY-BUILDING **1158-23**

Now, as to the diet:

There has been the tendency to leave off those things that make for a better stimulation to the blood- and body-building forces. While vegetable juices are very good, these may be taken to extremes—as they have been at times here.

Noons—it is preferable that the vegetable juices, both cooked and raw, be taken at the noon meal, instead of at other meals.

As to the quantity of raw vegetable juices at a time—this would depend upon what would be included with same. Not more than two ounces, you see. This would include lettuce, celery, carrots and the like.

8/2/40
F. 20 yrs.
NERVE-BUILDING **2154-2**

Each day have at least an ounce of vegetable juices; such as a combination of lettuce and carrots especially, and at times including celery juice—to strengthen the general nerve forces of the body. These would be the raw juices, of course.

11/3/42
F. Adult
ANEMIA **2843-3**

In the matter of the diet, for the strength of the body, use vegetable juices; not raw juices but cooked combinations; beans, lentils, peas, cabbage and the like; a little meat, but not large quantities of same.

1)—Beet Juice

ARTHRITIS **3/31/43**
ASSIMILATIONS: ELIMINATIONS: INCOORDINATION **F. 48 yrs.**
CIRCULATION: LYMPH: ARTHRITIS **2946-1**

In this body there should be taken, at least three times each week, at least half an ounce to an ounce of pure beet juice. This may include the leaves also. Possibly it may be preferable from the cooked beets, by themselves. But the beet juice should be extracted, or prepared as in a juicer; or, if this is not practical for the body, then drink the juice in which the beets are prepared—the water in which they are boiled. But the pure juice is needed, not only the salts but those elements that are within; which will tend to alleviate these pressures and tendencies.

Also we would use the low vibrations from the violet ray (hand machine, bulb applicator), when there is the tendency towards tiredness in the limbs, through the shoulders, and the heaviness through the abdominal area. Do not give it too strong, but for a minute and a half apply the bulb applicator along the spine—when ready to retire. It will make those centers corrected (by the mechanical means, or osteopathically) coordinate with the juices, especially of beets, in the body.

Q. Do you think I can avoid an operation by following these directions?

A. We are sure you may avoid an operation. For these will cause a balance to be created in the vibratory forces of the body, as well as the elimination and assimilation through the system.

Q. Will that take care of the arthritis?

A. The beet juice itself will take care of that, as well as the other disturbance—if there are the corrections made in the cerebrospinal system.

4/23/43
M. 4 yrs.
ACIDITY: KIDNEYS: INCOORDINATION **2542-3**

Q. What can be done to help control the kidneys?

A. We would give the body beet juice.

2/18/44
F. 35 yrs.
CANCER **3672-1**

Drink plenty of beet juice. Prepare this preferably by cooking the beets in Patapar paper, so that all the salts and juices that come from the beets may be taken; about two ounces of this juice each day.

2/22/44
F. 26 yrs.
TUBERCULOSIS 3687-1

As to the diet, take quantities of beet juice, not so much at a time but often. Prepare this with the beets and with the tops cooked in Patapar paper so that all the juice is cooked from these and may be taken by the body; not necessarily the beets themselves, but the juices that will cook out of same in the Patapar paper.

4/30/40
ASSIMILATIONS: POOR M. 49 yrs.
CIRCULATION: LYMPH 2183-1

Each day also—throughout the afternoon, for instance—we would sip an ounce of beet juice. This would be the juice from cooked beets and the beet tops cooked with same, in their own juices—not cooked in water, but as in Patapar paper. Preferably use the young, tender beets, so that the tops are tender. If it is preferable to take the full amount at once, take at least fifteen to twenty minutes to sip same.

4/30/40
M. 36 yrs.
MYASTHENIA GRAVIS 2207-1

Each day with the evening meal take one ounce of beet juice, from cooked beets—but cooked in their OWN juice, as in Patapar paper, and using only the juice that comes from same. They may be cut and placed in the Patapar paper, for this will allow more of the juice to be released. Only use the beets themselves, not the beet tops in this instance; for this disturbance here is not of the nature that requires the influences from the beet tops, but only from the beets themselves—prepared each day; not pickled beets or the like, but the fresh beets cooked in their own juices.

Only use a little salt as seasoning for the beet juice—just sufficient to make same palatable. Make or prepare the juices fresh each day, you see.

i)—Beet and Carrot Juice

7/2/40
ARTHRITIS: TENDENCIES M. 56 yrs.
ELIMINATIONS: POOR 462-13

The inclinations for a hardening or a filling of portions of the digestive tract becomes the greater disturbance to the body, in hindering the eliminations through the activity of the excretory functionings of the liver as well as the kidneys.

As we find, here the combination of two juices taken alternately would be preferable for this body, and for this particular body both should be cooked—but in Patapar paper.

One day take about an ounce of beet juice; this means the tops also.

The next day an ounce of carrot juice; this does not include the tops.

The juices from these are to be prepared fresh each day. Do not attempt to keep them from one day to the next—it would be injurious rather than helpful; but the activities of this combination upon the system, with the general activities of the body, will be MOST beneficial.

Preferably take these before retiring, or at the evening meal; one taken one day, the other the next.

Take them for at least a month. Leave off then for a few days, and then take them again; but the beneficial effects from these will make the body desire to keep them pretty regularly.

In the preparation of these, of course, it would be very well that they be cut just before they are wrapped in the Patapar paper, instead of remaining cut very long beforehand.

Q. What causes the rectal irritation and itching, and what will relieve and finally cure same?

A.. These come from the hemorrhoids, which is a part of the general effect from lack of proper eliminations. These will be materially aided by the use of those juices.

Q. What causes the headaches?

A. Worry! and the general nervous conditions from the stomach! These should be materially aided with these juices as indicated for the body to be taken regularly, one used one day, the other the next.

2)—Carrot Juice

4/30/40
ASSIMILATIONS: POOR **M. 49 yrs.**
CIRCULATION: LYMPH **2183-1**

Also each day we would take an ounce of carrot juice—the juice extracted from fresh, raw carrots, by the use of a juicer. Do not take this whole quantity at once, to be sure, but sip it—take fifteen to twenty minutes to take this amount; or it may be sipped in smaller quantities but often through the day. Or, this quantity might be taken in small doses, sipped, throughout the morning of each day.

4/23/43
M. 4 yrs.
ACIDITY: KIDNEYS: INCOORDINATION **2542-3**

Q. What can be done to help control the kidneys?

A. We would give the body carrot juice.

4/26/40
F. 54 yrs.
ASSIMILATIONS: ELIMINATIONS: INCOORDINATION **2180-1**

Take an ounce of carrot juice EACH DAY. Use a juice extractor to obtain the juice from fresh, raw carrots. Take this each day for at least a month, then leave off for a week; then begin all over again.

These are for the better eliminations, you see. Especially the carrot juice, in combination with the rest of the diet, is to aid in dissolving the poisons and eliminating them.

4/25/40
CATARACTS **F. 3 yrs.**
EYES: INJURIES **2178-1**

We would have plenty of carrot juice; at least an ounce or ounce and a half every other day—or this much taken in two days, see? Use a juice extractor for securing the juice from fresh, raw carrots.

5/7/40
ARTHRITIS **M. 33 yrs.**
BODY-BUILDING **849-50**

Then, as to the diets—keep these in the regular order as we have indicated. These are the sources, to be sure, from which more body-building forces are to come.

Do not tire out the body with any food, of course—alternate it as much as practical, but:

Each day give the body at least an OUNCE—during the day—of carrot juice! Get a juicer, and MAKE carrot juice! Even if this tends to gag the body, DRINK IT!

Of course, keep up the citrus fruit juices.

4/20/40
F. 74 yrs.
ARTHRITIS **1224-3**

Noon meals—Raw vegetables (fresh)—especially carrots. At such a meal take also at least an ounce of pure fresh carrot juice. This also will aid, and prevent toxic forces being reformed when the organs have been stimulated to activity, and will aid also in reducing the blood pressures in the system.

4/30/40
M. 36 yrs.
MYASTHENIA GRAVIS **2207-1**

Then begin taking one ounce of carrot juice, from raw fresh carrots, at or with the noon meal. Use a juicer to extract the juice from the raw, fresh carrots. Do this each day.

Only use a little salt as seasoning for the carrot juice—just sufficient to make same palatable. Make or prepare the juices fresh each day.

1/12/40
F. 27 yrs.
NEURASTHENIA **2076-1**

Throughout this period the diet should consist more of the forces as in vitamin B-1. Plenty of carrot juice.

3)—Onion Juice

9/7/34
CANCER: TENDENCIES **F. 12 yrs.**
BLOOD-BUILDING **632-3**

And at one portion of the meal each day give quantities of the juice of onions. Cook these in Patapar paper—*boil* them in same, preserving the juices, and give in small quantities. This will strengthen the body.

6/20/34
M. Adult
TUBERCULOSIS **572-2**

Q. How is the best way for onions to be cooked in order to get the juice?

A. Steamed.

Q. Would cooking them in Patapar paper be a good way?
A. This is an *excellent* way; then you would have the juice *only.*
[Gladys Davis's note: Prepare onions for boiling and tie up in paper with strong cord, tightly; then place in water and boil for about an hour; strain off juice. Paper may be washed out and used again and again.]

8/1/34
M. 36 yrs.
BRONCHITIS **555-4**
We would prepare about six large onions, you see, steamed preferably in Patapar paper. Squeeze out the juice and sweeten just a bit. Begin with small doses of same taken about every two hours apart. This will change the condition for the stomach, change the condition in the respiratory system.

6/5/34
M. Adult
TUBERCULOSIS **572-1**
Also we find that the beef juice would be well, and especially *onion* juice—the juice squeezed from onions that are *steamed,* you see; this taken two or three times a day in small quantities—the *juices* from same.

4)—Sauerkraut Juice

9/4/41
BABY CARE **F. 2-1/2 yrs.**
ELIMINATIONS **1521-5**
Q. Any suggestions to help increase or make eliminations more normal?
A. The changing in the diet, with fruits and vegetables of the form and prepared in the manner indicated, will aid in this direction, or if there is the desire to use especially kraut juices, this would be well—even though there's a small quantity taken once or twice a day.

7/16/35
F. 64 yrs.
ARTHRITIS **950-1**
Noons . . . And drink about half a glass of the juice from *kraut.*

9/28/41
CONSTIPATION **M. 8 yrs.**
ASSIMILATIONS: POOR **2595-1**
Be very mindful of the diet. This is the diet to follow:
Small quantities of kraut juice would be well, but this taken of evening, not of morning.

5)—Spinach Juice

9/9/31
F. Adult
PSYCHOSOMATICS **5470-1**
Q. Would raw spinach juice be beneficial to body?

A. Rather that as has been outlined, as for corrections in the physical body, with a well-*balanced* diet that is both blood- and nerve-building. Spinach, to many an individual, is as a name. More oft are the effects, or good effects, overexaggerated; yet this, in its proper place, gives and offers that of *one* means of adding many elements to the body that are *often* not assimilated through other means. Better, then, that there be those corrections, and a well-*balanced* diet; spinach in its various modes or manners of being prepared for assimilation, used in a moderate way and manner, and through the regular ways.

6)—Tomato Juice

4/12/27
ASSIMILATIONS: ELIMINATIONS **F. 22 yrs.**
ASTHENIA **5714-2**

Then, the juices, the *active* principles of vegetable forces, especially of tomato juices. These *should* assimilate, and these *should* be given, for they carry the *necessary* vitamins for the body, and *in* their *proper* manner *to* be used for *this* body. Those that have been canned, or those that are fresh. These may be *changed* from one to the other, just to meet the needs of the body; or tomato soups, with small amount of the milk with same.

7/30/27
DERMATITIS **M. 5 mos.**
BABY CARE **5520-1**

Tomato juice would be better at present, were this given in small quantities. The tomato juice may be given at present—preferably that which has been canned *without* benzoate of soda.

As is seen, the tomato juice carries all of the vitamins for body in their regular order, and will not produce undue fermentation—if given in moderation, to be sure.

3/16/36
ANEMIA **F. 38 yrs.**
DEBILITATION: GENERAL **954-2**

Noons—Tomato juice, with whole wheat crackers or brown breads.

7/16/35
F. 64 yrs.
ARTHRITIS **950-1**

Evenings—We would have tomato juice; preferably the preserved tomato juice, not from the fresh tomatoes.

6/9/27
F. 1 yr.
BABY CARE **608-1**

Give foods that are of easy digestion. Tomato juice—especially that of canned tomatoes, that are canned good. Tomato juice or soups that are with beans, peas, tomatoes, potatoes.

1/8/30
F. 29 yrs.
BLOOD-BUILDING: VITAMINS: DEFICIENT **5615-1**

As much of the tomato juices, for these carry that *necessary* vital force to meet the needs of that that may be created *in* the blood as to *combat* the conditions existent, and *build* vital forces.

12/31/37
DEBILITATION: GENERAL **M. 41 yrs.**
ACIDITY & ALKALINITY **1476-1**

Mornings—Alter at times with tomato juice—this may be taken in preference to the citrus fruit juices.

5/29/34
F. 57 yrs.
OBESITY **1309-4**

Q. Should I take tomato juice? If so, at what time of day and how much?

A. As we find, if taken occasionally—a small quantity at various times—through the day, as the activities of the body are carried on—they should be helpful to the body.

2/5/36
F. 38 yrs.
TUBERCULOSIS **1045-6**

Tomato juice in moderation may be taken; just little sips, will be most helpful. Preferably not just the canned juice, but the juice taken from the canned tomatoes—and not those canned with any preservative. Libby's is a good brand.

4/2/36
BRAIN: CLOTS: TENDENCIES **F. 60 yrs.**
MALNUTRITION **1137-1**

While the food values should be body-building, in the first they should not be so rich in vitamins or calories or replenishing forces as not to be able to be handled by the digestive forces or the katabolism of the system. First we would have two to three times each day an ounce and a half to two ounces of tomato juice.

5)—Vegetable Soups & Broths

1)—Vegetable Broth: General

9/6/33
ASSIMILATIONS: POOR **F. 3 yrs.**
MALARIA: TENDENCIES **402-1**

Noons—Vegetable broths. Strained vegetable juices, as Gerber's are very good, provided they are not overly weighted with salt, see? Not too much salt.

2)—Vegetable Soup: General

12/1/30
M. Child
COLD: COMMON: SUSCEPTIBILITY: WORMS **203-1**

Beware of sweets for some time. Preferably would be as this: Noon—Preferably soups, or salads with soups that are not too greasy.

10/3/40
ACIDITY: ANEMIA **F. 19 yrs.**
COLD: COMMON: SUSCEPTIBILITY **2374-1**

Noons—Rather the vegetable soups; at least two to three times a week have a warm lunch, as of the vegetable soups, you see.

Do these, and as we find we will bring bettered conditions for this body; not only making for the corrections but improving the vitality, the strength, and increasing the weight.

7/5/41
F. 41 yrs.
SCLERODERMA **2526-1**

In the matter of the diet throughout the period—we would keep those foods that are easily assimilated and that are body-building. Have a great deal of vegetable soups, but not with meats or fats in same. These should be seasoned rather with butter. And ALL the vegetables should be cooked in Patapar paper, eating the juices of same with the vegetables, see?

12/12/31
F. 46 yrs.
ULCERS: STOMACH **482-3**

Noons—A little soup, but *never* any canned soup for *this* body, or any that has had any form of preservative with same. Always make same, the broth, of either the fresh vegetables or fresh meats and vegetables, but *none* of the meat. Particularly none of hog meat, unless later there is taken those that are of the gluten nature, to produce in the system more of that in the blood supply as aids in coagulation.

3/16/43
ASSIMILATIONS: POOR **F. 21 yrs.**
BODY-BUILDING **2937-1**

Do give vitamin-rich foods; such as vegetable soups—more than the vegetables themselves. Not that these should be strained from the preparations, but more of soup than vegetable, see? Season all with butter or the like, rather than with other forms of greases.

ANEMIA **1/28/44**
ACIDITY: EYES **F. 63 yrs.**
ASSIMILATIONS: ELIMINATIONS: INCOORDINATION **3607-1**

Not too much of soups, though vegetable soups with quantities of vegetables in same will be very well—but these should be thick.

Q. What can be done for my eyes?

A. Do these things and we will get rid of this acid throughout the system and relieve the stress upon the kidneys, which will help the eyes.

6/29/42
F. 25 yrs.
ANEMIA **2376-2**

Do have one meal each day consisting principally of raw vegetables; not all of the meal, but the greater portion, while the other part should be preferably soups, stews or the like. The vegetable soups or the condensed soups, or tomato or cream of tomato, or any of those kinds.

12/22/43
DEBILITATION: GENERAL **F. 66 yrs.**
NEURITIS: TENDENCIES **1409-9**

Begin to build up the body with good soups—vegetable soups; not canned soups but make them.

10/17/27
M. 8 mos.
BABY CARE **5520-2**

Q. Should he have any cooked vegetable juices? If so, *how soon?*

A. We *would* cook the spinach, or beans, lentils, or any of those that grow above the ground. The soups would be better—yet be sure there is very little or no grease in same. Seasoning, if any grease, would be only that of butter.

5/3/22
F. 49 yrs.
TOXEMIA **5647-1**

Of noon, would be those of vegetable soups, but the vegetables should be strained or cooked so well that they may pass through those of a colander that may be made by pressing out of same, with a green vegetable in a salad, as of tomatoes, lettuce, spinach, or the like.

i)—Celery Soup

6/9/27
F. 1 yr.
BABY CARE **608-1**

Q. What foods may be given the child besides the Mellin's Food?

A. Any foods that are of easy digestion. Celery soup may be given when properly prepared—not with a lot of fat meat in any, but any of those conditions that supply the proper building to the body are well.

ii)—Potato Soup

12/22/43
DEBILITATION: GENERAL **F. 66 yrs.**
NEURITIS: TENDENCIES **1409-9**

Begin to build up the body with good soups—not canned soups but make them. Even potato soup would be well, but take quantities of it.

iii)—Salsify Soup

10/11/37
DIABETES: TENDENCIES **M. 67 yrs.**
ACIDITY **1454-1**

Hence we would have the stimulating foods such as salsify soups.

XV

Miscellaneous

1)—Acclimation

5/3/40
M. 70 yrs.
ENVIRONMENT: LOCALITY **2094-2**

As we have oft indicated, where an individual is allergic to certain influences, vegetables, activities, or any form of foods carrying the various calories, proteins and vitamins—it will be found that these will vary in various sections. But adjust self to those that are grown the more in the section in which the individual resides at the time—this is the preferable way, when practical.

4/1/44
M. 36 yrs.
ENVIRONMENT: CLIMATE: GENERAL: SINUSITIS **4047-1**

Q. Is the climate of——— satisfactory and should I remain here?

A. The climatic conditions here are not the basis of the trouble. The body can adjust itself. As we have indicated bodies can usually adjust themselves to climatic conditions if they adhere to the diet and activities, or all characters of foods that are produced in the area where they reside. This will more quickly adjust a body to any particular area or climate than any other thing.

Q. Is a diet composed mainly of fruits, vegetables, eggs, and milk the best diet for me?

A. As indicated, use more of the products of the soil that are grown in the immediate vicinity. These are better for the body than any specific set of fruits, vegetables, grasses or whatnot. We would add more of the original sources of proteins.

Q. Are daily heavy chocolate malted milks detrimental?

A. Chocolate that is prepared in the present is not best for ANY diet. Take plenty of milk—you will find some of that around———.

2)—Cooking Utensils

1/6/42
HEMORRHOIDS **M. 57 yrs.**
INTESTINES: COLON: PROLAPSUS **462-14**

Q. Consider also the steam pressure for cooking foods quickly. Would it be recommended and does it destroy any of the precious vitamins of the vegetables and fruits?

A. Rather preserves than destroys.

3/28/39
F. 66 yrs.
ASSIMILATIONS: ELIMINATIONS: INCOORDINATION **1852-1**

Q. Is it all right to use club aluminum waterless cooker for preparing my food?

A. This is very well, but PREFERABLY Patapar paper* is the better manner for preparing food, especially for this body during the periods that the properties or foods and the medicinal applications are being administered.

Of course, there are some foods that are effected in their activity by aluminum—especially in the preparation of certain fruits, or tomatoes, or cabbage. But most others, it is very well.

3/30/37
ELIMINATIONS: INCOORDINATION **M. 58 yrs.**
TOXEMIA **1196-7**

Q. Is food cooked in aluminum utensils bad for this system?

A. Certain characters of food cooked in aluminum are bad for *any* system, and where a systematic condition exists—or a disturbed hepatic circulation or assimilating force, a disturbed hepatic eliminating force—they are naturally so. Cook rather in granite, or better still in Patapar paper.

7/18/36
KATABOLISM: METABOLISM **F. 29 yrs.**
INCOORDINATION **1223-1**

Cook not in aluminum but rather in enamel or glassware. *Not* in aluminum. For with this condition, aluminum becomes poisonous to the system. Do not use aluminum ware in *any* form where this body takes food from!

7/17/43
M. 31 yrs.
ALLERGIES: METALS: ECZEMA **2518-3**

Do keep away from the dust of aluminum. For this body, foods should not be cooked in aluminum, but rather in enamel or glassware.

---

*Patapar paper, now known as "parchment paper," may be purchased in any health food store.

8/15/38
M. 54 yrs.
COOKING UTENSILS: ALUMINUM: NOT RECOMMENDED 843-7

Q. Do I have aluminum or arsenate of lead poisoning?

A. Neither of these; though the effect of aluminum—or effect upon the body by foods being cooked in same—adds to rather than detracts from the activities in the system.

Hence, as we have indicated for many who are affected by nervous digestion or an overactivity of the nerve forces during the state of digestion taking place, the body should be warned about using or having foods cooked in aluminum. For this naturally produces a hardship upon the activities of the kidneys as related to the lower hepatic circulation, or the uric acid that is a part of the activity of the kidneys in eliminating same from the system.

11/18/33
ACIDITY: ALKALINITY: TOXEMIA F. 62 yrs.
INTESTINES: COLON: PROLAPSUS 445-2

Q. Is there any trace in the body of deposits of elements from aluminum, due to cooking the food in aluminum?

A. Where aluminum is used as the cooking vessels, and the food is directly in contact with same, there are produced those elements ever in the human system that become detrimental; unless there are certain characters of vitamins that make for the activity of certain glands in the body. In this body, as we find, there are certain traces; yet these having been changed or altered do not leave other than indications in the eliminating areas—as indicated.

6/13/44
ASSIMILATIONS: POOR F. 51 yrs.
COOKING UTENSILS 5211-1

The body has found such in regard to those conditions in which food is prepared. Some it will never hurt to have prepared in aluminum, but in most people it gradually builds something not compatible with the better conditions in the body forces. This is with certain types of food. Those which are acid will take particles of aluminum into the body.

5/7/40
LACERATIONS: STOMACH F. 34 yrs.
POISONING: COPPER 2188-1

Q. Was this poisoning caused from foods cooked in aluminum or copper utensils?

A. It was caused from pieces of copper being accidentally cooked in aluminum vessels with food.

3)—Condiments: General

1/25/34
F. 22 yrs.
ACIDITY & ALKALINITY 499-1

The foods that are most harmful are those that make for too great a quantity of the potashes in the system, as those that are of too high an acidity—as condiments.

8/3/34
F. 18 yrs.
PELVIC DISORDERS **625-1**

Very little if ever any of the condiments for the body; even salt should be refrained from to a great measure—that is, not seasoning things with salt, other than that which is, of course, cooked in foods. No peppers, no condiments that are as seasonings.

6/16/30
M. 28 yrs.
PERITONITIS: AFTEREFFECTS **102-3**

Not too much of the potash nor condiments, which would produce or bring about the tendency to produce too much weight in *places*, and not general. Let's build it up all over. Be a pretty good size man!

1)—Salt: General

7/10/30
BLOOD-BUILDING **M. 65 yrs.**
MENU: ASSIMILATIONS **4806-1**

We would be mindful of the diet, that there are those of the full rebuilding—especially of those that build for the blood supply, and more of that in the vegetable forces than in meats—though the *juices* of meats may be taken occasionally. Let these, *when* taken, not have *too much* of the condiments, but especially as much *salt* as the body can well take, or that is palatable.

5/23/43
F. 42 yrs.
ARTHRITIS **3014-1**

Keep away from foods with very much salt in same, or use very small quantities of salt.

1/5/36
F. 46 yrs.
COLITIS: TENDENCIES **404-6**

Q. Is salt harmful?

A. In excess, harmful. That there is salt in the blood, in the tears, in every secretion of the body, indicates that it becomes a necessary element—in moderation; unless those properties are taken that *produce* same in its activity through the system.

3/23/40
F. 12 yrs.
EPILEPSY **2153-1**

Each evening, as the body is prepared for sleep, put a pinch (that is, between the thumb and forefinger) of plain table salt (dry) on the tongue. Let this dissolve and be swallowed; *then* a drink of water would be taken. Do this once each day, at bedtime.

8/28/41
M. 56 yrs.
ASSIMILATIONS: POOR **619-10**

Q. Are my teeth causing any ailments?

A. No, these as indicated in the throat and mouth—are more from the disturbance of the glandular forces, or the thyroid activity in relationship to the metabolism. Thus the needs for the supplying those foods that carry quantities of iodine and calcium or the use of kelp salt upon other foods, or the use of iodized salt and the like in the seasoning of foods. These are the measures and means by which such elements are carried, and in which much of these influences as helpful forces will be found.

3/30/44
F. 32 yrs.
SPINE: SUBLUXATIONS **4031-1**

Use only kelp salt or deep sea salt, or the health salt, rather than plain calcium chloride that is mined internally in portions of the country.

i)—Iodized Salt

5/2/27
F. 25 yrs.
GOITER **4600-1**

In the diet, keep only those that have sufficient of the salt properties that keep elimination in the system. Do not use any salt that is not the iodized, or salt with iodine in same, for the lack of iodine is one of the things that has caused disturbance in the system, or from improper water supply, which first started these conditions.

10/1/38
M. 11 yrs.
ANEMIA **536-2**

Q. Is "Sea Kelp" of any food value to his body?

A. Not particularly. If iodized salt would be used it is just as well—or the foods prepared with same.

9/5/42
F. 33 yrs.
EYES: ELIMINATIONS: POOR **2582-2**

Q. What has caused the recent feeling of strain in eyes?

A. The tendencies for the drawing or straining on the system, as tending towards an acidity through the body. Hence, as indicated, we would increase the eliminations—when such occurs—by the use of some saline solution; or the taking of salt of mornings—about a quarter teaspoonful of table salt (preferably iodized salt) in warm or hot water, before the morning meal. Take it for at least three mornings in succession, leave it off, and then take it again if necessary. This would adjust this condition.

ii)—Kelp Salt

6/7/37
DEBILITATION: GENERAL **F. 65 yrs.**
ACIDITY & ALKALINITY **658-15**

The sea salt should be preferably used from the kelp rather than that from sea water. Kelp, to be sure, is a plant that carries all the properties of same; and this taken as seasoning for corn bread or seasoning of certain characters of vegetables *after* they are prepared is good in the diet.

ARTHRITIS: PREVENTIVE **8/31/41**
BODY: GENERAL **F. 51 yrs.**
GLANDS: INCOORDINATION **1158-31**

To help the glandular balance better now we would use the kelp salt in the food preparations. Just used as seasoning, not as a medicine; for this carries sufficient iodines and such activity to aid the body in the present.

Q. Would occasional taking of Atomidine be wise?

A. Not if you use the kelp salt.

8/11/36
ANEMIA **F. Adult**
CIRCULATION: INCOORDINATION **1247-1**

Throughout the whole period we would be mindful that the diet is ever that which is easily assimilated. *Especially* use as the seasoning the kelp or sea salt as is from kelp—this will add to the vibrations of the body.

5/12/44
F. 16 yrs.
DERMATITIS **2084-16**

Do use only the health salt or kelp salt or deep sea salt. All of these are of the same characters. But they are better than just that which has been purified, for the general health of many and this body in particular.

5/26/44
F. 37 yrs.
ARTHRITIS: RHEUMATOID **5150-1**

Do eliminate most of the calcium chloride or salt from the diet, or use kelp salt, deep sea salt or what is called health salt.

5/13/39
F. 40 yrs.
GOITER: TENDENCIES **1657-4**

Q. Is sea kelp good for me?

A. This is very well, if it is not taken in excess—but as a regular portion of diet or in the preparation of other foods.

Q. Should I take Atomidine?

A. Not if kelp is taken or used.

12/14/38
F. 45 yrs.
GLANDS: THYROID **1620-3**

Q. Have I a thyroid deficiency?

A. A little. This as we find is indicated by not a skip exactly, and yet a little irregularity in the metabolism of the system. This arises partially from a calcium AND thyroid activity deficiency.

As we find, the use of the iodized salt or kelp—as a sea salt—would be beneficial in the general meal.

Q. Do I have low blood pressure?

A. This may be materially aided if those properties are taken as indicated to supply more iodine in kelp or the like as a part of the salt or iodine content, AND the use of Calcios to raise the efficiency of the blood supply. Some little condition there needs those corrections.

5/22/44
F. 56 yrs.
ARTHRITIS: TENDENCIES **1895-2**

Then we would cut down on the kind of salt which is being taken. In the food and the preparation use only kelp salt or health salt made from kelp or from the deep sea salt. There are calcium deposits which are causing the disturbances in the tendons and nerves.

5/4/44
F. 31 yrs.
ARTHRITIS **5034-1**

All salt is not to be entirely left out, but use only kelp or deep sea salt or the better grade of the kosher salt.

iii)—Vegetable Salt

4/15/44
M. 60 yrs.
ARTHRITIS **5026-1**

Do leave off a great deal of salt, or use only the vegetable salt. Don't use the regular table salt. Have an increased amount of fresh raw vegetables—these will be better for the body.

3/22/32
F. 42 yrs.
COLITIS **404-2**

Q. What is the difference in food value to the ordinary table salt and Nu-Veg-Sal?

A. Great deal of difference! One—that of the ordinary table salt—acts only as a condiment, or making more palatable for those of the gastric juices of the ducts that produce the saliva activity; while the Veg-Sal acts with the gastric juices of the stomach itself, and makes it more savory through the stomach digestion.

2)—Vinegar

7/6/43
ANEMIA **F. 30 yrs.**
DEBILITATION: GENERAL **2186-3**

Keep away from those foods that have acetic acid (or vinegar) in same.

Q. What else can I do to improve my digestion?

A. Do these things indicated CORRECTLY, and eat the things indicated, keeping away from those that sour!

11/21/36
M. 38 yrs.
TOXEMIA **555-11**

Q. Is vinegar good for the physical body?

A. Very *harmful* for the body!

4)—Gelatin

1/25/44
ARTHRITIS **M. 36 yrs.**
GENERAL **849-75**

Q. Please explain the vitamin content of gelatin. There is no reference to vitamin content on the package.

A. It isn't the vitamin content but it is ability to work with the activities of the glands, causing the glands to take from that absorbed or digested the vitamins that would not be active if there is not sufficient gelatin in the body. See, there may be mixed with any chemical that which makes the rest of the system susceptible or able to call from the system that needed. It becomes then, as it were "sensitive" to conditions. Without it there is not that sensitivity.

ANEMIA: TENDENCIES **10/2/43**
ASSIMILATIONS: ELIMINATIONS: INCOORDINATION **F. 37 yrs.**
KIDNEYS **1695-2**

We would add the vital forces to the body as may be had from taking each day at least one quarter teaspoonful of gelatin (Knox gelatin). This will strengthen the body. Don't begin this until the glands are purified.

7/4/43
ANEMIA **F. 18 yrs.**
CIRCULATION: LYMPH **3070-1**

Also each day we would take half a teaspoonful of Knox gelatin stirred in two ounces of water, drinking this before it begins to jell, of course. This, with any form of Jello, or the component factors of gelatin, will aid in stimulating the flow and secretions to those areas where there is the lack of these elements in the body forces themselves.

1/18/44
CIRCULATION: POOR **M. 72 yrs.**
DEBILITATION: GENERAL **3137-2**

Q. Any suggestions as to diet?

A. Keep close to those things that are easily assimilated by the body. Use plenty of gelatin products in the diet. These especially with raw vegetables will be beneficial. Even the gelatin just dissolved and taken immediately will be helpful, not in hot water but in cold—as half or a quarter of a teaspoonful about three to four times a week. Or prepare all forms of vegetables that may be grated raw and take with gelatin.

10/2/43
M. 36 yrs.

ARTHRITIS **849-73**

Do keep up more of those foods that tend to make muscle tendon, nerve tissue and the like—in the gelatin, see? Do keep that up.

11/29/43
M. 36 yrs.

ARTHRITIS **849-74**

Do occasionally take the vitamin forces that are added especially in gelatin. These will aid the body, but these must be so carried on as to make for their ability to be assimilated and used by those portions of the system that need same; else we may become unbalanced. But keep the regular balance.

Q. In view of the mineral and vitamin deficiencies in Florida food should the body be given mineral salts in colloidal form—those found in normal body metabolism, and vitamins such as A, B, B-1, C, D, E?

A. Are we not giving those very foods, most of those, in the gelatin?

12/7/43
F. 21 yrs.

ARTHRITIS **3389-1**

Do not leave off the gelatin. Do keep the vitamins that will add strength to the body.

Q. Should anything being done now be left off?

A. As indicated, only take the gelatin and those strengthening foods.

Do follow these suggestions if we will find ease. Be consistent and persistent with these, and we may heal this body.

5/22/42
M. 40 yrs.

CIRCULATION: INCOORDINATION **412-14**

Q. What causes the weak feeling throughout the entire body?

A. Owing to the lack of those coagulative forces, and these may be aided by taking half a teaspoonful of gelatin (Knox gelatin) dissolved in cold water, stirred in a glass of water, about three times a week; with the rest of those applications suggested, of course. These will all work together.

Q. Why does the least extra physical condition affect body's heart?

A. As has been indicated.

Q. Is it not natural for body at my age to have such a condition?

A. As just indicated, there are those pressures existent and affecting the circulation. But it is not in the circulation; rather the nerve and muscular force controlling same, by lack of sufficient of those energies to maintain the equilibrium.

10/6/43
F. 48 yrs.

DEBILITATION: GENERAL **3266-1**

As we find, there are disturbances which prevent the better physical functioning. These have to do with the chemical supply, the inability of the glandular system—from the chemical compositions of the body forces, and from the hormones in the blood supply—to re-create those energies necessary for correct stamina in nerves.

These cause those disturbances as related to structural portions of the body, the vertebrae being in a state of flux almost as to position, and the activities of the whole system—with the digestive forces—cause an upsetting of the body.

The organs of the sensory forces suffer under these distresses.

All of these arise from glandular disorders.

We would supply to the system those vital forces that may aid in producing in the body energies that necessary influence for the reviving and regenerating of the body forces. Hence we would take Knox gelatin. One day in the morning take about a teaspoonful thoroughly dissolved in warm water cooled just a bit but not so that it jells before drinking. The next day in the afternoon take about half a teaspoonful prepared in the same way.

If consistently kept, these should bring very soon much better conditions for this body.

12/15/43
F. 23 yrs.
PARKINSON'S DISEASE **3405-1**

In the diet include often those foods prepared with gelatin. Give gelatin by itself also at least three times each week, at regular periods, about half a teaspoonful dissolved in water and taken.

8/3/39
ARTHRITIS **M. 32 yrs.**
VITAMINS **849-41**

For the vital forces as needed in the body (that have been left out), use the gelatin now, provided wine is used in the afternoons—with brown bread; not as a drink but as medicine—red wine or heavy wine that will not be taken in a quantity but the quality of such as blood-building, and will combine with the gelatin. Not Jello, nor Royal—but gelatin itself.

Q. Should the gelatin be given each day, and how much?

A. Don't try to take it all at once, but take it—not so much as medicine, but if it is taken twice a day if he can assimilate it, it's all right—but don't turn the body against same!

Q. Is there a brand of plain gelatin that can be used?

A. There is a brand of just plain gelatin. Buy plain gelatin (Knox gelatin).

7/21/44
F. 60 yrs.
CANCER: LUNGS **5374-1**

Oft raw vegetables should be prepared with gelatin, or gelatin alone would be well.

4/17/44
F. 36 yrs.
MULTIPLE SCLEROSIS **5031-1**

In the diet there should be a great deal of raw vegetables, especially mixed with gelatin. Even vegetable juices taken with gelatin would be well; not set, however, but taken as soon as the gelatin is stirred in same, to act in and with the gastric flows of digestion.

1/24/35
M. Child
COLD: CONGESTION **738-2**

With the cold and congestion in the present, almost an entire liquid diet would be the better. Also gelatin, these are well for the body, making for the sweets sufficient and keeping the strength and vitality without the use of cane sugar, and ridding the system of the cold.

4/27/42
F. 33 yrs.
ASSIMILATIONS: ELIMINATIONS: INCOORDINATION **2737-1**

Also every day we would take gelatin as an aid to the quick pick-up for energy, aiding the system—from the assimilation of this, with the chemical changes in the body—in creating those activities through the assimilating and glandular force for the energies that create corpuscle tissue in body. This we would take about a third of a teaspoonful (Knox gelatin) stirred in a glass of COLD water—each day. If this is taken around two or three o'clock in the afternoon it will aid the more.

3/12/43
F. 35 yrs.
ANEMIA **2936-1**

Take those things of the gelatin nature. Gelatin itself will be beneficial, either taken in the foods or dry.

12/8/39
F. Adult
ELIMINATIONS **1779-4**

Also keep a great deal of vitamin B-1, especially. This as we find may be obtained in the Knox gelatin.

5)—Pickles

4/28/31
M. Adult
ULCERS: DUODENAL: TOXEMIA **719-1**

Beware of stimuli, especially of an alcoholic nature or content, but these as an example: no highly seasoned foods. No pickles or such.

11/21/36
M. 38 yrs.
TOXEMIA **555-11**

Q. Is pickle good for the physical body?

A. Very *harmful* for the body!

6)—Vegetable Oils: General

11/19/30
M. 55 yrs.
BLOOD: HUMOR **2371-1**

In the noon, should be those not of meats or of much greases—but rather that as will aid in the assimilation of the gastric forces as in the digestive system. *Oils* may be taken, but not as *greases.* Those of vegetable oils may be used as dressings, or taken for a lubrication in the system. Small doses, rather than large, will be found more effective. These taken more often, but not more than the system may assimilate—so that, in the active forces of the gastric juices—these are not acted upon as one that *produces* an excess, but as enlivens or stimulates the functioning of same.

2/10/38
F. 25 yrs.
CANCER: COXITIS: HIP EROSION (HEAD OF FEMUR) **275-45**

Noons—such as vegetable juices, or combined with a little meat juices and a combination of raw vegetables; but not EVER any acetic acid or vinegar or the like with same—but oils, olive oil or vegetable oils, may be used with same.

7)—Olive Oil

ACIDITY **9/21/34**
ANEMIA **F. 19 yrs.**
LACERATIONS: STOMACH **667-1**

At all times take *all* the olive oil the body *will* assimilate. This in *very* small doses. Do not take gobs or spoonsful at a time, but half or a quarter teaspoonful, but take it every two or three hours. Not during the night, but be consistent, be very persistent in this direction.

Q. Why have I lost so much weight, and how can I regain it?

A. The strain or the acidity in the system has made for the hardships upon the digestive system, as indicated, which has gradually eaten up not only the reserve supply but deficiency is created in the bloodstream that has made for the losing of weight, and as indicated when we have formed those positions and conditions in the system whereby we may rectify these conditions, so that digestion and assimilation takes place in the normal way, before there has been such an attack upon the organs themselves—or the glands of the body, we will find the body will return to its *normalcy* in weight—and it'll be very good!

Be consistent, then, and be patient and persistent—and *enjoy* well-being.

7/22/31
ASSIMILATIONS: DEBILITATION: GENERAL **F. 28 yrs.**
BLOOD-BUILDING **3842-1**

We would give a diet that is easily assimilated. We would take all the olive oil we are able to assimilate, in very small doses. This may be taken two, three, four, five times each day—half a teaspoon.

6/30/26
SURGERY: TONSILLECTOMY: AFTEREFFECTS **M. 27 yrs.**
BLOOD-BUILDING **137-85**

Now the body only needs rest, plenty of food (as soon as the body can take it) that digests well with the system. Olive oil, and any condition that builds fat tissue in the system without taxing the digestive organism or overtaxing liver or kidneys, see? Any of these.

10/15/27
F. 42 yrs.
ACIDITY **482-2**

Oils a plenty—olive oil *well* for the body.

8/11/31
ELIMINATIONS: POOR **F. 42 yrs.**
BLOOD-BUILDING **484-1**

In the matter of the diet, keep those things that are . . . blood building . . . Olive oil should be taken with most of the foods.

2/24/35
ASSIMILATIONS: ELIMINATIONS: INCOORDINATION **M. 53 yrs.**
ACIDITY & ALKALINITY **843-1**

Very small doses of olive oil would be well to be taken. This should be taken often. Very small doses, meaning three to four drops to five drops at a time, not more than that. That is just enough to produce those activities in the gastric flow along throughout the esophagus and through the upper portion of the stomach, so that the activities with same will make for the enlivening or a food to the walls of the digestive force and system itself.

3/7/35
F. 43 yrs.
ELIMINATIONS: INCOORDINATION **846-1**

Q. Is olive oil and the yolk of eggs and mineral oil good to relieve the constipation?

A. These might be good, but we would find that the application of those things suggested will remove the cause—for they are not as those things that go with or for the alleviation without removing the causes. These, as we would give, would be the better. Olive oil in *small* quantities is *always* good for the whole of the intestinal system. *Quantities* are not advisable, unless taken as an emit—and then it would be under a different status entirely. The dosage should be about half a teaspoonful two to three to four hours apart, just as much as the body will assimilate. But these would *not* advise unless we are to have those corrections that have been indicated, stimulating the activity and those tendencies for the adhesions or congestions in the areas as indicated.

Q. Is it all right to take the olive oil and the yolk of eggs as food?

A. It's very good. These may be taken on the green vegetables if it is preferable to the body, for the taste of the body, but these taken in small quantities are always good for the system.

Q. How much olive oil on a salad at a meal?

A. Teaspoonful.

8/29/35
F. 45 yrs.
COLITIS **404-4**

Hence there should be a well-balanced diet, carrying more oils and fats—but only vegetable oils or those from fruits or nut fats—these would be more preferable to keep a balance for the system. The olive oils are well.

2/8/30
DEBILITATION: GENERAL: FLU: AFTEREFFECTS **F. 71 yrs.**
BLOOD-BUILDING **5604-1**

We would be first mindful or careful of the diet, that it consists of those foods that, while easily digested, are blood and nerve building in their nature. Be sure that olive oil, in as much quantity as will assimilate with the system, is taken—the pure olive oil, half a teaspoonful twice a day—this will aid digestion and the activity of the liver in aiding in blood building.

11/8/34
DEBILITATION: GENERAL **F. 12 yrs.**
BODY-BUILDING **632-6**

We find that the diet should continue to be of the body-building nature, with—of course—the olive oil that becomes food value to the intestinal system, taken internally. Not large quantities, but small quantities taken often for a period—then leaving it off for a period—would be the better and more effective; half to a quarter teaspoonful taken every two or three hours will be more effective with the activities of the system than in taking large quantities; for it will absorb and become active with the gastric flow, with the activities of the forces in the body, and will act as an intestinal food—which, in these conditions, becomes necessary. The olive oil makes for carrying certain vitamins for the building of the system.

8/6/34
F. 56 yrs.
DEBILITATION: GENERAL **626-1**

Begin with the activities in the diet that will make for the resuscitating of more vital forces. Do not overfeed, so that the body becomes a dross pit—as it were; but only take sufficient that the body does assimilate, does *use up* those forces that are taken into the system.

Also take, almost opposite from the beef juice periods, small quantities of olive oil, that will add to the vital forces of the digestive system so that—as the expansions are made in the activating forces of the organs that require food values (for we are going to build a good appetite!)—we will keep adding to the vital forces of the assimilating system; that we may meet all emergencies.

12/15/37
F. 29 yrs.
EPILEPSY **543-26**

Olive oil, in small quantities is rather beneficial, as it is a food for the intestinal system by absorption as much as by activity upon the organs of the assimilating forces; but the smaller doses are the better.

2/27/35
M. 26 yrs.
EPILEPSY **567-7**

Q. Would olive oil with meals help?

A. Olive oil, so it does not become rancid in the system, taken in small enough doses to assimilate, is helpful to any intestinal disturbance—which is a greater portion of the conditions as in this body. Where there have been tendencies for the caecum and the lacteal ducts and the connecting forces in the areas of the intestinal system to become dried, or lack of flow of the lymph, these produce such disturbances for the loss or lapse of the memory, or produces the falling conditions, see? These, then, need to be stimulated. Olive oil is well. The high enemas two or three times a week in the first, as we find, would be *most* helpful. Then later we would have these at least once a week, until we correct this colon and allow those influences that have disturbed the body from constipation to be entirely removed.

Q. Any indication of tapeworm?

A. No indication of tapeworm. There is an indication that there has been stomach worms and intestinal worms, as indicated from the walls of the intestines—especially in the caecum and lacteal duct areas; but not tapeworm. These indications are from those cohesions and adhesions, this drawing of tissue or tendency of tissue to be disturbed is from the infectious forces of such conditions, not from tapeworm.

Q. Any other advice for this body?

A. If there is the desire on the part of the body to test self for tapeworms, live for three days on raw apples only! Then take about half a teacup of olive oil, or half a glass of olive oil. And this will remove fecal matter that hasn't been removed for some time! But it will certainly indicate there is no tapeworm.

6/12/34
CANCER: TENDENCIES **F. 42 yrs.**
TUMORS **583-8**

It would be well for the body to take small quantities of olive oil in the afternoons; half a teaspoonful every two hours, beginning from about twelve o'clock and taking it until eight or nine o'clock in the evening, you see.

5/17/28
ENVIRONMENT: ALTITUDE: TUBERCULOSIS **M. 55 yrs.**
COLITIS **4874-3**

Well that as much of olive oil as is easily assimilated be taken. Be governed as to the quantity as to how same is assimilated—for this is detrimental when not being assimilated by the system, for it acts as an irritant to the gastric and to the juices of the intestines and digestion, when not assimilated.

8)—Yeast

11/10/42
ANEMIA **F. 37 yrs.**
CHILDBIRTH: AFTEREFFECTS **1505-7**

And we would take at least three days a week, the vitamin forces as found in the yeast cake with tomato juice. One cake of yeast—this, of course, the best yeast . . . the yellow label, and break same, dissolve in a small quantity of the juice and then stir in and drink a whole glass of the tomato juice with same, see?

2/2/34
INTESTINES: COLON: ENGORGEMENT **M. 50 yrs.**
ACIDITY & ALKALINITY **506-1**

Be mindful that all periods there are taken through the diet the activities in food values that have a greater amount of the alkaline than of acid reaction. Little or no stimuli of the alcoholic nature, though at times the food values as in yeast would be well to be taken. However, these will of necessity be rather far apart.

11/24/37
ANEMIA: TENDENCIES **F. 9 yrs.**
APPETITE: BODY-BUILDING **1179-3**

Q. Squibb's yeast tablets?

A. These are very well when there are the disturbances through eliminations. These carry foods into the system that make for activities in the intestinal forces of the system, which is very good. But these activities SHOULD be builded in the body! These tablets, though, we would use occasionally; or sufficiently often to keep the bodily forces in the proper eliminations through the alimentary system.

12/19/38
F. 58 yrs.
MENU: TOXEMIA **1762-1**

Evenings—For the most part leafy vegetables, and not too much of same. Before the evening meal a yeast cake AND then the vegetables taken afterward. Use the ironized yeast; this is preferable to the plain or just vitamin yeast.

This is to act as a cleanser for the alimentary canal, as well as a better balance for the fermenting and the eliminations of poisons from the system.

11/24/37
M. 48 yrs.
ELIMINATIONS: INCOORDINATION **1151-11**

Q. Should Squibb's yeast tablets be taken?

A. These are very well for the body occasionally, but do not become DEPENDENT upon them!

11/15/39
F. 20 yrs.
ACNE **1709-4**

As we find now, we would take the Fleischmann's Yeast; not the ironized, but that carrying the vitamins necessary for better activity through the eliminations, as well as the building or replenishing to the body. Two bars each day would be the correct amount. Take these for at least a week at a time, and then rest from same a week, and then take again; and repeat this procedure for at least three or four times.

3/31/27
F. 29 yrs.
ANEMIA **1713-4**

Before the evening meal is eaten, take at least a half cake of Fleischmann's Yeast, see? so that the system will be *cleansed* throughout, overcoming the constipation, overcoming those toxins as sap the vitality.

11/23/24
M. 5 yrs.
ASSIMILATIONS: ELIMINATIONS: BACILLOSIS **5454-2**

Then to give the correction for these conditions, we would first be *very* careful in the diet for the body, giving properties to the system that will produce the vitamins necessary to bring assimilation and the eliminations in system, giving more blood, giving the change in the hemoglobin, wherein the white and leucocyte and Iymph tissue exercise their functionings through the system; not overtaxing the body mentally or physically, using those restrictions that make more methodical in diet, and in rest, and in exercise, taking the properties as the vitamin builder—Fleischmann's Yeast.

Q. What quantity, and at what intervals, should the yeast be given?

A. At meal once each day, cake, half cake taken at a time, or cubes, as they are prepared.

Q. Have you anything further to say regarding this body?

A. Do this, as given. We will bring the normal conditions to this body.

3/30/27
M. 39 yrs.
CONSTIPATION: TOXEMIA **779-16**

Be more regular and more careful with the diet—and well, to overcome the constipation and the tendency of colon to absorb poisons, that the body use Fleischmann's Yeast at least once each day, until these conditions are corrected, see? Preferably, for *this* body, that the cake be used with warm milk, see? This will absorb poisons. It will also start eliminations, and will bring about the normal conditions for this body, [779].

Do that.

3/4/41
F. 61 yrs.
DEBILITATION: GENERAL **538-70**

We would now add the iron yeast tablets, as a means for adding strength—as well as the effluvium for better eliminations, as these are attempted to be set up by the local applications, see? As to make or brand, just so it is the yeast with the iron. The Ironized Yeast is one brand, see? We would begin with one tablet a day. Then after two or three days increase to two tablets. In two or three more days increase to three tablets. This should be sufficient, but it will depend upon the reaction upon the body.

Have plenty, or what the body will assimilate, of beef; not so much the meat itself but chew the meat well—as steak or roast—and swallow the juices but discard the meat. This is some preferable to using just the plain beef juice, if the yeast is taken; though the beef juice might be taken also if it is palatable to the body.

3/21/39
RELAXATION **F. 49 yrs.**
ELIMINATIONS **1158-21**

Q. What is best way to insure satisfactory daily bowel movements?

A. By the diet, and not by dependence upon ANY of the taking of laxatives or the like. But these are the better taken in the diet in those things indicated, such as yeast or the like. These if taken occasionally should keep the bowels in the proper condition.

11/19/37
F. 47 yrs.
ELIMINATIONS **1158-11**

Q. What about Squibb's yeast tablets for me?

A. There are occasions when these would be very well. These as we find are those that aid the activity of the plasm through the digestive system to produce sufficient activity for better eliminations.

Q. How often should I take them?

A. Whenever there is the feeling that there has not been sufficient activity through the colon.

This may be then every day for several days, left off for a few days and then repeated again. Take one after each meal, though, when taken.

7/6/42
F. 32 yrs.
TUBERCULOSIS: TENDENCIES **421-15**

Preferably mid-afternoon—half a cake of yeast in three to four ounces of the tomato juice.

8/29/40
M. 27 yrs.
PSORIASIS: TENDENCIES **641-5**

Q. Should I continue the yeast cakes?

A. Leave off the yeast cakes if the ADIRON is to be taken. If the ADIRON is not to be taken, keep up the yeast cakes.

12/15/37
F. 29 yrs.
EPILEPSY **543-26**

Q. Would it aid the body to eat yeast?

A. If this is taken periodically, and not just taken continuously, this would be very well. That means about a cake after each meal for a period of three to four days, then a rest period.

XVI

Mind Is the Builder

To every individual who requested a reading, no matter what the problem or illness, Cayce stressed the importance of "right thinking." Without self-control the body and mind will run rampant, he tells us. Every cell in the human body has a consciousness of its own which reacts according to what we eat and think. I have cited here a few quotations from the over 14,000 readings.

8/17/38
1662-1

Then, for the body-physical-mental self—the mind is the builder. The attitude individuals maintain, as an entity, towards conditions, individuals and activities, creates that atmosphere for the supplying of energies from that which has been taken as the material for supplying the physical body.

Thusly: If one partakes of the fruit of the vine, or of cereal or of whatnot, and then holds the attitude of fire or RESENTMENT or animosity or hate—what can the spiritual and mental self do with such an attitude in those environs created by the attitude for such an assimilation or digestion in a body active in material forces?

Thus, as has been indicated, what would be the practical application of the mental self respecting conditions, individuals, influences about it of every nature?

First—patience, love, long-suffering, gentleness, kindness; speaking not of anyone in a resenting manner. For know, as He hath given, all power that is in the influence of an individual, a nation, a country, is only lent of the Lord as an opportunity for the individual according to that it has once purposed—for to carry forward that He hath willed respecting each soul!

For ye know, ye understand—all stand as one before Him. There are no ones above another; only those that do His will. What is His will? "Thou shalt love the Lord with all thy heart, thy mind, thy body . . . and thy neighbor as thyself." This is the whole law the spiritual law, the mental law, the material law. And as ye apply same, thus ye become the LAW . . .

3/28/44
4008-1

Q. Spiritual foods?

A. These are needed by the body just as the body physical needs fuel in the diet. The body mental and spiritual needs spiritual food—prayer, meditation, thinking upon spiritual things. For thy body is indeed the temple of the living God. Treat it as such, physically and mentally.

7/14/32
5754-1

In purely physical, we find in sleep the body is *relaxed* and there is little or no tautness within same, and those activities that function through the organs that are under the supervision of the subconscious or unconscious self, through the involuntary activities of an organism that has been set in motion by that impulse it has received from its first germ cell force, and its activity by the union *of* those forces that have been impelled or acted upon by that it has fed upon in all its efforts and activities that come, then it may be seen that these may be shown by due consideration—that the same body fed upon *meats,* and for a period—then the same body fed upon only herbs and fruits—would not have the same character or activity of the other self in its relationship to that as would be experienced by the other self in its activity through that called the dream self.

7/8/29
5639-1

Worry will not gain for the body in *any* direction. Then, learn from within to cast the burdens of self and surrounding influence on Him who is able to bear, and who knows the heart of man in such a way and manner as to be *the* door through which man and woman may approach the creative element of all forces as are active in this material world; knowing that all force is of that Creative Energy and is sufficient to sustain one, will one but cast self upon the promises as have been for man's own understanding through the indwelling of the Divine within each individual, and is ever ready and willing to answer to the call for self and those dependent upon same.

11/5/43
3352-1

But take time to add something to your mind mentally and spiritually. And take time to play a while with others. There are children growing. Have you added anything constructive to any child's life? You'll not be in heaven if you're not leaning on the arm of someone you have helped. You have little hope of getting there unless you do help someone else.

Do that and live a normal life, and you'll live a heap longer. Be worth a heap more than the position you occupy. For it is not what you do but what you really are that counts. This shines through—what you really are—much more than what you say. You can say No, or you can say Yes, but do you ask

God to show partiality? Do you show partiality to others?

3/30/37
1196-7

Q. If I follow the treatment you outline, do you think I can get entirely well?

A. This depends entirely upon the attitude the body assumes toward same. As the body has experienced through many of its experiences, when you work towards a thing you do not allow little disturbing factors or a continual changing to this form or that form to interfere. Be sure you are on the right road, then go ahead—to that which will bring health, if properly applied.

Know that all healing forces must be within, *not* without! The applications from without are to create within a coordinating mental and spiritual force. Set the mind to believe in SOMETHING, and let that be creative—and as we find, and as we have indicated, it must be of a spiritual nature.

3/4/41
538-70

Q. Approximately how long will it take?

A. How long is it until tomorrow, or how long will it take for anything? It depends upon the attitude of the body and the response to the applications. It may be a week, it may be a month, it may be six months or it may be a year! Such depends upon other conditions.

Apply these, and set a time in your own mind as to how soon you want it done, and have it done then!

1/25/44
849-75

Q. Is the body getting rid of the poisons discharged into the bloodstream as well as can be expected?

A. As indicated, it is getting rid of some, but when there is the ruffling of your disposition when there is any anger, it prepares the system so that it blocks the flow of the circulation to the eliminating channels. Thus you can take a bad cold from getting mad. You can get a bad cold from cursing out someone else, even if it is your wife.

Q. Is the condition of the body such that the entity can adopt and hold to the mental attitude that no matter how lethargic or dull or weak or painful he feels he is nonetheless continually getting better?

A. Depends upon just those things indicated. One can get so in the habit of just being cross until he alone doesn't think there's anything wrong—everyone else knows there is.

849-74
11/29/43

Do keep the mental attitude better. Ye know, but don't lose hold. Don't lose the hold on His hand. In thy purpose, in thy aim, in thy prayers, walk closely with Him—who has promised that what ye ask "In my name believing," that ye have already—if ye will act like it, in thought, in deeds, in purpose.

849-73
10/2/43

And keep the spiritual attitude as for a purposefulness. This is very necessary. Don't become aggravated. You are about to pull over the hill—don't grow weary in well-doing.

6/7/37
658-15

First analyze self, get right with Creative Forces, with a purposefulness of self first. Not as selfishness, not as self-exaltation, not as self-indulgences; but know:

"I *know* my Redeemer liveth—I KNOW!"

How?

Because you believe what has been written, you believe what has been said. Has He not given to you, "Try me—know me—call and I will hear"? This means YOU, not someone else!

And this attitude of living, being a manifestation of that in thy dealings with thy fellow man, will aid the most in assisting the natural forces or creative energies to bring the physical body to normalcy.

4/28/31
719-1

In the mental and the associations, the mental outlook on life, the attitude of life that the world and the conditions and surroundings are at variance to self is *all wrong!* Rather do something for the *world,* than having the world do something for you! Act in a way and manner as that a *service* to *others* will be the highest service as may be rendered for self. That held in the mental forces of the body as grudge can only create *poisons,* can only create distrust, disruption, disorder, discouragement through the whole activities of self.

7/19/43
3134-1

Change the attitude. Don't take these applications merely expecting that they will correct conditions unless the attitude as to the usefulness of body, mind, and purpose is for creative forces.

Do not condemn others nor self most of all. Give thanks daily for the opportunity that you may have in this experience of being a manifestation of the glory and the work of God in the earth.

1183-2
3/8/37

Then the diet: This should be not so rigid as to appear that you can't do this or you can't do that, but rather let the attitudes be . . . everything that is eaten, as well as every activity . . . purposeful in conception, constructive in nature. Analyze that! Purposeful in activity, constructive in nature!

1/17/44
3564-1

Don't be afraid of having troubles this or that time—you won't! Know that whatever you want you can have. For the Lord loveth those who love Him and He will not withhold any good thing from such.

Q. Is there likelihood of bad health in March?

A. If you are looking for it you can have it in February! If you want to skip March, skip it—you'll have it in June! If you want to skip June, don't have it at all this year.

5/1/36
906-2

Keep the mental attitude in the constructive forces that make for knowing that the body is not only good but good for something. And apply self in those ways and manners that are known to the mental body, and we will find the physical forces, the mental reactions, continually helpful.

7/24/42
69-5

Q. Please advise how I can realize my desire for healing to come without physical remedies. Is it possible for me to demonstrate this?

A. Anyone can demonstrate that which is really desired, if the entity is willing to pay the price of same!

As we have indicated so oft, when there are disturbances in the physical that are of a physical nature, these need to be tended to or treated, or application made, through physical means. There is as much of God in the physical as there is in the spiritual or mental, for it should be one! But it was as necessary, when the Master demonstrated, to use that needed in the bodies of individuals as curative forces as it was in the mental. To some He gave, "Thy sins be forgiven thee." To others He applied clay. To others they were dipped in water. To others, they must show themselves to the priest, offering that as had been the mental and the material law.

These are one. Understand them as one yet do not attempt, at all times, to heal with word when mechanical or other means are necessary to attune some disturbed portion with the mental and the spiritual forces of the body.

3/8/35
631-6

Q. What is the proper method or medicines to apply to correct or eliminate all of these conditions?

A. Let's then, for the moment discard or disregard all that has been given. If there is the desire on the part of the body *first* in itself to have applied and to be consistent and persistent in the applications of those elements and influences necessary, first there must be a change in the mental attitude of the body. There must be eradicated that of any judgment or of condemnation on the part of self as respecting self or *any* associated with the body in *any* manner, either previously or in the present. This must be eradicated from the mind. How? By filling same with constructive loving influence towards self, towards others, and as these are raised within the consciousness of self by the proper thinking, with the less and less of condemnation to anyone, these create the proper surroundings, the proper attitude.

2/5/42
2067-9

Q. Will I be able to overcome this condition and keep my job?

A. If you'll do as has been indicated! If you half do it and then are still pessimistic about it, no! Remember the word of the psalmist, "That which I hated has come upon me."

12/11/37
849-23

Q. Is the present trouble to be expected as an aftermath of future illnesses, or will it be eradicated after the present attack is over?

A. This depends upon just those things as indicated to the body from the beginning! This is an acute condition, but the applications of coordinating the system in its eliminations of poisons, and of the causes and the effects, should ERADICATE the condition—and not to be expected to be returning! though if the body builds that consciousness that "I've got a weakness or a tendency and must give way to it," then if you look for that, and know you're going to have it, you'll certainly have it! for the mind builds it then, and it must be met! For remember, ever is the individual constantly—in the physical—meeting that it has builded in its mental AND physical forces of its body!

8/31/34
646-1

And keep an even mental balance. *Don't* worry! It is easy to say "Don't worry," but how may a person prevent it? By keeping control of the mind, not only through the very will of self but by keeping occupied in doing something for others.

12/26/38
1548-4

Then, there needs to be the general precaution taken. For as should be held in the attitude of the body, irrespective of what may be said locally or incidentally: Know that the body rebuilds itself (this is often said and then forgotten when there are improvements in a condition), and that as long as the conditions are on the IMPROVE these will CONTINUE to make for improvements in warding off, in replenishing, in building up. And as the mental and physical is improved, use it—the self, the time, the experience—in that of constructive thinking. Leave off animosities, hates, petty jealousies; and we will find it will make for more and more a constructive influence in the body-forces.

8/25/44
4021-1

Yes, here we have a disturbing condition with the body, and a very unusual mind to deal with. To be sure, attitudes oft influence the physical conditions of the body. No one can hate his neighbor and not have stomach or liver trouble. No one can be jealous and allow the anger of same and not have upset digestion or heart disorder. Neither of these is present here, and yet those attitudes have much to do with the accumulations which have become gradually the disorders that tend to produce those tendencies towards a neuritic-arthritic reaction.

12/18/36
1259-2

Q. What should I do about taking the hydrochloric acid internally? I seem to be much better when taking it.

A. If that is the desire of the body that these be added in this form, then take it! For the mental outlook has as much to do with the results as the material applications!

10/10/36
1102-2

Do not become as one dependent upon either the medicinal properties, the massages or corrections, or a specific diet; but *know* (and then act like it) that there *are* the properties within the physical organism—if a balance is kept—that will reproduce within itself the necessary forces and influences to keep the body building and the body replenishing and the body normal in its activity.

4/1/43
2948-1

Do keep sweet. Keep that attitude of expectancy. Do keep the attitude of hope. And KNOW that there is healing in the power and might of the love of God.

8/27/44
5401-1

A great deal will depend upon the mental attitude of the body. Music is that realm between sublime and the ridiculous. Do practice the sublime. Not merely in thought but in what you think of and say about others, and how you treat them personally.

Index